Orthopaedic
Radiography

BRUCE W. LONG, MS, RT(R)
JOHN A. RAFERT, MS, RT(R)
Department of Radiologic Science
Indiana University School of Medicine
Indianapolis, Indiana

W.B. SAUNDERS COMPANY
A Division of Harcourt Brace & Company
Philadelphia London Toronto Montreal Sydney Tokyo

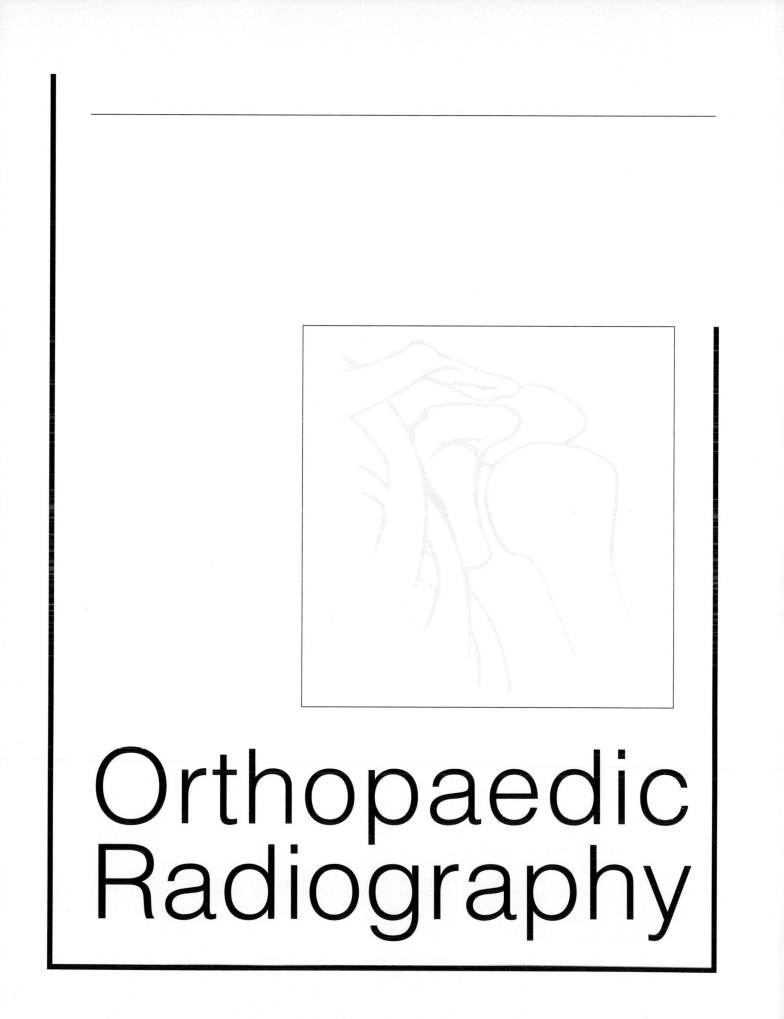

Orthopaedic Radiography

W.B. SAUNDERS COMPANY
A Division of
Harcourt Brace & Company

The Curtis Center
Independence Square West
Philadelphia, Pennsylvania 19106

Library of Congress Cataloging-in-Publication Data

Long, Bruce W.

Orthopaedic radiography / Bruce W. Long, John A. Rafert.—1st ed.

p. cm.

ISBN 0–7216–6649–3

1. Radiography in orthopedics.   I. Rafert, John A.   II. Title.
   [DNLM: 1. Musculoskeletal Diseases—radiography.   2. Bone and Bones—
   radiography.   3. Fractures—radiography. WE 141 L848o 1995]

RD734.5.R33L66   1995
617.3′0028—dc20

DNLM/DLC   94–14941

Orthopaedic Radiography   ISBN 0–7216–6649–3

Copyright © 1995 by W.B. Saunders Company

All rights reserved. No part of this publication may be reproduced or transmitted in any form or by any means, electronic or mechanical, including photocopy, recording, or any information storage and retrieval system, without permission in writing from the publisher.

Printed in the United States of America.

Last digit is the print number: 9   8   7   6   5   4   3   2   1

To Jeanne, the love of my life, for her encouragement, patience, and understanding during the two and a half years it took to prepare this book.

To my son, Michael, who had to share his dad with a book.

To my parents, Jack and Marianne Long, who taught me to do my best.

To my fourth grade teacher, JoAnn Bain, who taught me that I was responsible for my own learning.

To all the radiologic technologists I have been associated with, from whom I have learned a great deal of what I know about radiography.

—Bruce W. Long

To my wife Jayne and daughter Angela, for their support and encouragement during a long project.

To my son, Max, who was born during the preparation of this book.

To all my art teachers, professors, and friends in the art community, who taught that fine art is far more than an acquired skill.

To Emily Hernandez, Suetta Kehrein, Sarah Baker, Terry Whitson, and Jay Oakes, my professors and instructors of radiography, who taught me a whole new world of elegant science.

To all the fine professional radiographers with whom I have had the pleasure of working and learning over the years.

—John A. Rafert

Acknowledgments

We would like to thank the following groups and individuals for their support during the production of this book:

The Indiana University Department of Radiology and especially Ethan Braunstein, MD, Kenneth Buckwalter, MD, and Donald Kreipke, MD, for their advice and encouragement.

The Indiana University Department of Orthopaedic Surgery and in particular Robert Colyer, MD, Robert Huler, MD, and Alexander Mih, MD, for their input.

The Indiana University Department of Radiologic Sciences and especially our boss, Emily Hernandez, for the understanding, time, and patience necessary to allow completion of the book.

The radiography staff of the Outpatient Radiology Department of Indiana University Hospital in Indianapolis.

The radiography staff of the Outpatient Radiology Department of Regenstrief Health Center in Indianapolis.

The Emergency Room radiography staff of Wishard Memorial Hospital in Indianapolis.

Phil Wilson, of the Indiana University Department of Pharmacology and Toxicology, for his photographic assistance.

The following radiographers provided radiographs for the book:

Heather Alley, RT(R)   Trisha Scheible, RT(R)
Larry Robinson, RT(R)   Paula Gunning, RT(R)
Vickie Byers, RT(R)   Paula Shyko, RT(R)
Trina Roush, RT(R)   Michelle Hodosi, RT(R)
Susan Davis, BS, RT(R)   Julie Todd, RT(R).

A special thank you to Roger Strieski, RT(R), for providing sources of information and the benefit of his extensive research throughout the preparation of the book.

READ THIS FIRST!

Preface

This book is based on the premise that proper orthopaedic radiography requires the same depth of understanding and skill as any other area of practice in radiology. It was written to address the need for comprehensive coverage of specialized radiographic positions and projections applicable to orthopaedic practice. For years, we have listened to orthopaedists, radiologists, residents, and radiographers frustrated by their inability to find good descriptions of these radiographic positions/projections. The descriptions were available but were often difficult to find or to understand.

The book concentrates on joints because they are the most problematic to radiograph and because the majority of specialized positions/projections have been developed for these anatomical areas. The positions/projections included were gathered from experience and from the literature. The decisions regarding what to include were based on documented diagnostic value and reproducibility of each. Routine radiographic projections/positions were included for completeness. Radiography of diaphyses was excluded because the positioning poses few difficulties for the experienced radiographer.

The overviews of pathology related to each body part and the supplemental chapters are intended to aid in decision making regarding inclusion of radiographs that may be needed for accurate and complete diagnosis.

Positioning Guides

The positioning guides were written for *experienced* radiographers. The written explanations are brief and are intended to complement the position drawings, not to stand alone. The following icons are provided to facilitate use of the guides.

This icon represents the rationale for performing the position or projection.

This icon represents the position description.

This icon represents the image appearance and evaluation criteria.

This icon represents case studies illustrating application of the position or projection.

Position Drawings

Depiction of positioning is by line drawing rather than by photograph because more information can be included and non-essential details excluded. The following symbols/devices are used in the position drawings to graphically present or clarify specific details.

 This symbol indicates the central ray.

 This symbol indicates the direction and angulation of the central ray.

 This symbol indicates the entrance point for the central ray.

 This symbol indicates angulation of the body or part.

 This symbol indicates rotation of the body part.

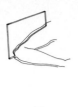

This imaginary plane is a device to aid in understanding central ray direction or body part orientation.

This inset (circle) is a device indicating central ray perspective and entrance point.

Anatomical Drawings

The anatomical drawings that accompany the radiographs were drawn from the radiographer's perspective during positioning. We believed that this would provide the orthopaedic radiographer with a better understanding of the spatial relationships of anatomical components in the radiograph. This understanding should, in turn, provide insight into the reason for changes in anatomical relationships resulting from central ray angulation and/or positioning variations. The anatomical drawings were based on radiographs and were developed from dry bone specimens.

Anatomy radiographed in the posteroanterior (PA) projection was drawn as it would be seen by the radiographer and not flipped left to right as it is customarily viewed. The accompanying radiographs were not flipped, so that comparison with the drawing could be made. Drawings of anatomy radiographed in anteroposterior (AP) projections should not result in confusion because these radiographs are not flipped when viewed.

The following drawing represents the process for creation of anatomy drawings accompanying PA projection radiographs.

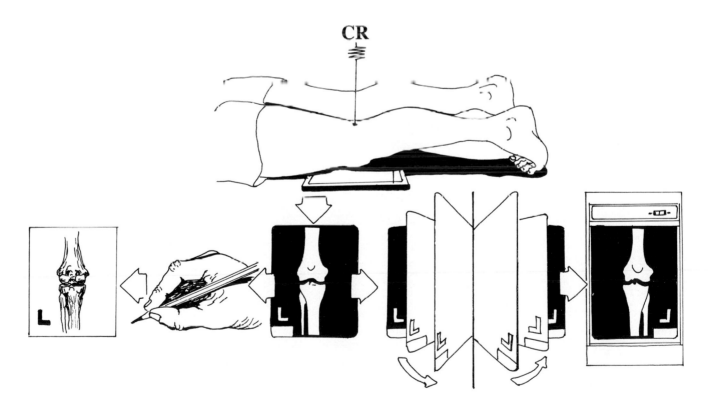

Anatomical Drawings

Request for Case Studies

This edition was intended to disseminate an accurate and complete description of the specialized orthopaedic positions/projections. Readily available case studies were included, but additional cases were not aggressively sought.

Our intention was to solicit case studies illustrating the diagnostic value of the specialized positions for the second edition. This is the request:

"We would be pleased to receive copies of case films illustrating the diagnostic value of a particular specialized position or projection. We need both the routine radiographs and the specialized position/projection. A written explanation of the case should also be included. The case studies included in this edition are examples of what we need.

"Individuals submitting usable cases will be acknowledged at the site of the radiographic case and in the front matter."

Position Guide Reference

POSITION/PROJECTION	FOR DEMONSTRATION OF	PAGE

Thumb

Hand

Wrist

Elbow

Shoulder

Acromioclavicular and Sternoclavicular Joints

Spine

Cervical Spine

Lumbar Spine

Abnormal Spine Curvature

Sacroiliac Joint

Pelvis and Hip Joint

Pelvis

Hip Joint

Knee

Ankle

Foot

Contents

THREE
The Wrist

FOUR
The Elbow

FIVE
The Shoulder

SIX
The Spine

SEVEN

The Pelvis and Hip Joint

EIGHT

The Knee

NINE
The Ankle

TEN
The Foot

2

ELEVEN
Fractures

TWELVE
Orthopaedic Hardware

THIRTEEN
Arthritides

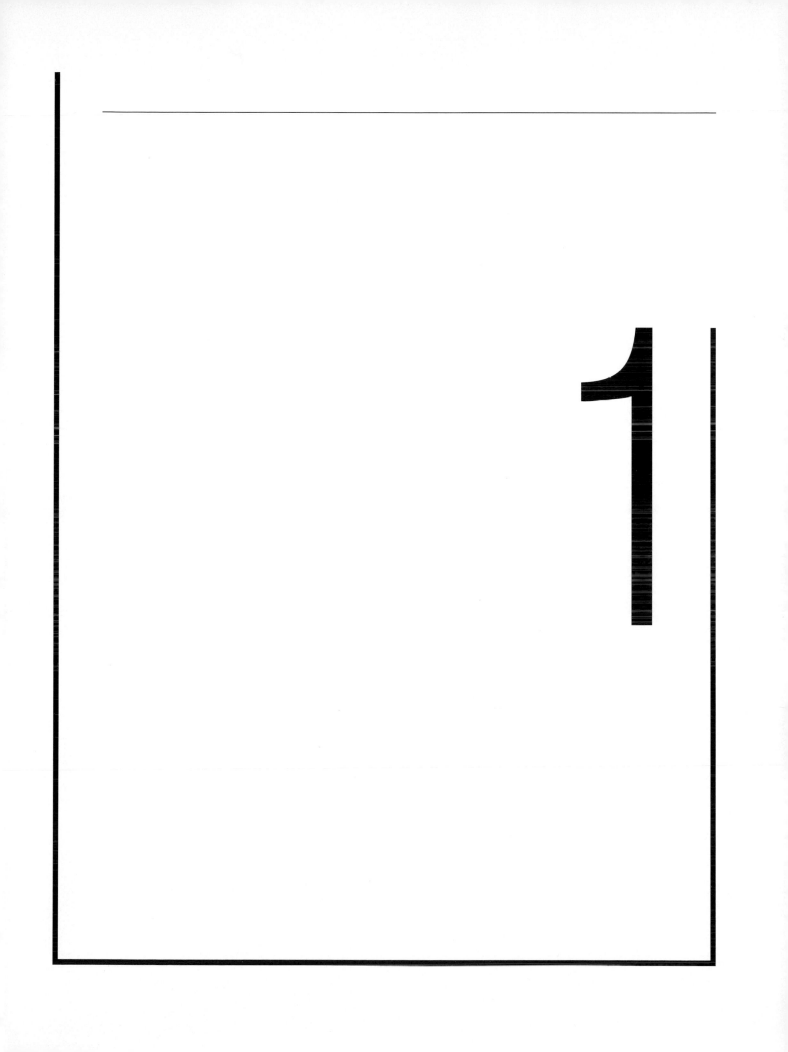

1

THE THUMB: AN OVERVIEW

ROUTINE THUMB RADIOGRAPHY

Routine AP Thumb Projection
Routine PA Thumb Projection
Routine Oblique Thumb Position
Routine Lateral Thumb Position

SPECIALIZED THUMB RADIOGRAPHY

Abduction Stress Thumb Position
Adduction Stress Thumb Position
Burman Thumb Position
Eaton Stress Thumb Position
Gedda-Billings Thumb Position
Modified Eaton Stress Thumb Position
Modified Roberts Hyperpronation Thumb Position

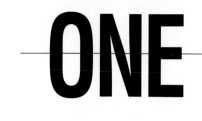

ONE

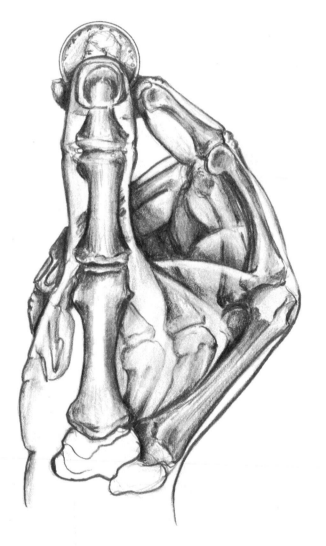

The Thumb

The Thumb: An Overview

The thumb is essential to proper function of the hand. With it, humans are able to manipulate the environment with fine dexterity. A variety of bone and soft-tissue conditions afflict the thumb, partly because of its exposed location. The most common conditions include fracture, ligament or tendon injury, and arthritis. These pathological conditions must be accurately assessed to ensure prompt treatment. Radiographic examination has an important role in this diagnostic process.

Fracture of the thumb most often involves the metacarpal base. The injury may result from a fall on the hand, hyperabduction, hyperextension, or a blow directed along the long axis of the bone. The fractures can be divided into intra-articular and extra-articular types. The predominant intra-articular type is a fracture-dislocation called **Bennett's fracture**.[1] It involves an oblique fracture through the joint surface of the metacarpal base with resultant proximal dislocation of the major fragment. Closed reduction is often possible, but Kirschner wire fixation is usually necessary.[2] A comminuted form of the Bennett's fracture is termed **Rolando's fracture**.[3]

Extra-articular fractures of the thumb metacarpal base are predominantly transverse. A small percentage are oblique and may be misinterpreted as Bennett's fractures if the relationship of joint to fracture line is not clearly imaged. Correct diagnosis is important, because most extra-articular fractures can be successfully treated only with closed reduction,[4] whereas Bennett's intra-articular fractures usually necessitate internal fixation.

As in adults, extra-articular fractures of the thumb metacarpal are the most common thumb fractures in children. They usually consist of a transverse metaphyseal fracture or a Salter-Harris type II fracture with a medial metaphyseal fragment.[5] The less commonly seen equivalent to Bennett's fracture is a Salter-Harris type III fracture with a medial epiphyseal fragment remaining attached to the trapezium.

A variety of ligament and tendon injuries involving partial or complete tears may occur in the thumb. Many of these conditions are readily apparent on physical examination. When the diagnosis is uncertain, radiographic examination may demonstrate joint incongruity or associated bone avulsion at attachment sites.

Dislocations of the interphalangeal (IP) or metacarpophalangeal (MCP) joints are usually evident on clinical examination, unless they have been reduced before examination. With hyperextension injuries, a deformity may not be readily apparent, especially at the IP joint. However, flexion may be impaired and an associated avulsion fracture on the volar aspect of the joint, demonstrated radiographically, will indicate the injury. Radiography should be performed on any suspected dislocation to demonstrate associated fracture. Radiographs of a dislocation, displaying joint space widening or the presence of sesamoids in the joint space, indicate probable soft-tissue entrapment.[6] This condition is considered an irreducible, or complex, dislocation and necessitates open reduction. Complex dislocation is more commonly associated with the MCP joint than with the IP joint.[7]

The posture of the thumb or alignment of its parts may indicate the injury location. A **mallet thumb** (baseball or dropped thumb) is characterized by flexion deformity of the IP joint. The deformity results from forcible flexion of the extended distal joint, causing disruption of the extensor mechanism of the IP joint. This may be caused by rupture of the extensor tendon or by intra-articular fracture of the distal phalangeal base involving the extensor tendon insertion. The equivalent injury in children results from physeal separation (Salter-Harris type I or II fracture) or epiphyseal avulsion (Salter-Harris type III fracture) of the distal phalanx.[5]

The abducted posture of the thumb provides opportunity for varus or valgus stress to be experienced, especially by the MCP joint. A significant injury of this type is the **gamekeeper's thumb** (skier's thumb). It is the result of injury to the ulnar collateral ligament of the thumb MCP joint, caused by excessive valgus (radial) stress. This type of injury is found in children as well as in adults. The injury was first reported in Scottish gamekeepers,[8] but this injury is currently seen most often in athletes in association with football, stick sports (hockey, snowskiing), and racket sports.[9] It is diagnosed primarily by clinical evaluation, but it may be demonstrated radiographically with stress images or by the presence of an evulsion fracture at the ulnar aspect of the MCP joint. Varus and valgus stress positions, recommended by Downey and Curtis,[10] have been included in this chapter to assist in diagnosis of injury to the thumb MCP collateral ligaments.

The thumb is also afflicted by both degenerative and inflammatory arthritides. Primary osteoarthritis predominantly affects the trapeziometacarpal (TMC) joint in the thumb. The early radiographic signs in this area may be limited to ligamentous laxity with minimal osteophyte formation. As the degeneration progresses, ligamentous laxity increases, and more extensive osteoarthritic changes (joint space narrowing, subchondral sclerosis, subchondral cysts, margin osteophytes) become evident on radiographs.[11] Eaton and Glickel[12] suggested the addition of a posteroanterior (PA) stress projection to the routine radiographic examination to document the presence and degree of ligamentous laxity. Several projections that assess laxity at the TMC joint are described in this chapter. When degenerative changes are suspected to involve this area, the basal thumb positions (Gedda,[13] Burman,[14] modified Roberts' hyperpronation[15, 16]) described in this chapter should be used.

A high percentage of patients with rheumatoid arthritis in the hand have thumb involvement. The synovial hypertrophy, cartilage destruction, and tendon weakening associated with the condition may result in deformity of the digit. The **boutonnière deformity** manifests as flexion of the MCP joint and hyperextension of the IP joint. Stretching and volar slippage of the extensor tendon structures of the MCP joint cause the joint to remain in flexion. The IP joint hyperextends as a result of the MCP flexion imbalance. A reverse boutonnière posture of the digit is termed a **swan-neck deformity**. It is more commonly present in the other digits but may be found in the thumb. A mallet deformity may also occur. All of these deformities can be documented by a lateral thumb radiograph.

Routine Thumb Radiography

Routine AP Thumb Projection

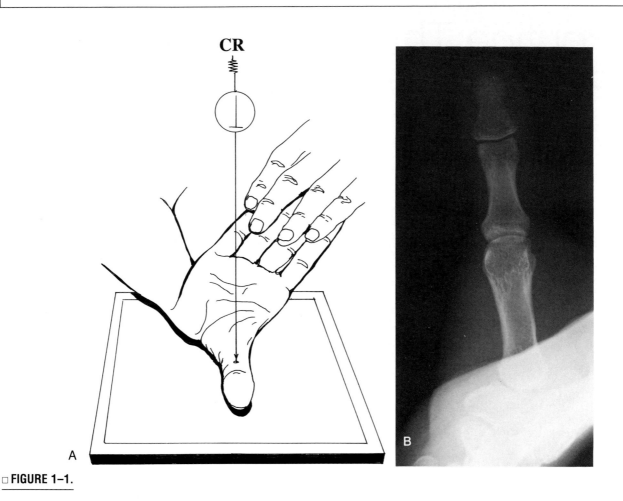

□ **FIGURE 1–1.**

POSITION DESCRIPTION

Part Position: The hand is hyperpronated to place the dorsal (thumbnail) surface of the thumb on the cassette, without obliquity. The remainder of the hand is dorsiflexed, and the patient may hold the fingers back with the other hand.

Central Ray: Perpendicular to the cassette, through the metacarpophalangeal (MCP) joint.

IMAGE EVALUATION

The entire thumb should be seen in AP projection, without rotation (obliquity), as evidenced by equal concavity of both margins of the metacarpal and phalangeal shafts. The interphalangeal (IP) and MCP joint spaces should be well visualized. The basilar thumb (trapeziometacarpal [TMC]) joint may be partially obscured by the thenar and hypothenar soft tissues.

Routine PA Thumb Projection

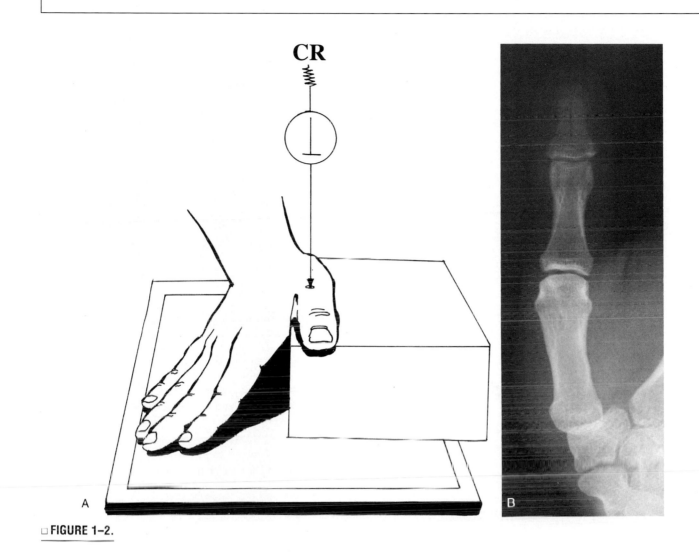

CR

A

B

☐ **FIGURE 1-2.**

POSITION DESCRIPTION

Part Position: The hand is placed on the cassette in an ulnar lateral position and adjusted by slight pronation to place the dorsal aspect of the thumb parallel to the cassette. A sponge may be used to support the thumb.

Central Ray: Perpendicular to the cassette, through the metacarpophalangeal (MCP) joint.

IMAGE EVALUATION

The entire thumb should be seen in PA projection, without rotation (obliquity), as evidenced by equal concavity of both margins of the metacarpal and phalangeal shafts. The interphalangeal (IP) and MCP joint spaces should be well visualized. The basilar thumb (trapeziometacarpal [TMC]) joint may be partially obscured by the thenar and hypothenar soft tissues.

Routine Oblique Thumb Position

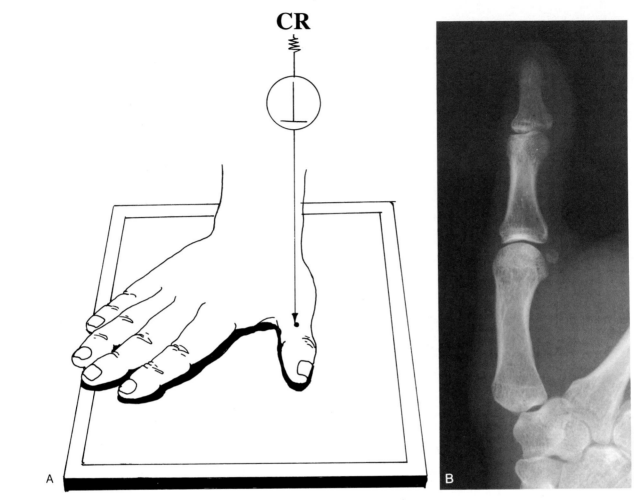

CR

A

B

□ **FIGURE 1–3.**

POSITION DESCRIPTION

Part Position: The hand is pronated on the cassette, with the thumb abducted slightly.

Central Ray: Perpendicular to the cassette, through the metacarpophalangeal (MCP) joint.

IMAGE EVALUATION

The entire thumb should be seen in an approximately 45° oblique position. The interphalangcal (IP), MCP, and trapeziometacarpal (TMC) joint spaces should be open.

Routine Lateral Thumb Position

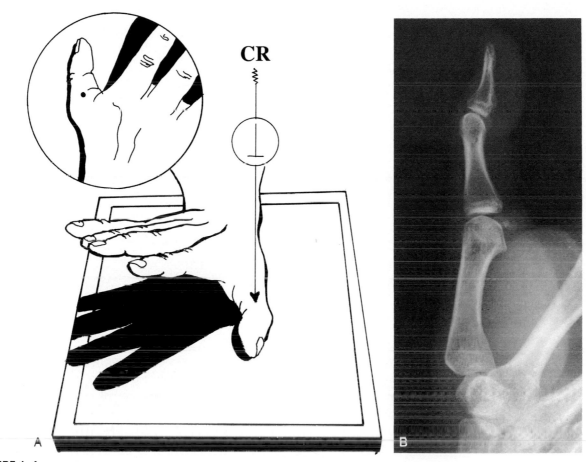

CR

□ **FIGURE 1–4.**

POSITION DESCRIPTION

Part Position: The fingers of the pronated hand are flexed to rotate the thumb into a lateral position. The thumb is abducted to prevent superimposition of the second phalanx and metacarpal.

Central Ray: Perpendicular to the cassette, through the metacarpophalangeal (MCP) joint.

IMAGE EVALUATION

The entire thumb should be seen in lateral position, without rotation (obliquity), as evidenced by concavity of the palmar (anterior) margin of the metacarpal and phalangeal shafts. The interphalangeal (IP), MCP, and trapeziometacarpal (TMC) joints should be well visualized.

Specialized Thumb Radiography

Abduction Stress* Thumb Position

RATIONALE FOR USE

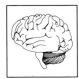

The abduction stress thumb position allows the demonstration of *joint widening under stress*, associated with ligamentous injury or laxity at the *ulnar (medial) aspect of the first metacarpophalangeal (MCP) joint*. This position is done bilaterally for joint comparison. The accuracy of diagnosis is dependent on the patient's willingness to apply adequate stress to the joint.

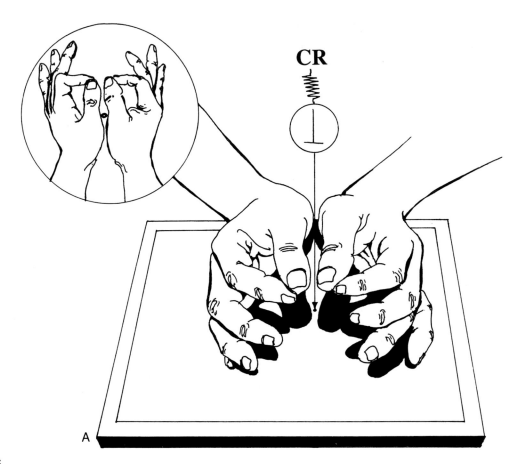

□ **FIGURE 1–5.**

POSITION DESCRIPTION

Part Position: Both hands are placed in the lateral position with the thumbs elevated, to place the dorsal surfaces parallel to the cassette. The tips of the index fingers are placed on the ulnar (medial) side of the distal portions of the thumbs, and stress is applied.

Central Ray: Perpendicular to the cassette, centered between the hands at the level of the first MCP joints.

Abduction Stress* Thumb Position *(continued)*

IMAGE EVALUATION

Both first MCP joints should be clearly demonstrated in PA projection for comparison. The distal soft tissues of the thumbs should be seen for determination of adequate stress pressure. Exposure factors should allow for good bone detail, as well as for demonstration of soft tissues.

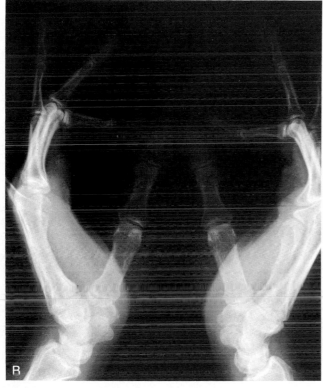
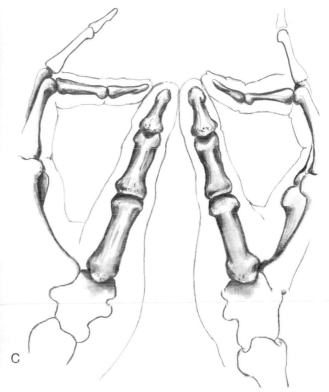

□ **FIGURE 1–5.** *(continued)*

---

*Downey EF, Curtis DJ. Patient-induced stress test of the first metacarpophalangeal joint: a radiographic assessment of collateral ligament injuries. *Radiology* 1986; 158:679–683.

Adduction Stress* Thumb Position

RATIONALE FOR USE

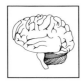

The adduction stress thumb position enables the demonstration of *joint widening under stress,* associated with ligamentous injury or laxity at the *radial (lateral) aspect of the first metacarpophalangeal (MCP) joint.* This position is performed bilaterally for joint comparison. The accuracy of diagnosis is dependent on the patient's willingness to apply adequate stress to the joint.

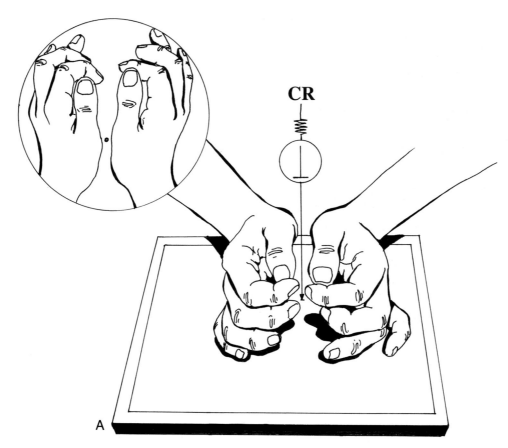

□ **FIGURE 1–6.**

POSITION DESCRIPTION

Part Position: Both hands are placed in the lateral position with the thumbs elevated, to place the dorsal surfaces parallel to the cassette. The tips of the index fingers are placed on the radial (lateral) side of the distal portions of the thumbs, and stress is applied.

Central Ray: Perpendicular to the film, centered between the hands at the level of the first MCP joints.

Adduction Stress* Thumb Position *(continued)*

IMAGE EVALUATION

Both first MCP joints should be clearly demonstrated in PA projection for comparison. The distal soft tissues of the thumbs should be seen for determination of adequate stress pressure. Exposure factors should allow for good bone detail, as well as soft tissue demonstration.

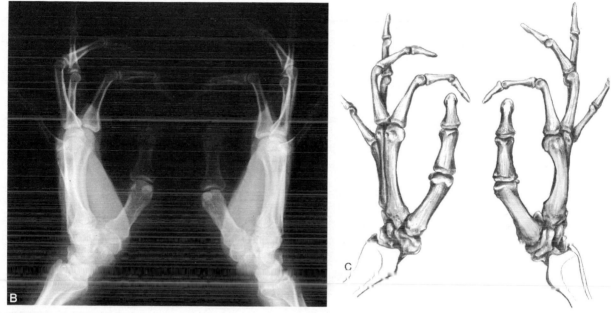

□ **FIGURE 1–6.** *(continued)*

---

*Downey EF, Curtis DJ. Patient-induced stress test of the first metacarpophalangeal joint: a radiographic assessment of collateral ligament injuries. *Radiology* 1986; 158:679–683.

Burman* Thumb Position

RATIONALE FOR USE

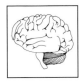

The Burman thumb position demonstrates the *trapeziometacarpal (TMC) joint* free of superimposition. Fractures and arthritic changes occurring at this site may be demonstrated with this position. Angulation distortion is radiographically prominent and may limit its use in some cases.

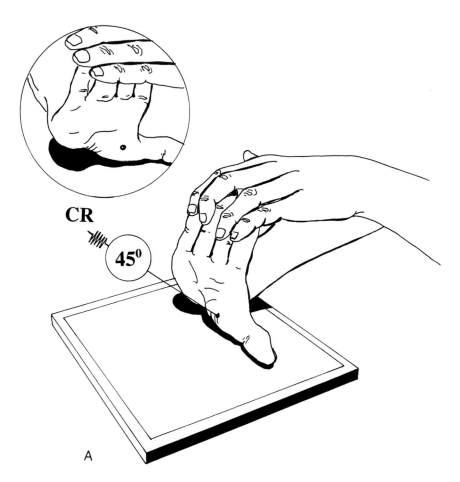

CR

45°

A

□ **FIGURE 1–7.**

POSITION DESCRIPTION

Part Position: The thumb is placed in the lateral position with the fingers fully extended and held with the opposite hand.

Central Ray: Angled 45° proximally and aligned with the long axis of the forearm, entering at the TMC joint.

Burman* Thumb Position *(continued)*

IMAGE EVALUATION

The trapezium and TMC joint should be clearly demonstrated and free of superimposition. The remainder of the carpus and the distal thumb are significantly distorted but are not important in this projection.

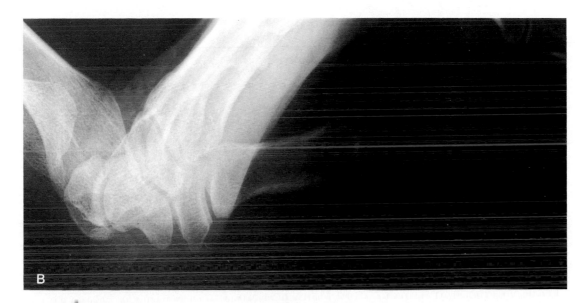

B

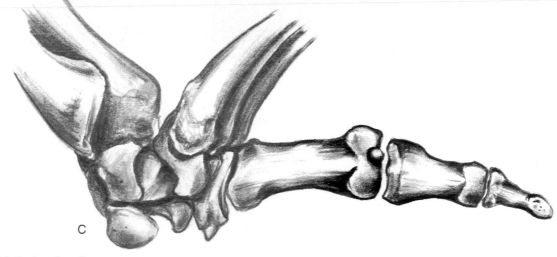

C

□ **FIGURE 1–7.** *(continued)*

Eaton* Stress Thumb Position

RATIONALE FOR USE

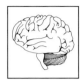

This projection demonstrates the *integrity of the trapeziometacarpal (TMC) joint under stress.* Injury or laxity of the surrounding ligaments may allow the thumb metacarpal to sublux or completely dislocate when stress is applied.

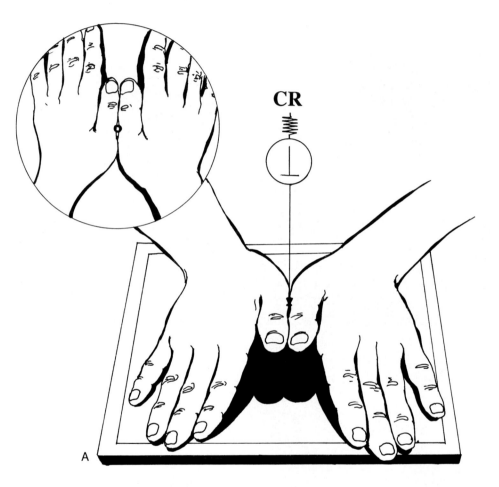

□ **FIGURE 1–8.**

POSITION DESCRIPTION

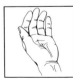

Part Position: Both hands are semi-pronated on the cassette with the radial (lateral) margins of the thumbs together. The patient is instructed to press the thumbs together with as much force as possible.

Central Ray: Perpendicular to the cassette, between the thumb metacarpophalangeal (MCP) joints.

Eaton* Stress Thumb Position *(continued)*

IMAGE EVALUATION

A PA projection of the TMC articulations of both thumbs should be clearly demonstrated. The exposure field should be limited to the area of interest.

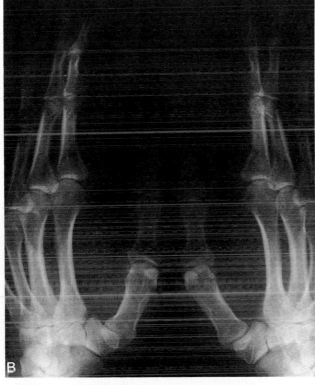

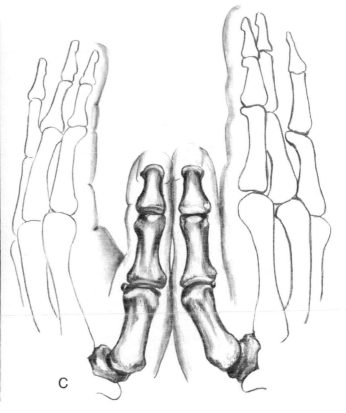

□ **FIGURE 1–8.** *(continued)*

(B courtesy of Paula Gunning, RT[R].)

---

*Eaton RG, Littler JW. Ligament reconstruction for the painful thumb carpometacarpal joint. *J Bone Joint Surg* 1973; 55A:1655–1666.

Gedda-Billings* Thumb Position

RATIONALE FOR USE

The Gedda-Billings thumb position accurately demonstrates the *first metacarpal base in lateral position*. This projection aids in diagnosis of fractures of the first metacarpal base.

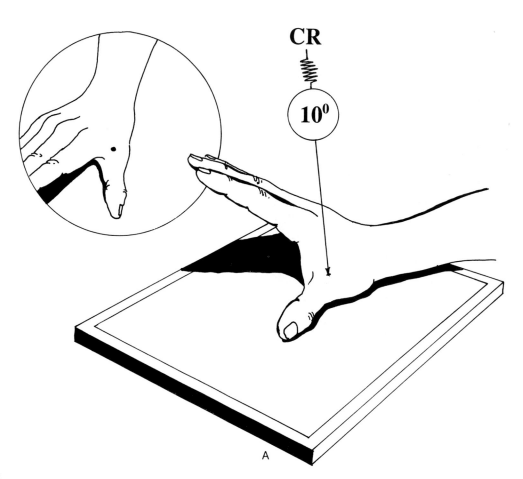

CR

10⁰

A

□ **FIGURE 1–9.**

POSITION DESCRIPTION

Part Position: The thumb is placed in the routine lateral position.

Central Ray: The central ray is angled 10° proximally along the long axis of the thumb, entering at the first metacarpal base.

Gedda-Billings* Thumb Position *(continued)*

IMAGE EVALUATION

The entire thumb is clearly demonstrated in lateral position, and the articular surface of the first metacarpal base is free of superimposition.

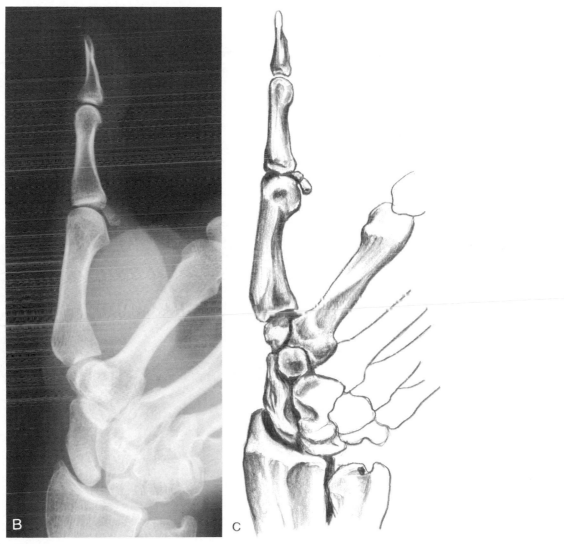

□ **FIGURE 1–9.** *(continued)*

*Billings L, Gedda KO. Roentgen examination of Bennett's fracture. *Acta Radiol* 1952; 38:471–476.

Modified Eaton Stress Thumb Position

RATIONALE FOR USE

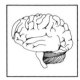

The modified Eaton stress thumb projection is performed to demonstrate the *integrity of the trapeziometacarpal (TMC) joint under stress*. Injury or laxity of the surrounding ligaments may cause the thumb metacarpal to sublux or completely dislocate when stress is applied. It has been suggested that this modification to the routine Eaton projection allows for greater axial force to the base of the metacarpal.

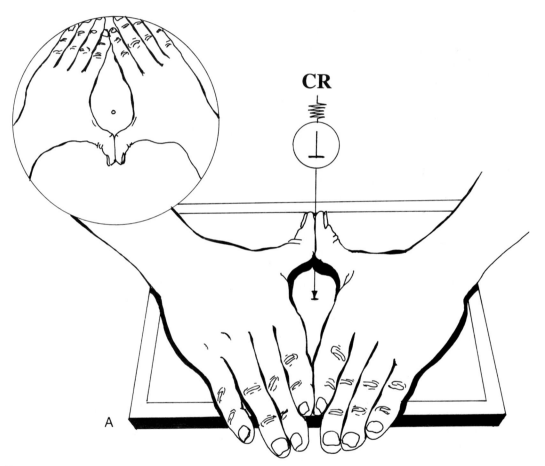

□ **FIGURE 1–10.**

POSITION DESCRIPTION

Part Position: Both hands are pronated and flat on the surface of the film. The palmar surfaces of the thumbs are placed together. The patient is asked to apply as much force as possible to the thumbs.

Central Ray: Perpendicular to the cassette, midway between and just distal to the thumbs.

Modified Eaton Stress Thumb Position *(continued)*

IMAGE EVALUATION

The TMC articulations of both thumbs should be clearly demonstrated. The exposure field should be limited to the area of interest.

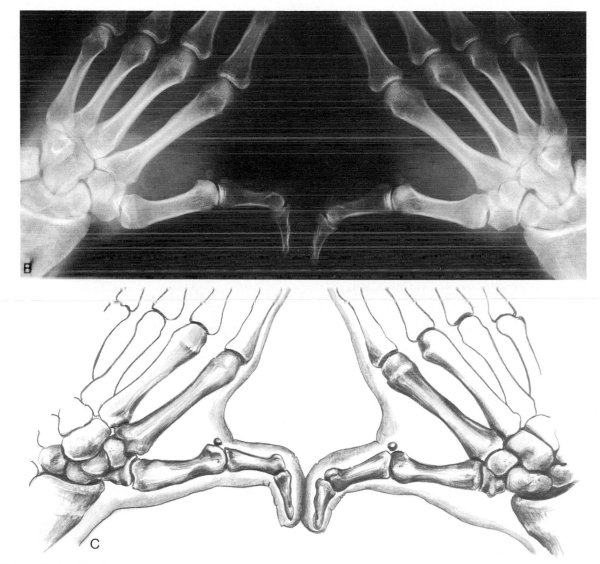

□ **FIGURE 1–10.** *(continued)*

(B courtesy of Paula Gunning, RT[R].)

Modified* Roberts Hyperpronation† Thumb Position

RATIONALE FOR USE

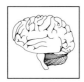

The modified Roberts hyperpronation thumb position results in an *AP projection of the trapeziometacarpal (TMC) articulation*, free of bone and soft-tissue superimposition. This projection aids in diagnosis of basilar fractures of the first metacarpal and arthritic changes in the TMC joint.

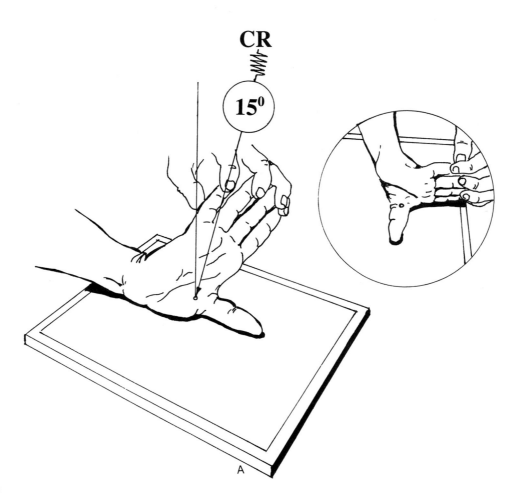

□ **FIGURE 1–11.**

POSITION DESCRIPTION

Part Position: The hand is hyperpronated to place the dorsal (thumbnail) surface of the thumb on the cassette, without obliquity. The remainder of the hand is dorsiflexed, and the patient may hold the fingers back with the other hand.

Central Ray: Angled 15° proximally, entering the base of the first metacarpal.

Modified* Roberts Hyperpronation† Thumb Position (continued)

IMAGE EVALUATION

The TMC articulation is clearly demonstrated in AP projection, without bone or soft-tissue superimposition.

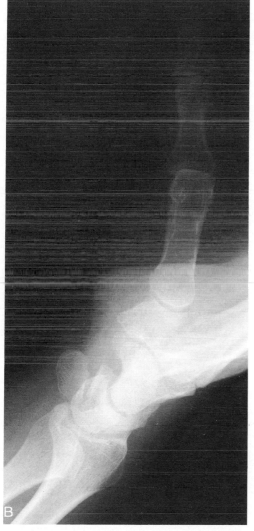

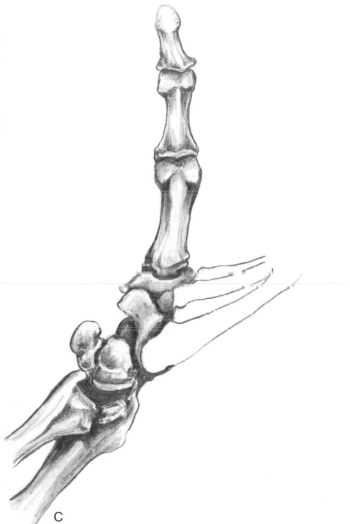

□ **FIGURE 1–11.** (continued)

*Lewis S. New angles on the radiographic examination of the hand—II. *Radiography Today* 1988; 54(618):29.
†Roberts P. La radiographie de l'articulation trapézo-métacarpienne. Les arthroses de cette jointure. *Bulletins et Memoires de la Societe de Radiologie Medicale de France* 1936; 24:687–690.

References

1. Bennett EH. On fracture of the metacarpal bone of the thumb. *Br Med J* 1886; 2:12–13.
2. Breen TF, Gelberman RH, Jupiter JB. Intra-articular fractures of the basilar joint of the thumb. *Hand Clin* 1988; 4(3):497.
3. Griffiths JC. Fractures at the base of the first metacarpal bone. *J Bone Joint Surg* 1964; 46B:712–719.
4. Wood MB, Berquist TH. The hand and wrist. *In* Berquist TH (ed). *Imaging of Orthopedic Trauma,* 2nd ed. New York: Raven Press; 1992:832.
5. O'Brien ET. Fractures of the hand and wrist. *In* Rockwood CA, Wilkins KE, King RE (eds). *Fractures in Children,* 3rd ed. Philadelphia: JB Lippincott; 1991:319–413.
6. Weissman BW, Sledge CB. *Orthopedic Radiology.* Philadelphia: WB Saunders; 1986:87.
7. Green DP, Terry GC. Complex dislocation of the metacarpophalangeal joint. *J Bone Joint Surg* 1972; 55A:1480.
8. Campbell CS. Gamekeeper's thumb. *J Bone Joint Surg* 1955; 37B:148.
9. Hankin FM, Peel SM. Sport-related fractures and dislocations of the hand. *Hand Clin* 1990; 6(3):446.
10. Downey EF, Curtis DJ. Patient-induced stress test of the first metacarpophalangeal joint: a radiographic assessment of collateral ligament injuries. *Radiology* 1986; 158:679–683.
11. Dray GJ, Jablon M. Clinical and radiologic features of primary osteoarthritis of the hand. *Hand Clin* 1987; 3(3):361.
12. Eaton RG, Glickel SZ. Trapeziometacarpal osteoarthritis: staging as a rationale for treatment. *Hand Clin* 1987; 3(4):459.
13. Billings L, Gedda KO. Roentgen examination of Bennett's fracture. *Acta Radiol* 1952; 38:471–476.
14. Burman M. Anteroposterior projection of the carpometacarpal joint of the thumb by radial shift of the carpal tunnel view. *J Bone Joint Surg* 1958; 40A(5):1156–1157.
15. Lewis S. New angles on the radiographic examination of the hand—II. *Radiog Today* 1988; 54(618):29.
16. Roberts P. La radiographie de l'articulation trapézo-métacarpienne. Les arthroses de cette jointure. *Bulletins et Memoires de la Societe de Radiologie Medicale de France* 1936; 24:687–690.

TWO

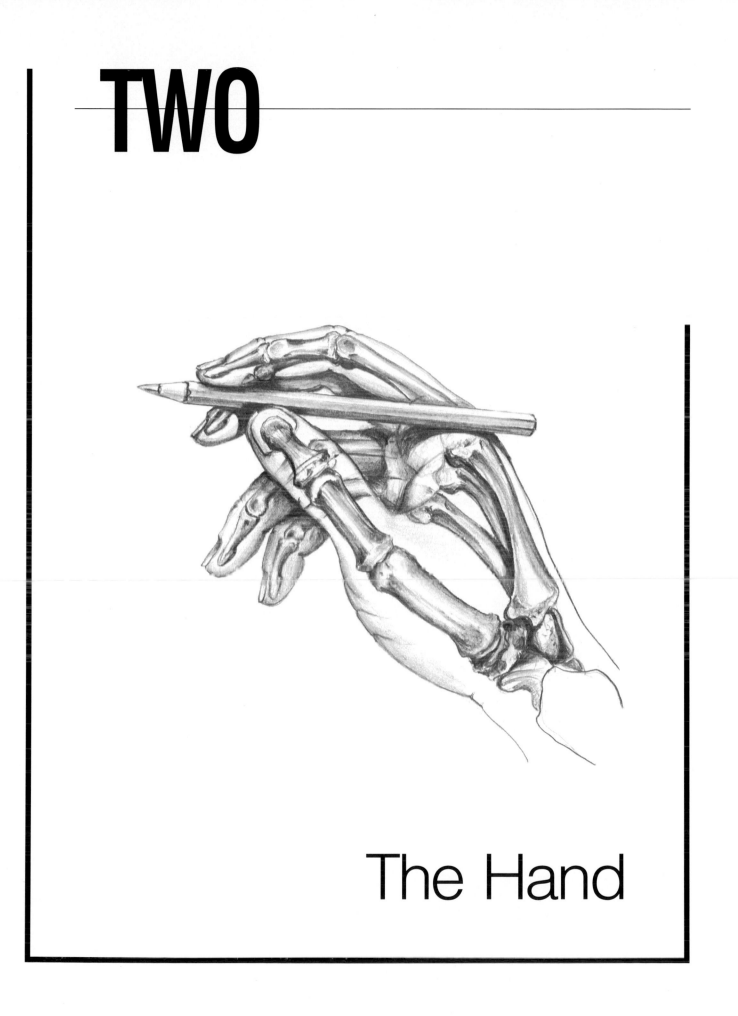

The Hand

THE HAND: AN OVERVIEW

ROUTINE HAND RADIOGRAPHY

Routine PA Hand Projection
Routine Oblique Hand Position
Routine Lateral Hand Position

SPECIALIZED HAND RADIOGRAPHY

AP Hand Projection
Bora Hand Position
Brewerton Hand Position
Extended Lateral Hand Position
Fourth and Fifth Metacarpal Oblique Position
Nørgaard (Ballcatcher) Hand Position
Relaxed Lateral Hand Position
True PA Hand Projection

The Hand: An Overview

The hand, with its apposable thumb, enables humans to manipulate their environment with great dexterity. Quality of life is based in part on its function. The location and extensive use of the hand frequently subject it to risk of injury. The phalanges and metacarpals are the most frequently injured components of the skeletal system. In addition, a number of arthritides affect the hands.

All phalanges and metacarpals are subject to fracture and dislocation to some degree. Those with the most exposure are injured most frequently. Fractures of the distal phalanges are involved in approximately half of all hand injuries; the middle finger is the most frequent site in adults.[1] The thumb ranks second in frequency of involvement. Crushed-eggshell, comminuted fractures of the ungual tuft are the most common injuries. They are usually nondisplaced and often accompanied by nail bed laceration. Transverse fractures through the proximal portion of the phalanx are less commonly seen and are associated with deformity (angulation and/or displacement) of the distal fragment. Crush injuries to the distal phalanges are common among young children, usually resulting from a door closing on the finger.[2]

The metacarpals are the second most frequently injured bones in adult hands. They are less commonly fractured in children. The fifth metacarpal is most likely to be fractured, followed by the first or thumb metacarpal.[3] The most common fifth metacarpal fracture is the **boxer's fracture**.[4] It is a transverse fracture through the metacarpal neck, resulting in volar angulation of the head. The fracture name is derived from the common mechanism of injury: punching a solid object with a bare fist. The majority of third and fourth metacarpal fractures occur in the midshaft, and these two bones are often fractured simultaneously. Fractures of the second metacarpal are more common at the distal end. In general, transverse fractures of the metacarpals tend to angle dorsally, whereas oblique fractures result in shortening or rotation. Fractures involving the thumb metacarpal are discussed in Chapter 1.

In adults, the proximal phalanges are injured less often than the metacarpals but more often than the middle phalanges. Half of all proximal phalanx fractures involve the thumb.[1] The index finger is next in frequency of injury. A fall on or a direct blow to the hand is the common mechanism of injury. Transverse or oblique fractures of the proximal or midportion of the shaft are most frequently seen. As in the metacarpal, transverse fractures tend to angulate, and oblique fractures to rotate or overlap. Radiographs of the entire hand are not sufficient to demonstrate these injuries because of the overlapping of phalangeal structures. The injuries are best demonstrated on radiographs of the individual finger or fingers.

In children, the proximal phalanges are fractured more often than the metacarpals. The thumb, fourth finger, and fifth finger are most frequently involved. In contrast to adults, shaft fractures are uncommon in children. A Salter-Harris type II fracture is most common and results from a hyperextension or torsion force.[2]

The middle phalanges are the least commonly injured components of the hand both in adults and in children. Fractures are most commonly seen in the distal shaft and result from crushing injuries or direct blows. Volar plate avulsion fractures are commonly seen at the base of the middle phalanx[5] and are the result of hyperextension injury. Radiographs of the individual finger or fingers involved are necessary in order to ensure that small bone fragments are not missed as a result of overlapping of other phalanges. Oblique and lateral images best demonstrate the avulsion fracture. In the absence of a bone fragment, a properly exposed radiograph aids in diagnosis by demonstrating associated soft-tissue swelling.

When the extremes of joint motion in the hand are exceeded, ligament or tendon injury can occur. The result of the injury may be pain, reduced function, or deformity. Much of the diagnosis is made on the basis of clinical presentation. Radiographs may demonstrate the presence of associated avulsion fractures or dislocation of the joint. When the metacarpophalangeal (MCP) joints are involved, radiography is helpful to determine whether the dislocation is simple or complex (irreducible).

The distal interphalangeal (DIP) joint may be involved in flexion or hyperextension injuries. Forced flexion of an extended DIP joint may cause extensor tendon avulsion or rupture in adults and result in a flexion deformity called **mallet finger** (baseball or drop finger). This injury is also seen in adolescents involved in sports, and it results from physeal separation (Salter-Harris type I or II fracture) or epiphyseal avulsion (Salter-Harris type III fracture) of the distal phalanx.[2] In some cases, an avulsion fracture on the dorsal aspect of the distal phalanx base is demonstrated on a lateral radiograph. Flexion injury can cause anterior dislocation of the DIP joint, but such dislocation is uncommon. Dorsal dislocation of the DIP joint results from hyperextension with rupture or avulsion of the volar plate. Hyperextension injury at the DIP joint may also cause avulsion or rupture of the flexor tendon. There is often no deformity, but the patient is unable to flex the joint. In either case, a volar avulsion fracture may be evident on a lateral or an oblique radiograph.

The flexion injury that causes mallet finger in the DIP joint may cause an equivalent injury to the proximal interphalangeal joint (PIP). When the PIP joint is involved, the injury is termed **trigger finger**. A dorsal avulsion fracture may be evident on the lateral radiograph. As in the DIP joint, excess flexion forces can cause anterior dislocation of the PIP joint, but such dislocation is uncommon. If an anterior dislocation were to occur at the PIP joint, rupture of the extensor tendon slip would favor development of a boutonnière deformity (see Chapter 1 for description). Hyperextension is the most common mechanism of injury at the PIP joint and is often caused by a fall on the outstretched hand. The injury may result in dorsal dislocation, volar plate rupture without dislocation, or damage to the flexor mechanism. The addition of axial force can result in fracture-dislocation.

MCP joint injuries often result from hyperextension forces, such as a fall on the outstretched hand. The border digits (thumb, index finger, and little finger) are most susceptible to MCP hyperextension injury.[6] A resulting dorsal dislocation is clinically evident, but radiography is needed in order to differentiate between a simple dislocation and a complex dislocation. The lateral radiograph may demonstrate overriding of the proximal phalanx against the dorsal aspect of the metacarpal head, joint space widening, or sesamoids within the joint space when the dislocation is complex.[7]

The carpometacarpal (CMC) joints are not commonly injured. When such injuries occur, they are present most often in the more mobile first (thumb) and fifth (little finger) CMC joints. Dislocation of CMC joints is often associated with crushing injury, direct lateral or dorsal blows, or punching a solid object with a closed fist. Injury is more commonly isolated to a particular joint, but extremely traumatic injuries tend to result in multiple dislocations or fracture-dislocations. A CMC dislocation may be associated with displaced fracture to an adjacent metacarpal.[8]

Of the routine hand radiographs, the lateral position best demonstrates the metacarpal base displacement of CMC dislocation. Posteroanterior (PA) hand radiographs must be performed with the palm flat in order to result in true representation of the second to fifth CMC joints. If the fingers cannot be extended, an anteroposterior (AP) projection should be substituted. This enables the metacarpals to lie approximately parallel to the film and better demonstrates small fractures of the base.[9] Loss or widening of the CMC joint space, on the PA or AP radiograph, may be the first indicator of a dislocation. When routine projections are inconclusive, they may be augmented. Green and Rowland[10] advocated use of 60° supinated and pronated ulnar oblique positions (rotated 30° off lateral). The Bora[11] hand position described in this chapter is a 30° supinated ulnar oblique position. Kaye and Lister[12] espoused the Brewerton[13] hand projection, also described in this chapter, for demonstration of occult metacarpal base fractures.

A significant number of conditions involving the joints manifest in the hands and wrists. Radiography of the hand and wrist is commonly performed when an arthritis is suspected. These radiographs may aid in initial diagnosis and documentation of disease progression. Exposure and positioning must be precise because early radiographic signs are often subtle. Differential diagnosis, on the basis of hand radiographs, is often possible because many arthritides have characteristic radiographic features.

Primary osteoarthritis is a degenerative joint condition most commonly involving the DIP joints of the fingers. The PIP and thumb CMC joints are next in frequency of involvement.[14] The radiographic features include joint space narrowing, marginal osteophytes, subchondral sclerosis, subchondral cysts, and alteration in the shape of bone ends.[15]

Rheumatoid arthritis is the most common inflammatory arthritide. It often begins in the hands and most commonly affects the MCP joints.[16] The PIP joints are also frequently affected. The earliest radiographic sign of the disease is often soft-tissue swelling involving the affected joints. According to Nørgaard,[17, 18] early bone changes involve the bases of the proximal phalanges and consist of cortical irregularity on the dorsoradial aspect. He advocated use of the Nørgaard[17] (ballcatcher) half-supinated ulnar oblique position, described in this chapter, to best demonstrate the abnormality.

Rheumatoid arthritis can cause significant deformity in the hand. Hypertrophy of the synovium causes stretching or rupture of the ligaments and tendons of the joint, as well as destruction of articular cartilage. These changes result in characteristic postures of the digits. The two most common postures are the swan-neck deformity and the boutonnière deformity. The **swan-neck deformity** consists of hyperextension of the PIP joint with flexion of the DIP joint.[19] Either joint may precipitate the deformity. It begins at the DIP joint with a mallet finger deformity, which is caused by stretching or rupture of the extensor tendon. The PIP joint hyperextends to compensate for the alignment imbalance. It begins at the PIP joint with hyperextension caused by stretching or rupture of the flexor tendon, or distention of the volar capsule. The DIP flexes to compensate for the imbalance. The **boutonnière deformity** is characterized by extension of the DIP joint, flexion of the PIP, and extension of the MCP joint. The deformity is caused by synovitis of the PIP joint, resulting in stretching of the central portion (slip) of the extensor tendon. This is accompanied by volar slippage of the lateral bands of the extensor tendon and contracture of the retinacular ligaments.[20]

A number of other arthritides affect the hand. Although important, they are less common. For the sake of brevity in this chapter, these arthritides are discussed in Chapter 13.

Routine Hand Radiography

Routine PA Hand Projection

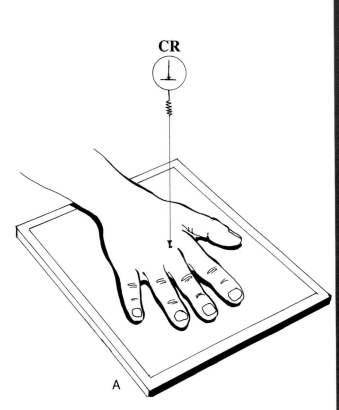

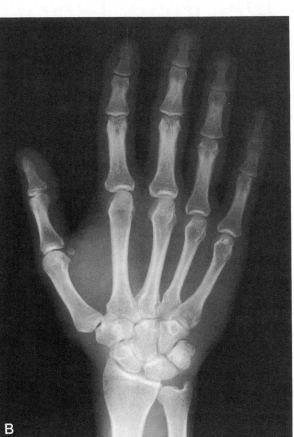

□ **FIGURE 2–1.**

POSITION DESCRIPTION

Part Position: Hand pronated on cassette with fingers slightly separated.

Central Ray: Perpendicular to the cassette, through the third metacarpophalangeal (MCP) joint.

IMAGE EVALUATION

A PA projection of the entire hand and wrist joint should be demonstrated without rotation (obliquity), as evidenced by equal concavity of both margins of the second to fifth metacarpal and phalangeal shafts. The interphalangeal (IP) and MCP joint spaces should be open when the hand can be placed flat on the cassette.

Routine Oblique Hand Position

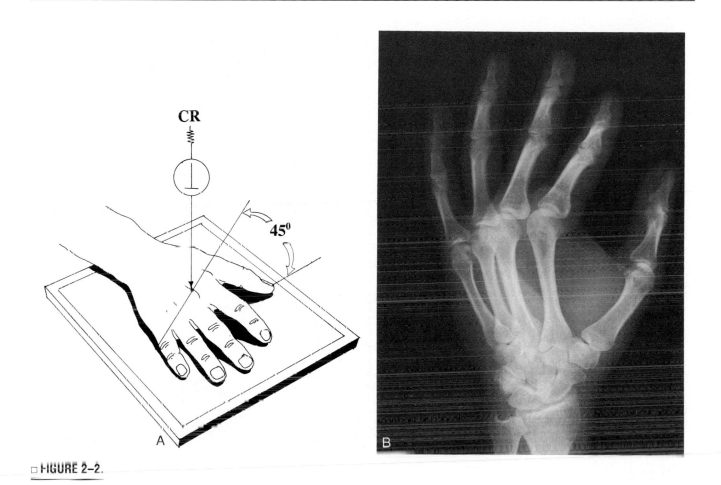

□ FIGURE 2–2.

POSITION DESCRIPTION

Part Position: The hand is semi-pronated to place the coronal plane (metacarpophalangeal [MCP] joints) at a 45° angle to the plane of the cassette. An oblique hand sponge should be used if the digits are to be evaluated.

Central Ray: Perpendicular to the cassette, through the third MCP joint.

IMAGE EVALUATION

The entire hand and wrist joint should be demonstrated in a semi-pronated ulnar oblique position. The interphalangeal (IP) joint spaces should be open when an oblique hand sponge is used. The metacarpal heads and bases will be slightly overlapped. The third and fourth metacarpal shafts will be slightly overlapped, but the second and third metacarpal shafts should be separated.

Routine Lateral Hand Position

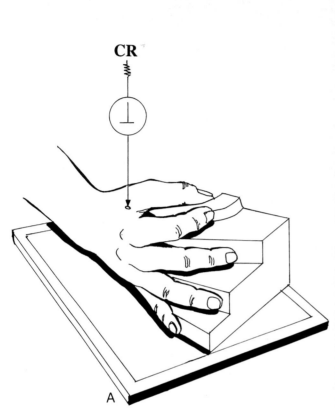

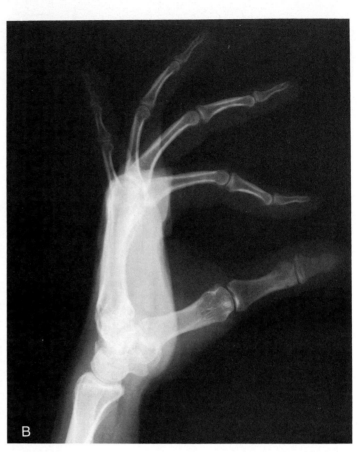

□ **FIGURE 2–3.**

POSITION DESCRIPTION

Part Position: The hand is placed on the cassette in lateral position, with the fingers separated in a "fan" configuration and the dorsal surface of the thumb parallel to the plane of the cassette. Forearm rotation is adjusted to superimpose the metacarpals, resulting in slight pronation of the wrist. Use of a fan lateral hand sponge is recommended for ease and consistency of positioning.

Central Ray: Perpendicular to the cassette, entering the second metacarpophalangeal (MCP) joint.

IMAGE EVALUATION

The second to fifth metacarpals should be superimposed, and all phalanges should be relatively free of superimposition. The metacarpals and phalanges should be seen in lateral position, as evidenced by concavity of the palmar margin of the metacarpal and phalangeal shafts. The thumb should be seen in PA projection, as evidenced by equal concavity of both margins of the first metacarpal and phalangeal shafts. The carpus and distal radius/ulna will appear slightly pronated, and the ulna will be seen just dorsal to the middle of the radius.

Specialized Hand Radiography

AP Hand Projection

RATIONALE FOR USE

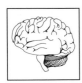

The AP hand projection is used as a *substitute for the PA hand projection*, when the *patient's condition does not allow extension of the fingers*. This position enables the metacarpals to be placed parallel to the cassette, in spite of the flexed fingers.

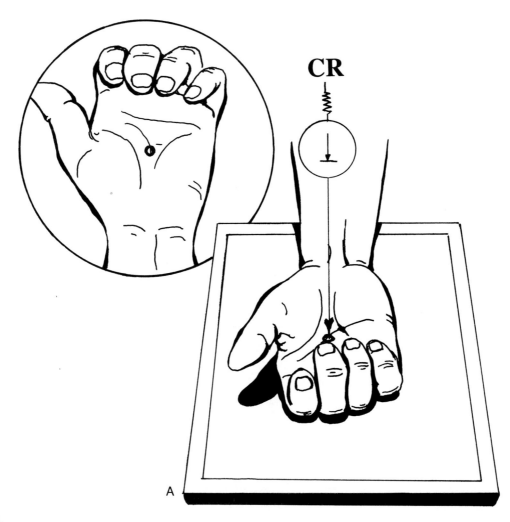

CR

A

□ **FIGURE 2–4.**

POSITION DESCRIPTION

Part Position: The hand is supinated and the dorsal surface placed on the cassette. Rotation is adjusted so that the palmar surface of the hand is placed parallel to the cassette.

Central Ray: Perpendicular to the cassette, through the center of the palm.

AP Hand Projection *(continued)*

IMAGE EVALUATION

The metacarpals, carpus, and distal radius/ulna should be seen in AP projection without rotation, as evidenced by equal concavity of both margins of the second to fifth metacarpal shafts. The ulnar styloid should be superimposed over the middle of the ulnar head.

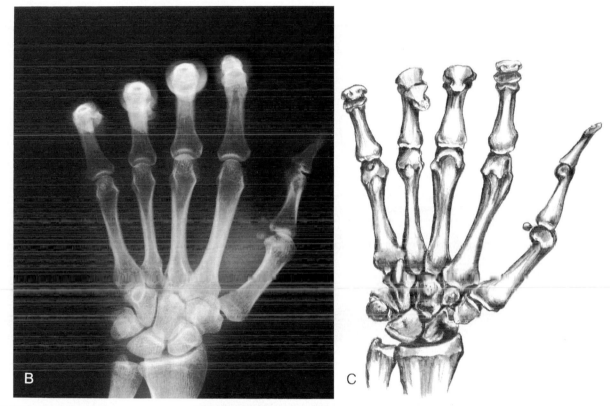

□ **FIGURE 2–4.** *(continued)*

Bora* Hand Position

RATIONALE FOR USE

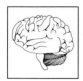

The Bora hand position demonstrates the *bases of the fourth and fifth metacarpals and the carpometacarpal (CMC) articulation with the hamate.* This may aid in the diagnosis of trauma and bone changes from arthritis.

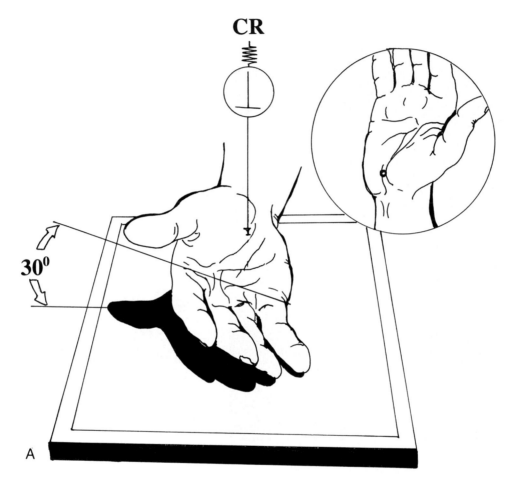

□ **FIGURE 2–5.**

POSITION DESCRIPTION

Part Position: The hand is placed in a 30° semi-supinated ulnar oblique position.

Central Ray: Perpendicular to the cassette, entering at the fourth CMC joint.

Bora* Hand Position *(continued)*

IMAGE EVALUATION

The bases of the fourth and fifth metacarpals and the articulations of the metacarpals and the hamate should be clearly seen. The exposure field should be limited to the area of interest for best detail.

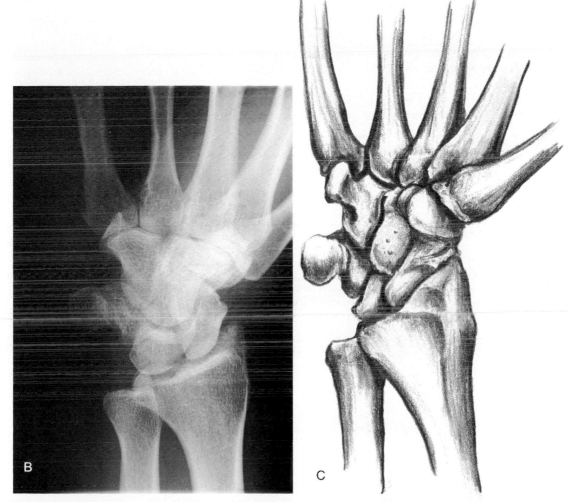

□ **FIGURE 2–5.** *(continued)*

*Bora FW, Didizian NH. The treatment of injuries to the carpometacarpal joint of the little finger. *J Bone Joint Surg* 1974; 56A:1459–1463.

Brewerton* Hand Position

RATIONALE FOR USE

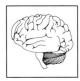

The Brewerton hand position results in a *tangential AP projection of the second to fifth metacarpal heads*. The contour and articular surface of the metacarpal heads are evaluated for early arthritic changes.

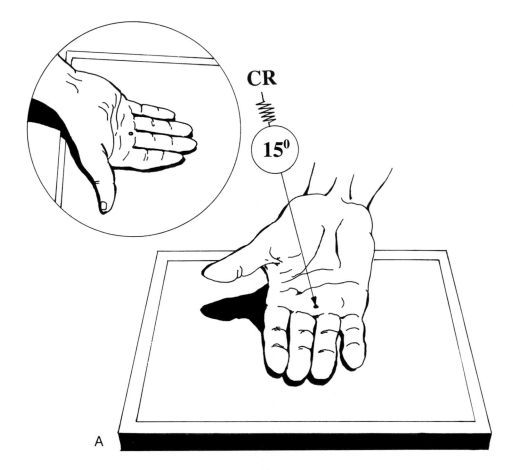

CR

15⁰

A

□ **FIGURE 2–6.**

POSITION DESCRIPTION

Part Position: The dorsal surfaces of the phalanges are placed in contact with the cassette. The hand is flexed at the metacarpophalangeal (MCP) joints, to result in a 65° angle between the dorsum of the hand and the cassette.

Central Ray: Angled 15° toward the ulnar (medial) aspect of the hand, entering at the third MCP joint.

Brewerton* Hand Position *(continued)*

IMAGE EVALUATION

The distal articulating surfaces of the second to fifth metacarpals should be clearly demonstrated. The MCP joint spaces should be open.

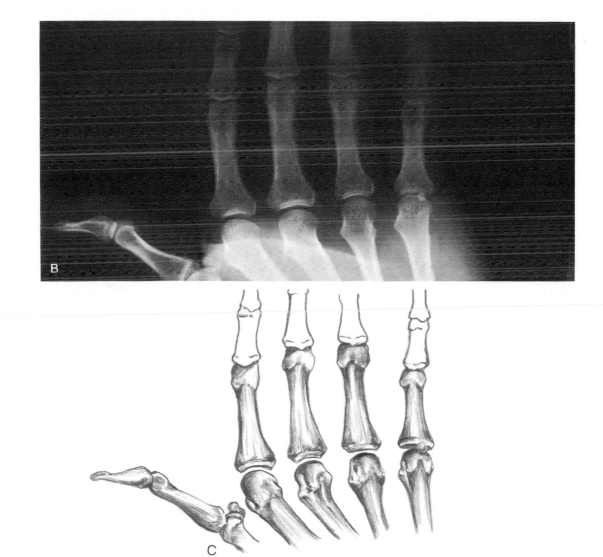

□ **FIGURE 2–6.** *(continued)*

---

*Brewerton DA. A tangential radiographic projection for demonstrating involvement of the metacarpal head in rheumatoid arthritis. *Br J Radiol* 1967; 40:233.

Extended Lateral Hand Position

RATIONALE FOR USE

The extended lateral hand position is used to *demonstrate suspected foreign bodies in the soft tissues of the hand.* The extended position results in optimal superimposition of the metacarpals and phalanges.

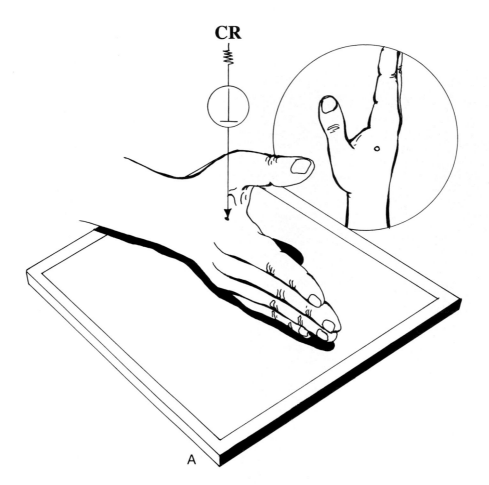

□ **FIGURE 2–7.**

POSITION DESCRIPTION

Part Position: The hand is placed in lateral position with the ulnar surface against the cassette. The fingers are extended, and the dorsal surface of the thumb is positioned parallel to the plane of the cassette. Forearm rotation is adjusted so that the metacarpals are superimposed, resulting in slight pronation of the wrist.

Central Ray: Perpendicular to the cassette, entering the second metacarpophalangeal (MCP) joint.

Extended Lateral Hand Position *(continued)*

IMAGE EVALUATION

The second to fifth metacarpals and phalanges should be seen in lateral position without rotation, as evidenced by concavity of the palmar margin of the metacarpal and phalangeal shafts. The thumb should be seen in PA projection, as evidenced by equal concavity of both margins of the first metacarpal and phalangeal shafts. The carpus and distal radius/ulna will appear slight pronated, and the ulna will be seen just dorsal to the middle of the radius.

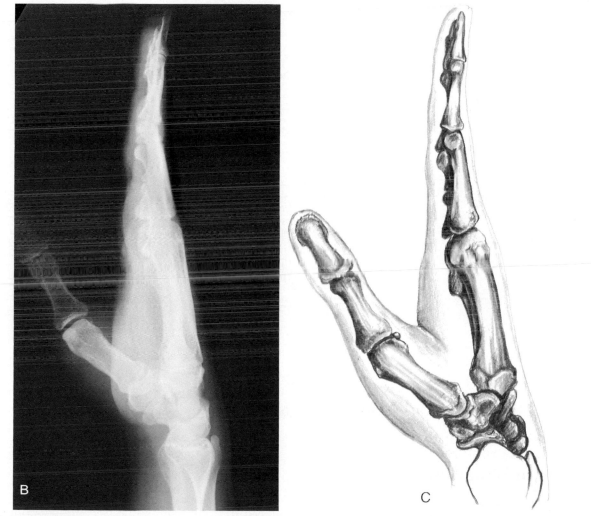

□ **FIGURE 2–7.** *(continued)*

Fourth and Fifth Metacarpal Oblique Position*

RATIONALE FOR USE

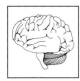

This position results in a *near lateral projection of the fourth and fifth metacarpals*, with minimal superimposition by the second and third metacarpals. The hook of the hamate is also well demonstrated in its broadest aspect and with minimal superimposition.

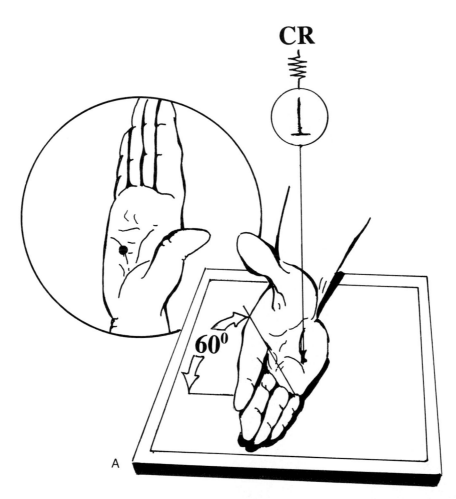

□ **FIGURE 2–8.**

POSITION DESCRIPTION

Part Position: The hand is placed in a 60° semi-supinated ulnar oblique position with the fingers extended. The thumb is abducted to prevent superimposition over the area of interest.

Central Ray: Perpendicular to the cassette, entering the middle of the palm (mid-shaft of the third metacarpal).

Note: If the hamate hook is the structure of interest, centering is through the midcarpus.

Fourth and Fifth Metacarpal Oblique Position* *(continued)*

IMAGE EVALUATION

The hand and wrist should be seen in a steep oblique position. The fourth and fifth metacarpals should be relatively free of superimposition by the second and third metacarpals. The hook of the hamate should appear in its broadest aspect, just proximal to the fifth metacarpal base.

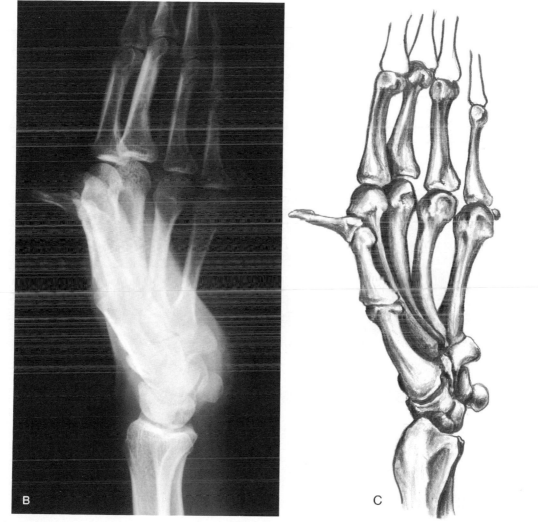

□ **FIGURE 2–8.** *(continued)*

---

*Green DP, Rowland SA. Fractures and dislocations in the hand. *In* Rockwood CA, Green DP, Buckholz RW (eds). *Rockwood and Green's Fractures in Adults.* Philadelphia: JB Lippincott; 1991:527.

Nørgaard* (Ballcatcher) Hand Position

RATIONALE FOR USE

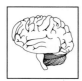

The Nørgaard (ballcatcher) hand position is useful to demonstrate *early arthritic changes at the dorsoradial aspect of the second to fifth proximal phalangeal bases.* The examination is performed bilaterally.

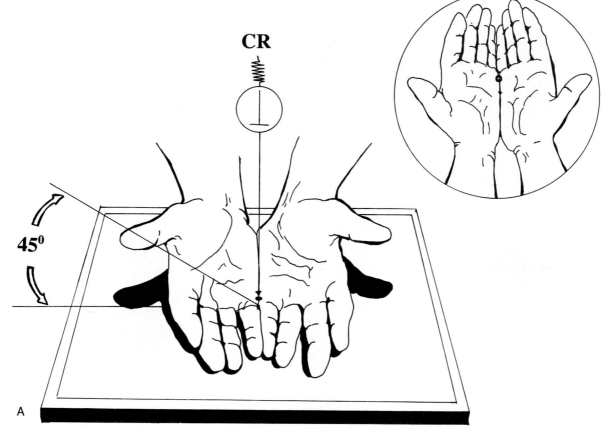

A

□ **FIGURE 2–9.**

POSITION DESCRIPTION

Part Position: The ulnar (medial) aspects of the hands are placed in close proximity, and both hands are adjusted in a 45° semi-supinated oblique position. The thumbs should be abducted to avoid superimposition.

Note: Nørgaard recommended resting the patient's hands on wedge sponges to prevent motion artifacts.

Central Ray: Perpendicular to the cassette, centered between the hands and at the level of the fifth metacarpophalangeal (MCP) joint.

Nørgaard* (Ballcatcher) Hand Position *(continued)*

IMAGE EVALUATION

The second to fifth proximal phalangeal bases of both hands should be clearly demonstrated. The MCP joint spaces should be open. The articulation between the fourth and fifth metacarpal bones may be demonstrated, as may that of the pisitriquetral joint. The exposure field may be limited to the area of the MCP joints, to improve visibility of image details.

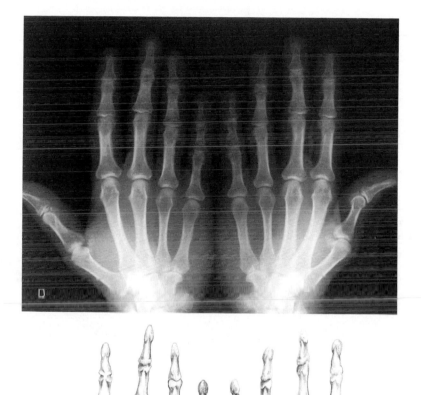

□ **FIGURE 2–9.** *(continued)* C

---

*Nørgaard F. Earliest roentgenological changes in polyarthritis of the rheumatoid type: rheumatoid arthritis. *Radiology* 1965; 85:325–329.

Relaxed Lateral Hand Position

RATIONALE FOR USE

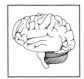

The relaxed lateral hand position is used to *evaluate anterior or posterior displacement of metacarpal fractures or dislocations*. The relaxed position allows the metacarpals to assume their natural relationships and is less painful for the patient.

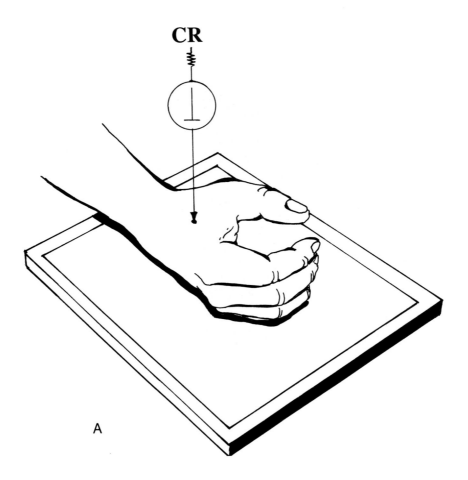

A

□ **FIGURE 2–10.**

POSITION DESCRIPTION

Part Position: The hand is placed in lateral position with the ulnar surface against the cassette. The fingers are allowed to relax and assume their normal flexed position. The dorsal surface of the thumb is positioned parallel to the plane of the cassette. Forearm rotation is adjusted to superimpose the metacarpals, resulting in slight pronation of the wrist.

Central Ray: Perpendicular to the cassette, entering the second metacarpophalangeal (MCP) joint.

Relaxed Lateral Hand Position *(continued)*

IMAGE EVALUATION

The second to fifth metacarpals and phalanges should be seen in lateral position without rotation, as evidenced by concavity of the palmar margin of the metacarpal and phalangeal shafts. The phalanges will appear flexed. The thumb should be seen in PA projection, as evidenced by equal concavity of both margins of the first metacarpal and phalangeal shafts. The carpus and distal radius/ulna will appear slightly pronated, and the ulna will be seen just dorsal to the middle of the radius.

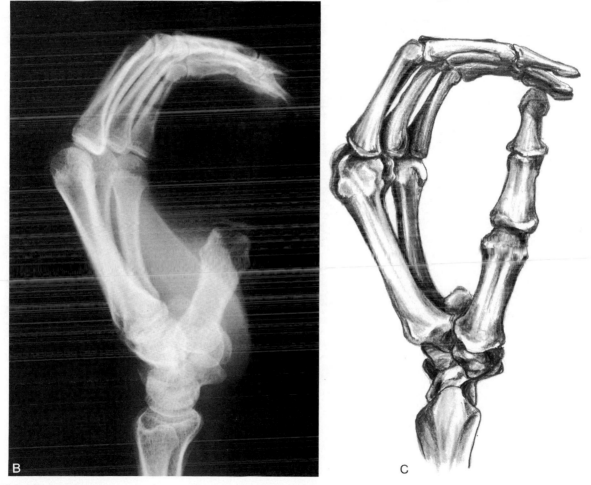

□ **FIGURE 2–10.** *(continued)*

True PA* Hand Projection

RATIONALE FOR USE

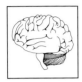

This position results in a *true PA projection of the second to fifth metacarpals and phalanges*. Superimposition of the scaphoid articulations is reduced, and the thumb is placed in a true lateral position.

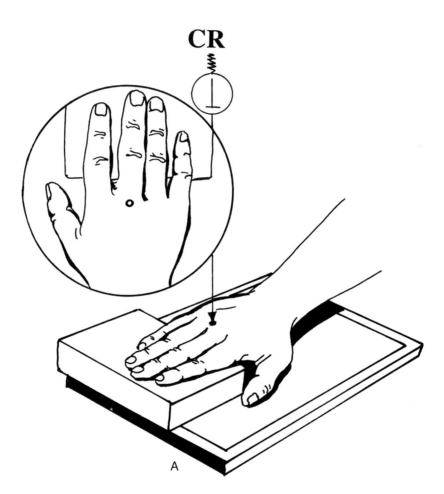

□ **FIGURE 2–11.**

POSITION DESCRIPTION

Part Position: The hand is pronated on a cassette; the ulnar aspect of the hand is raised to place the dorsum of the hand parallel to the cassette and is then supported with a sponge. The phalanges are adjusted parallel to the cassette and supported on another sponge. The thumb should be in a lateral position.

Central Ray: Perpendicular to cassette, through the third metacarpal head.

True PA* Hand Projection *(continued)*

IMAGE EVALUATION

The second to fifth metacarpals and phalanges should be demonstrated in a true PA projection without rotation (obliquity), as evidenced by equal concavity of both margins of the shafts. The scaphoid should be seen with minimal superimposition. The central carpometacarpal (CMC) and intercarpal joints should also be open. The thumb should be seen in a true lateral position.

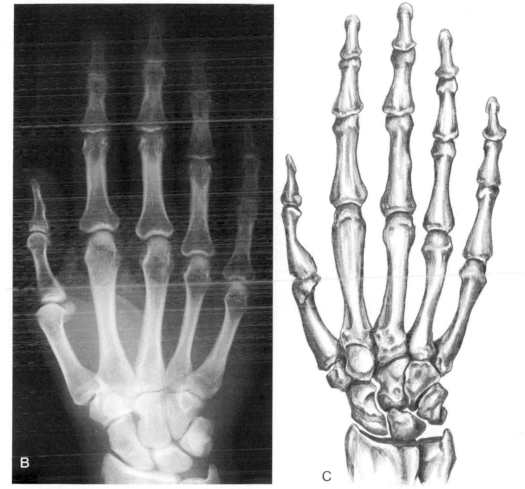

□ **FIGURE 2–11.** *(continued)*

---

*Lewis S. New angles on the radiographic examination of the hand—I. *Radiog Today* 1988; 54(617):44–45.

References

1. Butt WB. Fractures of the hand. *Can Med Assoc J* 1962; 86:731.
2. O'Brien ET. Fractures of the hand and wrist. *In* Rockwood CA, Wilkins KE, King RE (eds). *Fractures in Children,* 3rd ed. Philadelphia: JB Lippincott; 1991:319–413.
3. Rogers LF. *Radiology of Skeletal Trauma.* London: Churchill Livingstone; 1982:576.
4. Neviaser RJ, Eisenfeld LS, Weisel SW, Lewis RJ. *Emergency Orthopedic Radiology.* New York: Churchill Livingstone; 1985:144.
5. Nance EP, Kaye JJ, Milek MA. Volar plate fractures. *Radiology* 1979; 133:61.
6. Green DP, Terry GC. Complex dislocation of the metacarpophalangeal joint. *J Bone Joint Surg* 1973; 55A:1480–1486.
7. Kaplan EB. Dorsal dislocation of the metacarpophalangeal joint of the index finger. *J Bone Joint Surg* 1957; 39A:1081–1086.
8. Hsu JD, Curtis RM. Carpometacarpal dislocations on the ulnar side of the hand. *J Bone Joint Surg* 1970; 52A:927–930.
9. Murless BC. Fracture-dislocation of the base of the fifth metacarpal base. *Br J Surg* 1943; 31:402–404.
10. Green DP, Rowland SA. Fractures and dislocations in the hand. *In* Rockwood CA, Green DP, Buckholz RW (eds). *Rockwood and Green's Fractures in Adults.* Philadelphia: JB Lippincott; 1991:527.
11. Bora FW, Didizian NH. The treatment of injuries to the carpometacarpal joint of the little finger. *J Bone Joint Surg* 1974; 56A:1459–1463.
12. Kaye JJ, Lister GD. Another use for the Brewerton view (letter). *J Hand Surg* 1978; 3:603.
13. Brewerton DA. A tangential radiographic projection for demonstrating involvement of the metacarpal head in rheumatoid arthritis. *Br J Radiol* 1967; 40:233.
14. Buckwalter KA, Swan JS, Braunstein EM. Evaluation of joint disease in the adult hand and wrist. *Hand Clin* 1991; 7(1):135–151.
15. Dray GJ, Jablon M. Clinical and radiologic features of primary osteoarthritis of the hand. *Hand Clin* 1987; 3(3):351–367.
16. Wilson RL, Carlblom ER. The rheumatoid metacarpophalangeal joint. *Hand Clin* 1989; 5(2):223.
17. Nørgaard F. Earliest roentgenological changes in polyarthritis of the rheumatoid type: rheumatoid arthritis. *Radiology* 1965; 85:325–329.
18. Nørgaard FE. Diagnosis of arthritis. *Radiology* 1982; 142:807.
19. Nalebuff EA. The rheumatoid swan-neck deformity. *Hand Clin* 1989; 5(2):203–214.
20. Ferlic DC. Boutonnière deformities in rheumatoid arthritis. *Hand Clin* 1989; 5(2):215–222.

THREE

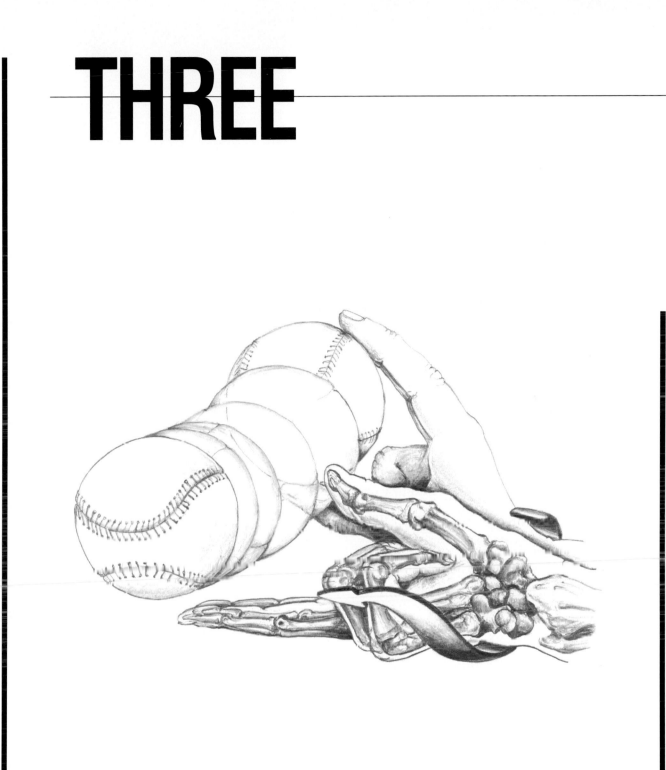

The Wrist

THE WRIST: AN OVERVIEW

ROUTINE WRIST RADIOGRAPHY

Routine PA Wrist Projection
Routine Oblique Wrist Position
Routine Lateral Wrist Position

SPECIALIZED WRIST RADIOGRAPHY

AP Wrist Projection
Capitate Position
Carpal Boss Position
Carpal Bridge Position
Clements-Nakayama Trapezium Position
Clenched-Fist AP Wrist Projection
Clenched-Fist PA Wrist Projection
Extension Lateral Wrist Position
Flexion Lateral Wrist Position
Gaynor-Hart Carpal Tunnel Position
Holly Pisiform Oblique Position
Holly Trapezium Position
Modified Stecher Scaphoid Position
Multiple-Angle Scaphoid Series
Papilion Hook of the Hamate Position
Radial Deviation (Flexion) PA Wrist Projection
Ulnar Deviation (Flexion) PA Wrist Projection
Zero-Rotation Lateral Wrist Position
Zero-Rotation PA Wrist Projection
Zero-Rotation–Ulnar Deviation PA Wrist Projection

The Wrist: An Overview

The wrist and forearm allow a great variety of controlled movements of the hand. The eight irregular bones of the carpus, in combined interaction with the radius, ulna, and metacarpals, result in an extensive range of motions. The basic motions, usually occurring in combination, include dorsovolar flexion or extension, radioulnar deviation, and axial rotation (pronation-supination). The majority of the motion in the wrist occurs at the radiocarpal and midcarpal joints. Pronation-supination of the hand is produced by forearm rotation. Motion in the carpometacarpal joints is primarily restricted to the thumb and the ulnar fourth and fifth fingers, which contribute to hand grip. Injury or disease that affects the wrist may limit the manipulative abilities of the hand. For this reason, prompt diagnosis of pathology is essential in order to reduce the likelihood of chronic instability in this joint.

Wrist fractures are the most common skeletal injuries and may involve the carpus or distal forearm. The most common mechanism of injury is a fall on the outstretched hand, resulting in hyperextension. The type and extent of injury are related to age, physical condition, direction and magnitude of force, degree of hyperextension, and amount of axial rotation and/or radioulnar deviation. For example, Weber and Chao[1] determined experimentally that scaphoid fractures tend to occur with hyperextension (dorsiflexion) greater than 95° and when the force is concentrated on the radial aspect of the corpus.

The most common injuries of the wrist involve fractures of the distal radius and ulna. They occur approximately 10 times more frequently than fractures of the carpals.[2] Colles'[3] fracture is the most common in adults, especially in elderly women. It consists of a dorsally and radially angulated, transverse fracture of the distal radial metaphysis. The fracture is frequently comminuted, may extend into the joint surface, and may be accompanied by an associated ulnar styloid fracture or distal radioulnar joint dislocation. The less frequently seen reverse Colles' fracture, or **Smith's**[4, 5] **fracture**, is characterized by volar angulation of the radial fragment. Colles' and Smith's fractures have a very similar appearance on the posteroanterior (PA) radiograph. The essential interpretation of dorsal or volar angulation is made from the lateral radiograph.

The distal radius is also the most common site of injury in children.[6] The fracture may involve the metaphysis or physis. A complete fracture of the distal radial metaphysis with a greenstick fracture of the distal ulna is frequently seen. The physeal fracture is usually a Salter-Harris type I or II fracture.[7] Distal radius fractures in children are seldom intra-articular.

A significant intra-articular fracture of the adult radius is **Barton's**[5, 8] **fracture**. It consists of a radiocarpal fracture-dislocation involving the anterior (volar) or posterior (dorsal) rim of the distal radius. The carpus is displaced dorsally or volarward, depending on which rim is fractured. The classic type involves dorsal dislocation. Again, the lateral radiograph is most useful in determining the type and extent of injury. Another intra-articular distal radius fracture is the **chauffeur's (Hutchinson's) fracture**. It is characteristically a nondisplaced, oblique fracture of the radial styloid resulting from avulsion by the medial collateral ligament, direct blows, or impaction by the scaphoid. The fracture line is sagittally oriented and is best demonstrated on the PA projection.

Isolated fracture of the ulnar styloid is uncommon and most often results from avulsion by the ulnar collateral ligament or triangular fibrocartilage. The fracture is best demonstrated on the PA projection, because pronation of the forearm results in location of the ulnar styloid on the lateral margin of the ulna. The anteroposterior (AP) projection should not be performed because supination of the forearm results in superimposition of the ulnar styloid and ulnar head.[9]

Radioulnar joint dislocation occurs as an isolated hyperflexion or hyperextension injury, or it may be associated with fractures of the distal radius. **Galeazzi's**[10] **fracture** is a fracture of the distal radial shaft at the junction of the distal and middle third with an associated distal radioulnar joint dislocation. The ulna may dislocate dorsally or volarward, and this is best appreciated on the lateral radiograph. A Galeazzi's fracture equivalent also occurs in children.

The mechanism of carpal injury is essentially the same as that of injury to the distal radius and ulna: a fall on the outstretched hand. The actual injury, whether bony or ligamentous, depends on the magnitude of force, point of impact, and posture of the forearm, wrist, and hand. In addition, carpal injuries tend to be age dependent. Scaphoid fractures are most likely to occur in persons aged 17 to 40 years.[2] In the young, distal radial metaphysis fracture or epiphyseal separation predominates over carpal injury.[11, 12] Fractures of the distal radius and ulna are more common than carpal injuries in patients over 40, especially the elderly, osteopenic population.

Most carpal injuries occur in the "vulnerability zone": an arc including the radial styloid, trapezium, scaphoid, proximal capitate, proximal hamate (tail), proximal triquetrum, and the midcarpal joint (scapholunate, capitolunate, triquetrolunate).[13] Fracture of the scaphoid waist accounts for approximately two thirds of carpal injuries. Dunn[14] found that the scaphoid was involved in up to 80% of all carpal fractures. It is believed that this may be due to the role of the scaphoids as a connecting rod between the proximal and distal carpal rows. It is tightly bound to each carpal row at the ends, and as the rows rotate away from each other during hyperextension, the scaphoid poles are forces in opposite directions. This may result in a stress fracture at the scaphoid waist.[15] In addition, Mayfield[16] demonstrated experimentally that the scaphoid may be fractured by impingement on the dorsal rim of the distal radius during hyperextension. Considerable attention has been given to radiography of the scaphoid, and so several scaphoid positions/projections are described in this chapter, including PA ulnar deviation, Stecher's,[17] and the multiple-angle series.[18]

The lunate is next most frequently fractured in the carpus.[19] As with most carpal injuries, the usual mechanism of injury is a fall on the outstretched, dorsiflexed hand. The fracture is thought to result from compression of the lunate between the capitate and radius, although avulsion and chip fractures are also seen. The compression-type fracture is significant in that it may lead to vascular compromise of the lunate. The resulting osteonecrosis or lunatomalacia was initially described in 1910 by Kienböck[20] and is commonly referred to as **Kienböck's disease**. Lunate injury is difficult to diagnosis radiographically at the time of injury because the fracture line is often obscured by surrounding structures, especially on the lateral radiograph. Also, trauma sufficient to cause Kienböck's disease may not be visible on a radiograph. When a lunate injury is suspected, a significant radiographic consideration is performing the PA projection without rotation of the forearm. This enables evaluation of the wrist for negative ulnar variance—a decrease in ulnar length in comparison with the radius—which has been linked to increased incidence of Kienböck's disease.[21] The zero-rotation wrist positions, from Epner and Bowers,[22] are described in this chapter to aid in evaluation of ulnar length in treatment of Kienböck's disease (ulnar lengthening) and settled Colles' fracture (ulnar shortening) and diagnosis in repetitive motion disorders.

The triquetrum is the third most commonly fractured carpal bone.[23] Dorsal chip fractures and body fractures are the most frequent; they result from hyperextension with ulnar deviation. The usual mechanism of injury for dorsal chip fractures is impingement by either the hamate or a long ulnar styloid.[24] Fractures of the body frequently result from impingement or a direct blow to the dorsum of the carpus.[25] Avulsion fractures can also occur because of the strong ligamentous attachments on the triquetrum. These may be dorsal (in hyperflexion injury) or volar (in association with perilunate dislocation).[23] The dorsal chip and avulsion fractures are best demonstrated on semi-pronated ulnar oblique and lateral radiographs. Fractures of the body are visualized on the PA and oblique radiographs.

The most common fracture of the trapezium is a radial margin shear fracture, commonly caused by compression between the thumb metacarpal and radial styloid during a fall on the hyperextended hand in radial deviation.[26] Fracture can also occur as a result of a direct blow to the dorsum of the wrist.[27] It is usually visualized on the PA and semi-pronated ulnar oblique radiographs. In some instances, specialized projections such as Roberts hyperpronation (described in the chapter on the thumb), the trapezium axial oblique of Holly[28] (described in this chapter), and the Clements-Nakayama position[29] (described in this chapter) may be needed to clearly demonstrate the basilar thumb joint and trapezial articulations. Cordrey and Ferrer-Torells[27] recommended a 20° semi-pronated ulnar oblique position to best demonstrate the trapezium. The trapezial volar ridge is occasionally fractured by a direct blow or forced distraction of the palmar arch during a fall on the outstretched palm.[30] The trapezial ridge may be demonstrated on the carpal tunnel projection.

Fractures of the hamate may involve the body or the hamulus (hook). Fracture of the body often results from direct crushing injury or indirect forces transmitted through the fifth metacarpal during a fist punch to a solid object.[25] The fracture is usually visible on the PA radiograph. The hamate hook is fractured either by a fall on the dorsiflexed wrist or, more commonly, during sports involving the use of clubs (golf), bats (baseball), or rackets (tennis). The sports-related fractures are thought to occur when these objects hit the hypothenar eminence or transverse carpal ligament during a missed strike.[31] The hamate hook is not well seen on routine wrist radiographs. Several positions and projections that demonstrate the hamate hook have been included in this chapter.

The pisiform is considered a sesamoid bone in the flexor carpi ulnaris tendon. Its position and relation to the triquetrum is maintained by the pisimetacarpal, pisihamate, and pisitriquetral ligaments. Fractures usually result from a fall on the outstretched hand or direct trauma. The most common fracture is linear and divides the bone approximately in half.[27] Avulsion, comminuted, and osteochondral (pisitriquetral joint) compression fractures may also occur, either as an isolated injury or in combination with other wrist injuries.[32] The pisiform is usually adequately demonstrated on the PA projection of the wrist. However, a 60°–70° semi-supinated ulnar oblique position is necessary to visualize the pisiform without superimposition of other carpals.[32, 33] The carpal tunnel projection may also be useful.

The capitate is infrequently fractured because of its protected central location. The most common mechanism of injury is forced hyperextension of the wrist, resulting in a transverse fracture of the waist (neck) or head.[25] The fracture may be associated with a scaphoid fracture (scaphocapitate syndrome) or a perilunate dislocation.[34] Direct, crushing injuries to the dorsum of the wrist may also result in capitate fractures. These fractures are usually visualized on a routine radiographic examination of the wrist.

The trapezoid is the least frequently injured carpal. Dislocation of this bone is more common than fracture. The most common mechanism of injury is a blow to the dorsal aspect of the index finger, resulting in a dorsal dislocation.[35] Fracture or dislocation of the adjacent metacarpal base may accompany the trapezoid dislocation. This dislocation or fracture-dislocation is best demonstrated on the PA and semi-supine ulnar oblique radiographs. The lateral radiograph is of less value because of superimposition.

The carpals are subject to a number of dislocations, most commonly during hyperextension injury. Many such dislocations are believed to be part of a continuum from the mildest, a series of perilunate dislocations, to the most severe, lunate dislocation. The most common classifications of carpal dislocation are dorsal perilunate, volar lunate, dorsal transscaphoid perilunate, and transradial styloid perilunate.[36] The dorsal perilunate dislocation is characterized by dorsal displacement of the capitate in relation to the lunate, with maintenance of lunate contact on the radial articular surface. In a volar lunate dislocation, the lunate is displaced anterior to the articular surface of the radius and the distal articular surface of the lunate faces palmar. The transscaphoid perilunate dislocation is basically a dorsal perilunate dislocation with a scaphoid waist fracture. The distal scaphoid fragment displaces dorsally with the capitate, but the proximal fragment remains with the lunate. The transradial styloid perilunate dislocation consists of a radial styloid fracture combined with a lunate or perilunate dislocation.[37] Other classifications of carpal dislocations occur, but are not as frequent. Volar perilunate and dorsal lunate dislocations are seen. In addition to lunate dislocation, other isolated carpal dislocations may occur. The most common is rotary subluxation or dislocation of the scaphoid.[36] Carpal dislocations are often evident on the routine PA and oblique wrist projections. However, the true nature of the dislocation is better appreciated on the lateral wrist radiograph.

In addition to the aforementioned fractures and dislocations, the wrist can exhibit carpal and radiocarpal instability patterns. These instability patterns result from new or old fractures, ligament ruptures (often associated with perilunate dislocation), or congenital ligamentous laxity. The instability may be present upon initial examination or may develop over time.[38] Radiographically, the normal relationship of the involved structures appears disrupted: malaligned, separated, or rotated. The most frequently encountered pattern of carpal malalignment is **dorsiflexion instability,**[39] sometimes called dorsal intercalated segment instability (DISI).[40] This instability pattern is best demonstrated on the lateral wrist radiograph as a slight palmar displacement of the lunate with its distal articular surface facing more dorsal than usual. This results in loss of the normal linear relationship among the radius, lunate, and capitate, with the distal capitate tilted palmar. The dorsiflexion instability pattern is most commonly associated with old and new fractures of the scaphoid, because stability between the two carpal rows (intercarpal joint) is maintained by the scaphoid.[38, 41] When no fracture is present, the dorsal instability pattern is commonly caused by a **scapholunate dissociation**. This loss of normal relationship between the scaphoid and lunate is due to disruption of the scapholunate interosseous ligament, and sometimes the ventral radiocarpal ligaments, during hyperextension injury to the radial side of the ulnarly deviated wrist.[42] This condition may result in widening of the scapholunate joint, often with palmar rotation of the long axis of the scaphoid when the ventral radiocarpal ligaments are disrupted. It is demonstrated radiographically as a widening of the scapholunate joint on a PA wrist projection. When a suspected scapholunate dissociation is not visualized on the routine radiographs, a PA or an AP clenched-fist or PA ulnar deviation position should be used.[43]

A **palmar flexion instability** or volar intercalated segment instability (VISI) is also seen. It may also be caused by scapholunate dissociation but is more commonly associated with **lunotriquetral dissociation**. This loss of normal relationship between the triquetrum and lunate is due to disruption of the interosseous lunotriquetral ligament, during hyperextension injury to the ulnar side of the radially deviated wrist.[19] Viegas and associates[44] demonstrated that a palmar flexion instability would not develop unless the lunotriquetral ligament tear was accompanied by disruption of the volar radiolunotriquetral and dorsal radiotriquetral ligaments.

This instability pattern is demonstrated on the lateral wrist radiograph, with the distal articular surface of the lunate facing more palmar than usual. The linear relationships of the radius, lunate, and capitate are disrupted, with the distal capitate tilted dorsally. Infrequently, the lunotriquetral joint may appear widened on a PA wrist radiograph.

The most common radiocarpal instability pattern is **ulnar (translation) translocation**, in which the carpus migrates ulnarward.[19] Upon visual inspection, the hand and carpus appear offset toward the ulna. This radiocarpal instability pattern is most often associated with radiocarpal ligament injury or perilunate dislocation.[45] It may also be seen in rheumatoid arthritis or Madelung's congenital deformity of the distal radius. Ulnar translation is best demonstrated on the routine PA wrist radiograph. **Dorsal subluxation** also occurs, often in association with collapse of a distal radius fracture.[46] This condition is demonstrated on a lateral wrist radiograph as dorsal migration of the carpus. **Palmar subluxation** occurs most commonly with rheumatoid arthritis and appears on the lateral radiograph as palmar displacement of the carpus.

Radiographic diagnosis of carpal and radiocarpal instability patterns is dependent on evaluation of changes in normal anatomical position and joint relationships. Routine positioning must be precise because wrist rotation, deviation, and flexion-extension affect radiocarpal and intercarpal relationships. The PA projection should be performed with the wrist in zero rotation and neutral deviation. The lateral position should be performed with zero rotation and neutral flexion-extension. These techniques are included in the routine and specialized radiographic positioning sections of this chapter. In addition, all or part of the "wrist instability" series of Gilula and Weeks[46] may be performed when instability is suspected but not evident on routine radiographs. The full series consists of three PA projections (neutral, radial, and ulnar deviation); AP clenched-fist projection; routine 45° semi-pronated ulnar oblique position; pisiform oblique (70° semi-supinated ulnar oblique) position; and four lateral positions (neutral flexion-extension, full flexion, full extension, and neutral flexion-extension with clenched fist).

In addition to fractures and instability patterns, the wrist is commonly affected by a number of arthritides. The pattern of wrist involvement often aids in clarifying the differential diagnosis. Primary osteoarthritis does not extensively involve the wrist; it is usually limited to the articulations of the trapezium.[47] The radiographic findings are non-uniform cartilage destruction, joint-space narrowing, sclerosis, subchondral cysts, and osteophyte formation. Secondary osteoarthritis is not as selective; it is most often related to previous trauma or repetitive motion injury, or it occurs in association with a crystal-deposition arthritis. The radiographic findings are similar to those of primary osteoarthritis, with the joint-space narrowing in regions of stress or weight-bearing.[48] Osteoarthritic changes are often evident on routine wrist radiographs. However, trapezial involvement is best visualized by use of the trapezium axial oblique of Holly[28] or the Clements-Nakayama position[29].

Rheumatoid arthritis commonly affects the hand and wrist. The earliest change is soft-tissue swelling, rather than osteochondral erosion. This swelling is most prevalent around the ulnar styloid in the wrist, but the synovitis progresses to involve the radiocarpal and intercarpal joints.[49] The earliest joint-space narrowing occurs at the radiocarpal joint and later progresses to the capitolunate joint.[50] The earliest bone erosions associated with rheumatoid arthritis in the wrist occur at the ulnar styloid.[51] The progressive osteochondral destruction and ligamentous laxity may result in wrist instability patterns. The patterns most commonly seen are ulnar translocation, palmar subluxation, and palmar flexion instability.[52] A scapholunate gap, as well as rotary subluxation of the scaphoid, may also result.[47]

Other arthritides also affect the wrist. Some of these include psoriatic arthritis, Reiter's disease, calcium pyrophosphate dihydrate deposition (CPPD) disease, and gout. However, space does not allow their full discussion in this chapter; they are discussed in Chapter 13.

Radiography plays an important role in the diagnosis and follow-up of arthritides. The presence and extent of the disease may be ascertained. Success of therapy, complications of the disease, and need for surgery may also be assessed.[53] Effective radiography depends on appropriate selection of exposure factors and imaging equipment to allow accurate visualization of both soft-tissue and osteochondral changes associated with early arthritis.

Routine Wrist Radiography

Routine PA Wrist Projection

CR

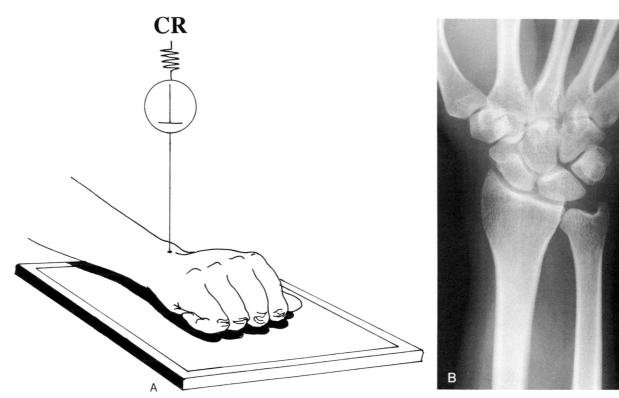

□ **FIGURE 3–1.**

POSITION DESCRIPTION

Part Position: The entire arm is parallel to the floor, with the elbow flexed 90°. The hand is pronated and the fingers flexed in order to place the volar (anterior) surface of the carpus in contact with the cassette.

Note: The appearance of carpal orientation changes with forearm rotation or with radial or ulnar deviation; both must be neutral.

Central Ray: Perpendicular to the cassette, through the midcarpus.

IMAGE EVALUATION

The carpus, distal radius and ulna, and proximal metacarpals should be demonstrated in a PA projection, with zero forearm rotation and neutral radioulnar deviation. The radiocarpal and intercarpal joints should be clearly seen.

Routine Oblique Wrist Position

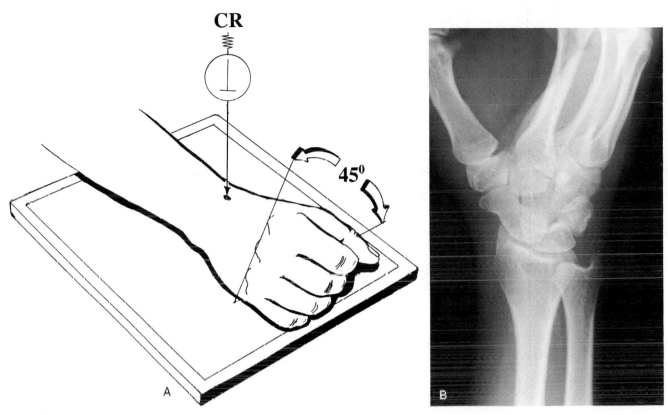

CR

45°

A

B

☐ **FIGURE 3–2.**

POSITION DESCRIPTION

Part Position: The hand is semi-pronated in order to place the coronal plane of the wrist 45° to the plane of the cassette.

Note: The appearance of carpal orientation changes with radial or ulnar deviation or radiocarpal flexion-extension; both must be neutral.

Central Ray: Perpendicular to the cassette, through the midcarpus.

IMAGE EVALUATION

The carpus, distal radius and ulna, and proximal metacarpals should be seen in a semi-pronate ulnar oblique position, with no radioulnar deviation or radiocarpal flexion-extension.

Routine Lateral Wrist Position

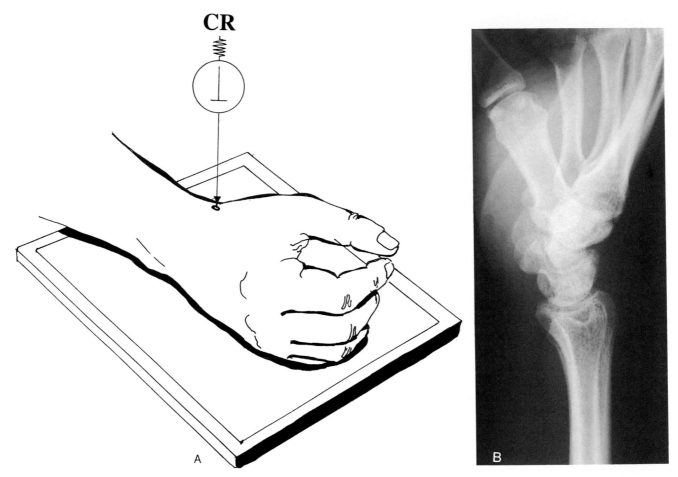

□ **FIGURE 3–3.**

POSITION DESCRIPTION

Part Position: The hand and wrist are placed on the cassette in an ulnar lateral position. Forearm rotation is adjusted to superimpose the radius and ulna, resulting in slight supination of the hand.

Note: Appearance of carpal orientation changes with forearm rotation or radiocarpal flexion-extension; both must be neutral.

Central Ray: Perpendicular to the cassette, through the midcarpus.

IMAGE EVALUATION

The carpus, distal radius and ulna, and proximal metacarpals should be demonstrated in lateral position, with no forearm rotation or radiocarpal flexion-extension.

Specialized Wrist Radiography

AP Wrist Projection

RATIONALE FOR USE

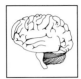

The AP wrist projection demonstrates the *carpals and intercarpal joints* more effectively than the PA wrist projection. This is because the x-ray beam divergence more effectively parallels the intercarpal joint spaces and also because of the position of the carpus.

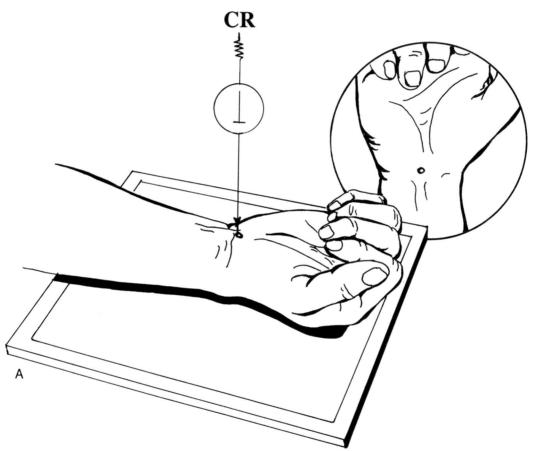

□ **FIGURE 3–4.**

POSITION DESCRIPTION

Part Position: The hand is supinated and elevated slightly on a sponge to place the dorsum of the wrist in contact with the cassette. Rotation of the forearm is adjusted in order to place the palmar surface of the wrist parallel to the cassette.

Central Ray: Perpendicular to the cassette, through the midcarpus.

AP Wrist Projection *(continued)*

IMAGE EVALUATION

The distal radius and ulna, the carpus, and the proximal portion of the metacarpals should be seen in AP projection, without rotation (obliquity) or radioulnar deviation. The carpals and intercarpal joint spaces should be well visualized. The ulnar styloid should appear superimposed over the middle of the ulnar head.

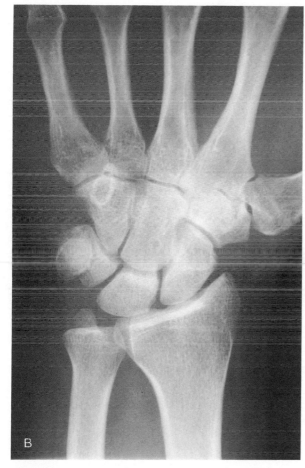

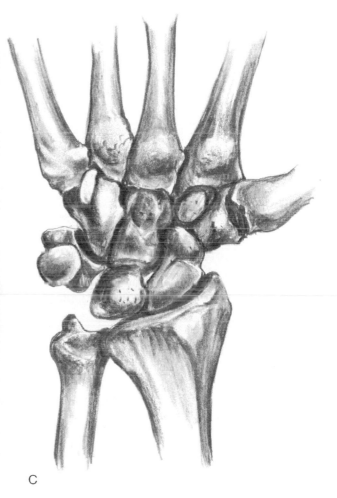

□ **FIGURE 3–4.** *(continued)*

Capitate Position

RATIONALE FOR USE

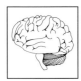

The capitate position allows visualization of the *entire capitate, with less foreshortening* than in the routine PA projection.

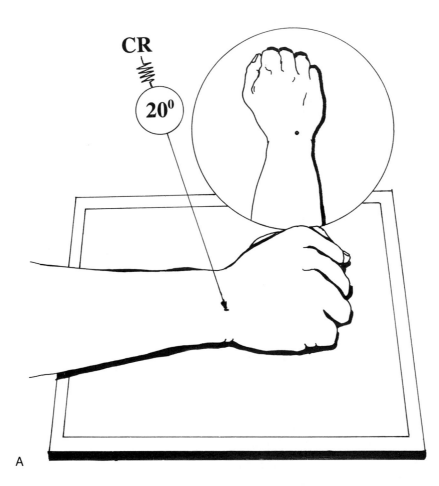

CR

20⁰

A

☐ **FIGURE 3–5.**

POSITION DESCRIPTION

Part Position: The wrist is positioned as for a routine PA projection.

Central Ray: Angled 20° distally, through the capitate (just proximal to the base of the third metacarpal).

Capitate Position *(continued)*

IMAGE EVALUATION

The capitate should be demonstrated with minimal foreshortening, as evidenced by visualization of the entire capitate waist. The lunatocapitate joint space should be open.

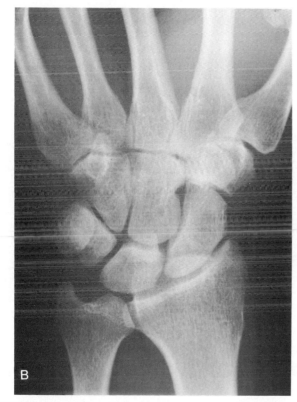

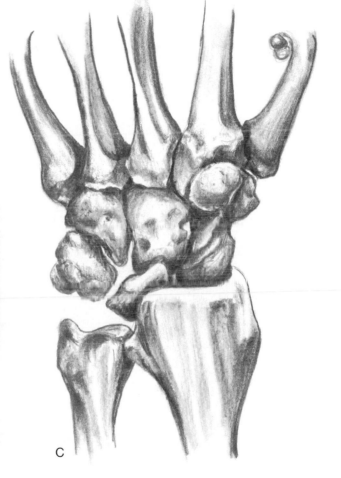

□ **FIGURE 3–5.** *(continued)*

Carpal Boss* Position

RATIONALE FOR USE

The carpal boss position allows *demonstration of a carpal boss*, which is a bony eminence on the posterior aspect of the wrist. This tangential projection visualizes the *dorsal aspect of the bases of the second and third metacarpals*, where there is the greatest likelihood of the presence of a carpal boss.

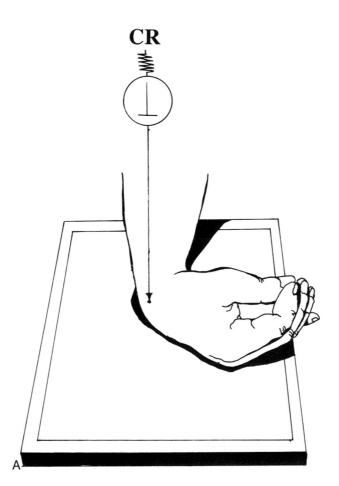

□ **FIGURE 3–6.**

POSITION DESCRIPTION

Part Position: The wrist is placed in a lateral position, with the hand in volar (palmar) flexion. A slight supination is added, by raising the forearm, to better visualize the bases of the second and third metacarpals.

Central Ray: Perpendicular to the cassette, through the base of the second metacarpal.

Carpal Boss* Position *(continued)*

IMAGE EVALUATION

The dorsal aspect of the second and third metacarpal bases should be seen in profile. The posterior aspect of the carpus should be clearly demonstrated, without overexposure. The remainder of the carpus may appear underexposed. The exposure field should be limited to the area of interest to improve image quality.

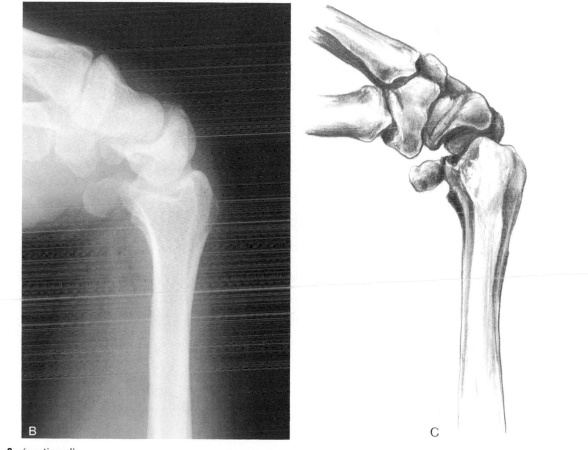

□ **FIGURE 3–6.** *(continued)*

*Fiolle J. Le carpe bossu. *Bull Soc Chir Paris* 1931; 57:1687.

Carpal Bridge* Position

RATIONALE FOR USE

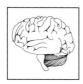

The carpal bridge position demonstrates the *dorsal aspect of the carpus, including the dorsal surface of the scaphoid, lunate, and triquetrum.* This tangential projection may be useful for evaluation of any injury or lesion in this area. In addition, the position may be more specific than the routine lateral position in localization of foreign bodies in the dorsal wrist soft tissues. The name "carpal bridge" was conferred supposedly because it is *over* the "carpal tunnel."

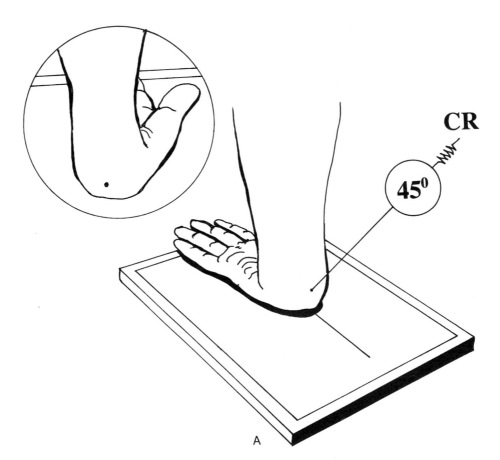

□ **FIGURE 3–7.**

POSITION DESCRIPTION

Part Position: The long axis of the forearm is vertical, and the wrist is flexed to place the dorsal surface of the hand in contact with the cassette.

Central Ray: Angled 45° distally, entering the distal forearm 2 inches above the cassette surface.

Carpal Bridge* Position *(continued)*

IMAGE EVALUATION

The dorsal aspect of the proximal carpal row should be demonstrated. The scaphoid will appear elongated, and the lunate and triquetrum will be seen in close proximity. The capitate may be seen, superimposed on the proximal portion of the scaphoid and lunate.

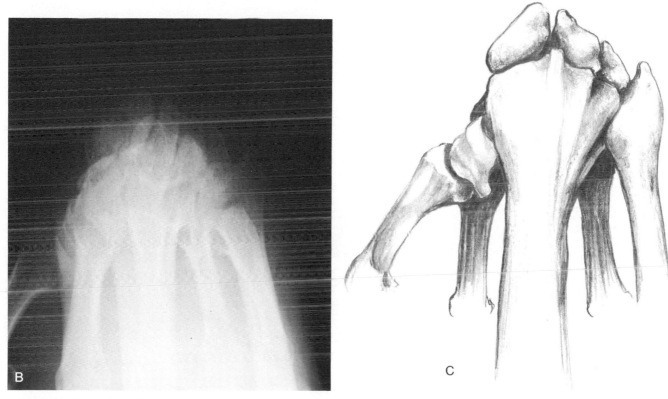

B

C

□ **FIGURE 3–7.** *(continued)*

*Lentino W, Lubetsky HW, Jacobson HG, Poppel MH. The carpal-bridge view: a position for the roentgenographic diagnosis of abnormalities in the dorsum of the wrist. *J Bone Joint Surg* 1957; 39A(1):88–90.

Clements-Nakayama* Trapezium Position

RATIONALE FOR USE

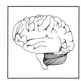

The Clements-Nakayama position enables visualization of the *trapezium, free of superimposition at its articulations.* The trapezium is commonly involved in osteoarthritis of the carpus, and this projection may be useful for evaluation of early bone changes. In addition, occult fractures may be diagnosed.

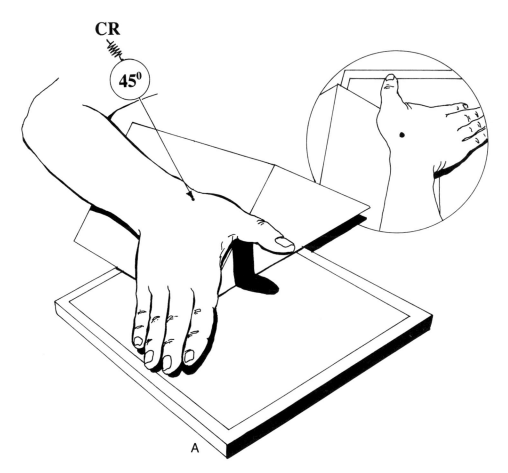

□ **FIGURE 3–8.**

POSITION DESCRIPTION

Part Position: The hand and wrist are placed in a 45° semi-pronated ulnar oblique position. Ulnar deviation of the wrist should be applied, if possible. A wedge sponge may be helpful in maintaining the position.

Central Ray: The central ray is angled 45° distally along the long axis of the forearm, entering the wrist at the snuff-box.

Clements-Nakayama* Trapezium Position *(continued)*

IMAGE EVALUATION

The trapezium should be demonstrated free from superimposition, and the surrounding joint spaces should be open. A significant amount of angulation distortion will be seen. Superimposition at the ulnar (medial) aspect of the trapezium often indicates too much wrist obliquity.

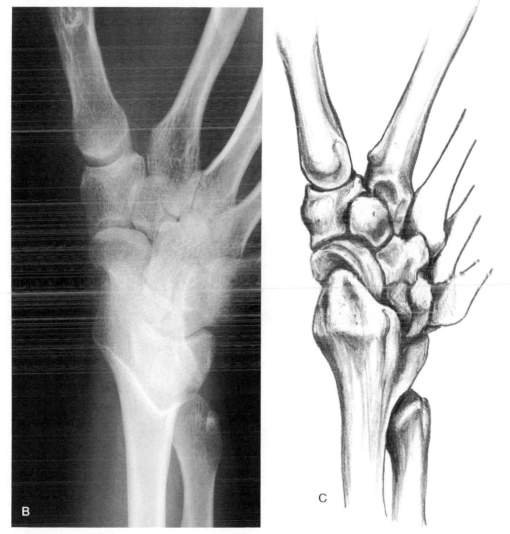

☐ **FIGURE 3–8.** *(continued)*

---

*Clements RW, Nakayama HK. Radiography of the polyarthritic hands and wrists. *Radiol Technol* 1981; 53(3):203–217.

Clenched-Fist AP Wrist Projection

RATIONALE FOR USE

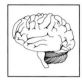

The clenched-fist AP wrist projection places *stress on the carpal and intercarpal ligaments, especially the scapholunate ligament.* Widening of the scapholunate joint space may indicate disruption of the scapholunate and radiocarpal ligaments. Choice of this projection over the clenched-fist PA projection is a matter of personal preference.

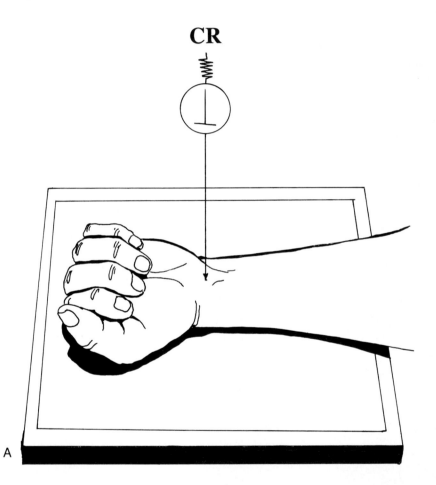

A

□ **FIGURE 3–9.**

POSITION DESCRIPTION

Part Position: The wrist is positioned as for an AP projection. The patient clenches the hand into a tight fist.

Note: An object, such as a wooden dowel, is often used for the patient to grip.

Central Ray: Perpendicular to the cassette, through the midcarpus.

Clenched-Fist AP Wrist Projection *(continued)*

IMAGE EVALUATION

The carpus, distal radius and ulna, and proximal portion of the metacarpals should be seen in AP projection, with minimal rotation (obliquity) or radioulnar deviation. The intercarpal joint spaces of a *normal* wrist will not appear significantly different than on a nonstressed AP projection.

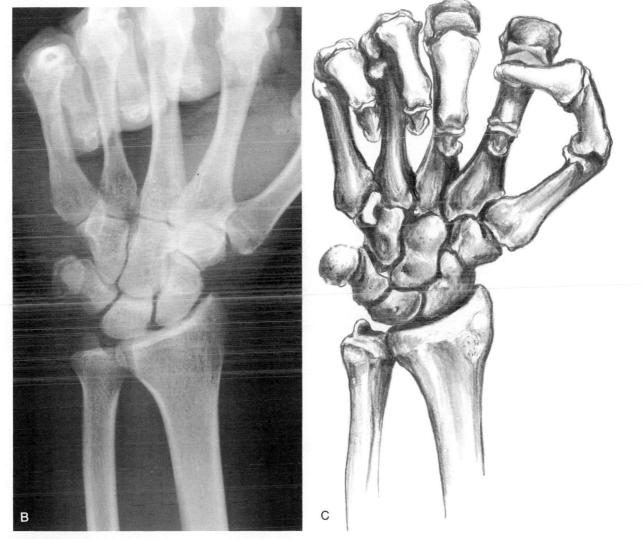

☐ **FIGURE 3–9.** *(continued)*

Clenched-Fist PA Wrist Projection

RATIONALE FOR USE

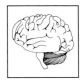

The clenched-fist PA wrist projection places *stress on the carpal and intercarpal ligaments, especially the scapholunate ligament.* Widening of the scapholunate joint space may indicate disruption of the scapholunate and radiocarpal ligaments. Choice of this projection over the clenched-fist AP projection is a matter of personal preference.

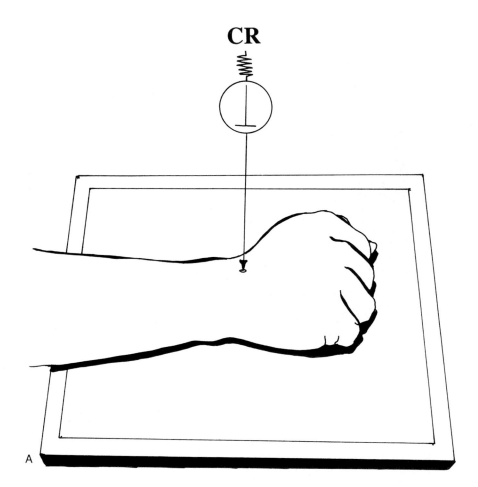

☐ **FIGURE 3–10.**

POSITION DESCRIPTION

Part Position: The wrist is positioned as for a PA projection. The patient clenches the hand into a tight fist.

Note: An object, such as a wooden dowel, is often used for the patient to grip.

Central Ray: Perpendicular to the cassette, through the midcarpus.

Clenched-Fist PA Wrist Projection *(continued)*

IMAGE EVALUATION

The carpus, distal radius and ulna, and proximal portion of the metacarpals should be seen in PA projection, with minimal rotation (obliquity) or radioulnar deviation. The intercarpal joint spaces of a *normal* wrist will not appear significantly different than on the routine PA projection.

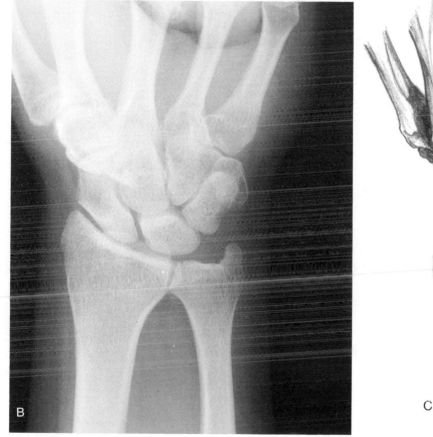

B

C

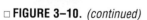

□ **FIGURE 3–10.** *(continued)*

Extension Lateral Wrist Position

RATIONALE FOR USE

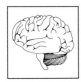

The extension lateral wrist position may be used to *evaluate loss of the normal relationships between the lunate, scaphoid, and capitate seen with carpal ligamentous instability.*

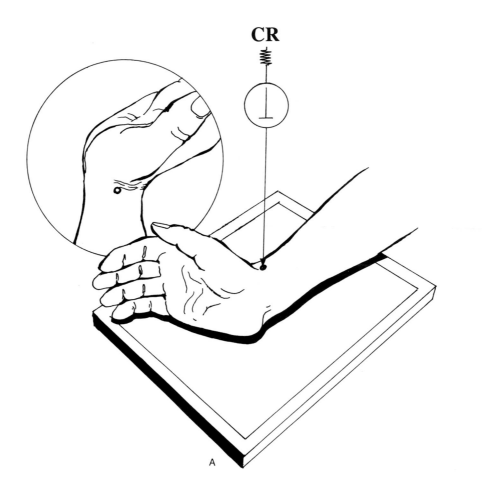

□ **FIGURE 3–11.**

POSITION DESCRIPTION

Part Position: The wrist is maximally extended (dorsiflexed) in the lateral position.

Central Ray: Perpendicular to the cassette, through the midcarpus.

Extension Lateral Wrist Position *(continued)*

IMAGE EVALUATION

The wrist should be seen in lateral position, with appropriate superimposition of the radius and ulna. The wrist should be seen in maximal extension (dorsiflexion).

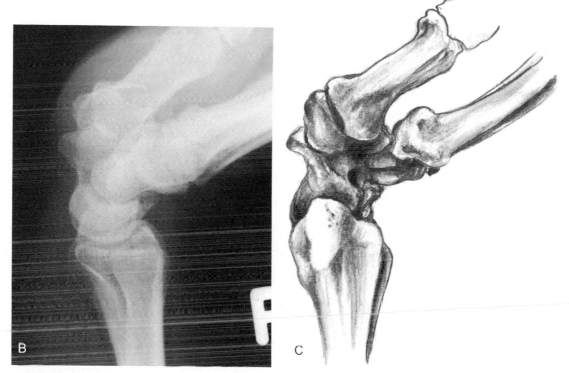

B

C

□ **FIGURE 3–11.** *(continued)*

Flexion Lateral Wrist Position

RATIONALE FOR USE

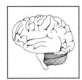

The flexion lateral wrist position may be used to *evaluate loss of the normal relationships between the lunate, scaphoid, and capitate seen with carpal ligamentous instability.*

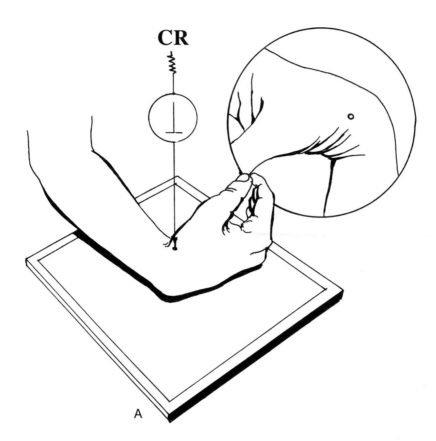

CR

□ **FIGURE 3–12.**

POSITION DESCRIPTION

Part Position: The wrist is maximally flexed in the lateral position.

Central Ray: Perpendicular to the cassette, through the midcarpus.

Flexion Lateral Wrist Position *(continued)*

IMAGE EVALUATION

The wrist should be seen in lateral position, with appropriate superimposition of the radius and ulna. The wrist should be seen in maximal flexion.

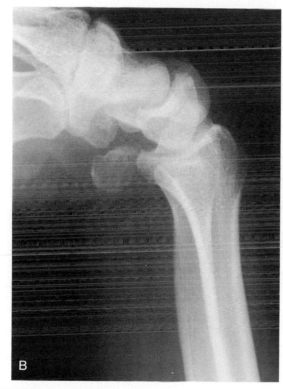

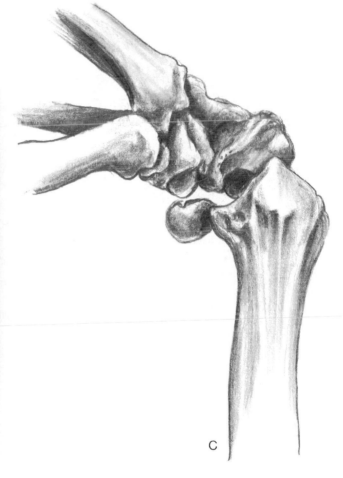

□ **FIGURE 3–12.** *(continued)*

Gaynor-Hart* Carpal Tunnel Position

RATIONALE FOR USE

The carpal tunnel position results in a *tangential projection of the palmar portions of the carpals (the "carpal tunnel")*. The position may be useful in demonstrating carpal fractures, as well as bone changes related to carpal tunnel syndrome.

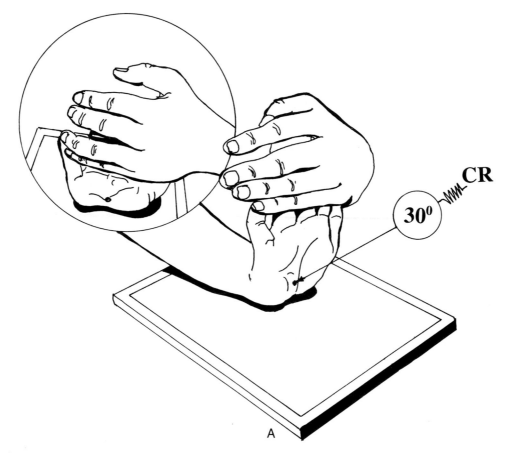

□ **FIGURE 3–13.**

POSITION DESCRIPTION

Part Position: The palmar aspect of the carpus is placed on the cassette, and the hand is extended as much as the patient's condition will allow. The patient may hold the hand in extension with the opposite hand.

Central Ray: Angled 30°–45° proximally, entering the palm 2 inches above the cassette.

Note: The less the patient is able to dorsiflex the hand, the greater the tube angle needed. This radiograph is very difficult to obtain on patients who cannot dorsiflex the hand at least 60° from horizontal.

Gaynor-Hart* Carpal Tunnel Position *(continued)*

IMAGE EVALUATION

The palmar portions of the carpal bones should be demonstrated in tangential projection. The metacarpals should be seen to radiate outward from the carpal bones. The hook of the hamate is usually visible.

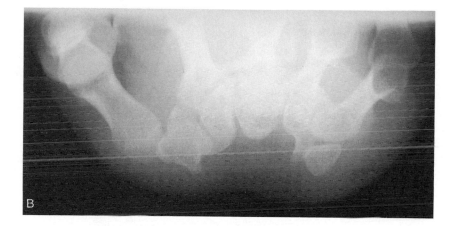

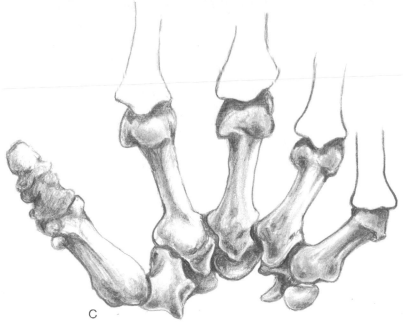

□ **FIGURE 3–13.** *(continued)*

*Hart VL, Gaynor V. Roentgenographic study of the carpal canal. *J Bone Joint Surg* 1941; 23(2):382–383.

Holly* Pisiform Oblique Position

RATIONALE FOR USE

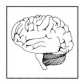

This position demonstrates the *pisiform without superimposition of the triquetrum* and opens the pisitriquetral joint space.

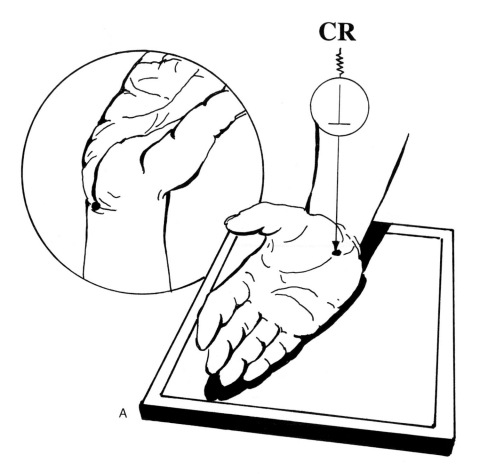

□ **FIGURE 3–14.**

POSITION DESCRIPTION

Part Position: The hand is placed in a 60° semi-supinated ulnar oblique position.

Central Ray: Perpendicular to the cassette, entering just ulnar (medial) to the midcarpus.

Holly* Pisiform Oblique Position *(continued)*

IMAGE EVALUATION

The pisiform should be seen without superimposition of the triquetrum and the pisitriquetral joint space should be open.

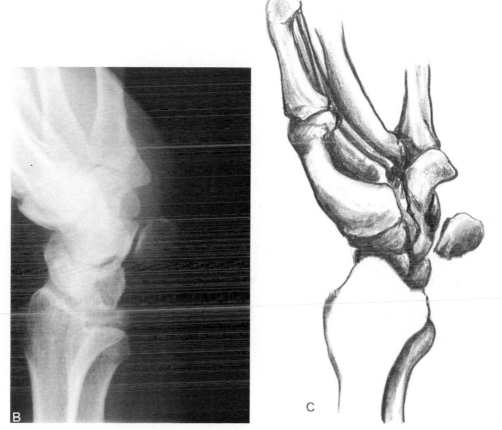

☐ **FIGURE 3–14.** *(continued)*

---

*Holly EW. Radiography of the pisiform bone. *Radiog Clin Photog* 1945; 21(3):69–70.

Holly* Trapezium Position

RATIONALE FOR USE

This position results in projection of the *entire trapezium, free of superimposition.* The trapezium is commonly involved in osteoarthritis of the carpus, and this position may be useful for evaluation. In addition, occult fractures may be diagnosed.

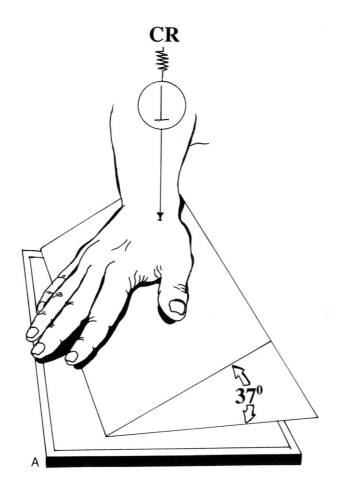

□ **FIGURE 3–15.**

POSITION DESCRIPTION

Part Position: The forearm is parallel to the plane of the film, resting on the peak of a 37° positioning sponge. The hand is in ulnar deviation (ulnar flexion), resting on the angled surface of the sponge. The fingertips just touch the cassette.

Central Ray: Perpendicular to the cassette, entering just proximal to the base of the first metacarpal.

Holly* Trapezium Position *(continued)*

IMAGE EVALUATION

The trapezium should be demonstrated free from superimposition, and the adjacent joint spaces should be open. Superimposition at the ulnar (medial) aspect of the trapezium often indicates too much wrist obliquity.

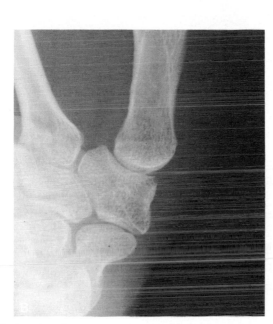

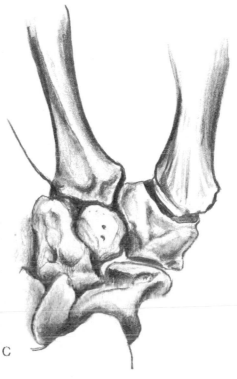

☐ **FIGURE 3–15.** *(continued)*

---

*Holly EW. Radiography of the greater multangular bone. *Med Radiog Photog* 1948; 24(3):79.

Modified* Stecher† Scaphoid Position

RATIONALE FOR USE

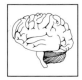

The modified Stecher scaphoid position clearly demonstrates the *entire scaphoid without foreshortening or bone superimposition.* Much of the palmar tilt of the distal scaphoid pole is reduced by the ulnar deviation. The elevation of the hand places the long axis of the scaphoid parallel to the cassette.

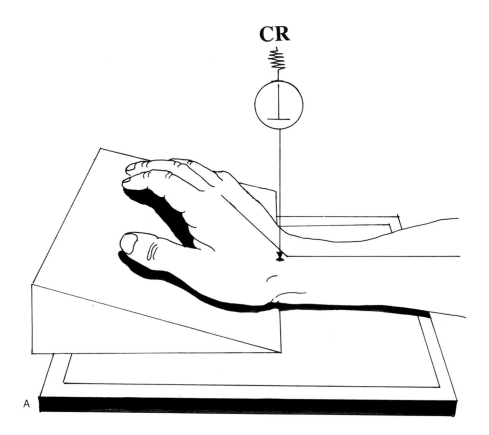

□ **FIGURE 3–16.**

POSITION DESCRIPTION

Part Position: The hand and wrist are pronated on the cassette. The hand is elevated on a 20°-angle sponge to place the palmar aspect of the wrist in contact with the cassette. The hand is placed in maximal ulnar deviation (ulnar flexion).

Note: Stecher recommended clenching the fist as an alternative to part or central ray angulation.

Central Ray: Perpendicular to the cassette, through the snuffbox (just radial to the midcarpus).

Note: The hand elevation may be replaced by a 20° proximal central ray angulation. However, the result is less satisfactory.

Modified* Stecher† Scaphoid Position *(continued)*

IMAGE EVALUATION

The entire scaphoid should be demonstrated without foreshortening or bone super-imposition.

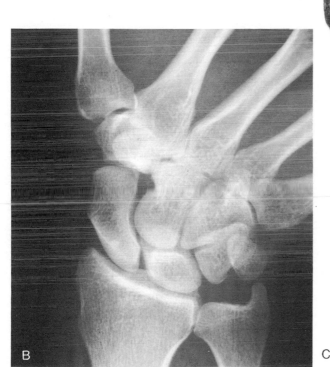

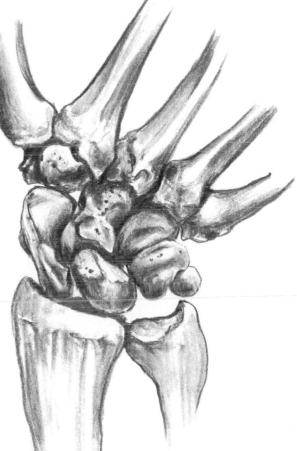

□ **FIGURE 3–16.** *(continued)*

---

*Bridgman CF. Radiography of the carpal navicular bone. *Med Radiog Photog* 1949; 25(4):104–105.
†Stecher W. Roentgenography of the carpal navicular bone. *AJR* 1937; 37:704.

Multiple-Angle Scaphoid Series*

RATIONALE FOR USE

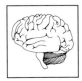

This four-exposure scaphoid series is designed to demonstrate *occult (obscure) fractures of the carpal scaphoid.* This type of fracture is more likely to be missed on a routine series. Delayed treatment may result in necrosis of the bone fragment, fracture non-union, or pseudoarthrosis.

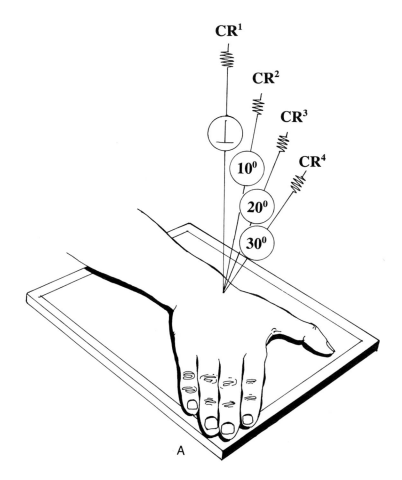

□ **FIGURE 3–17.**

POSITION DESCRIPTION

Part Position: The wrist is pronated as for a PA projection and then ulnar deviated.

Note: The wrist is maintained in this position for all four exposures.

Central Ray: Perpendicular to the cassette, and angled 10°, 20°, and 30° proximally along the long axis of the forearm, entering slightly to the radial side of the midcarpus.

Multiple-Angle Scaphoid Series* *(continued)*

IMAGE EVALUATION

The scaphoid should be demonstrated with minimal superimposition and minimal foreshortening. The degree of scaphoid elongation, because of angulation distortion, will increase as the tube angle is increased. The exposure field should be limited to the area of interest to improve image quality.

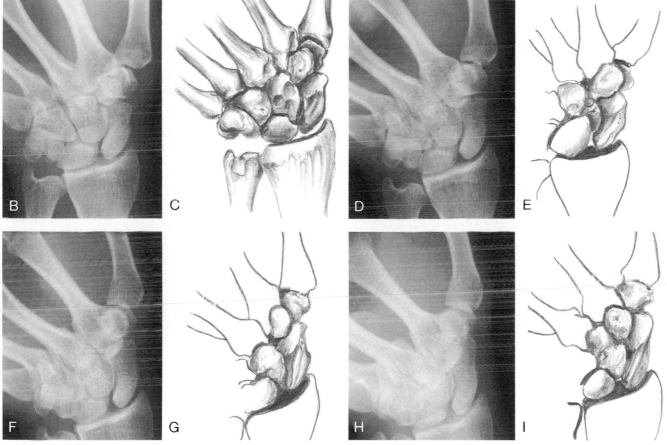

□ **FIGURE 3–17.** *(continued)*

B, — (0°); *D,* 10°; *F,* 20°; *G,* 30°; *H,* 30°.

---

*Rafert JA, Long BW. Technique for diagnosis of scaphoid fractures. *Radiol Technol* 1991; 63(1).16–21.

Multiple-Angle Scaphoid Series *(continued)*

CASE STUDY

The patient had fallen on the outstretched hand and presented with pain in the area of the anatomical snuffbox.

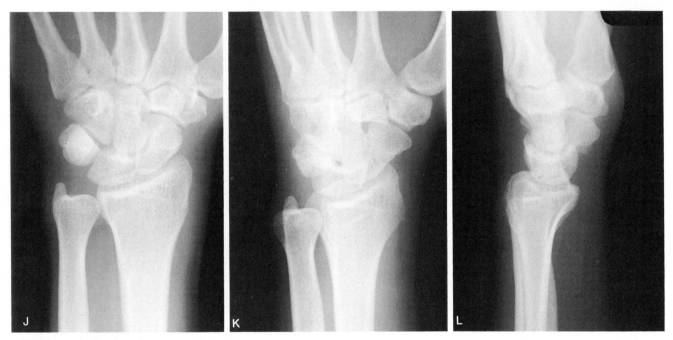

□ **FIGURE 3–17.** *(continued)*

Routine PA, oblique, and lateral wrist radiographs were taken. A lucency was noted in the area of the scaphoid waist on the oblique radiograph, but the findings were inconclusive.

Multiple-Angle Scaphoid Series *(continued)*

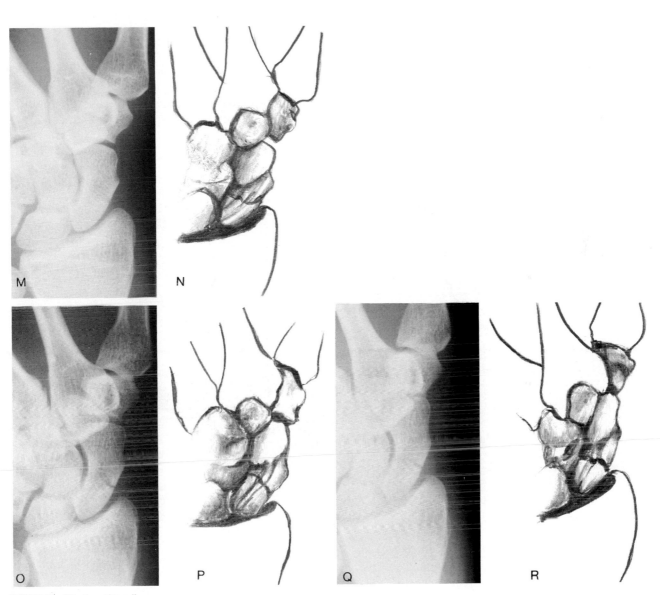

□ **FIGURE 3–17.** *(continued)*

M, 10°; *O*, 20°; *Q*, 30°.

The multiple-angle scaphoid series demonstrated a fracture of the scaphoid waist.

Papilion* Hook of Hamate Position

RATIONALE FOR USE

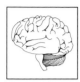

This position demonstrated the *hook of the hamate, in its broadest aspect.* This structure can be fractured, usually at the base, and is very difficult to radiograph. This position, along with the Gaynor-Hart carpal tunnel position, should enable the hook of the hamate (hamulus) to be visualized in the requisite two planes.

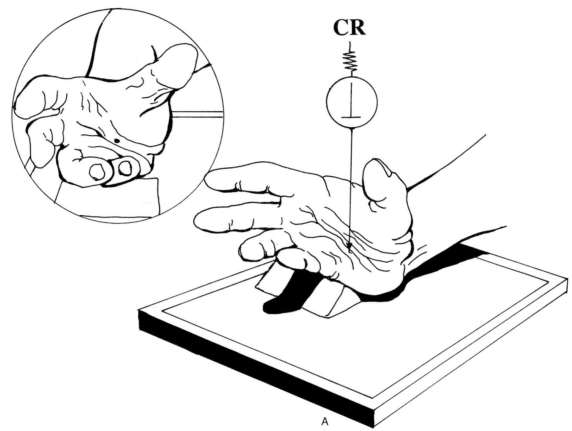

□ **FIGURE 3–18.**

POSITION DESCRIPTION

Part Position: The hand is placed in the lateral position with the ulnar aspect against the cassette and the wrist in maximum *radial* deviation (radial flexion). The hand is then supinated 10°, and the thumb is maximally abducted.

Note: A support, such as a wooden dowel, may be placed under the distal portion of the hand to aid in achieving maximal radial deviation.

Central Ray: Perpendicular to the cassette, entering midway between the first and second metacarpophalangeal (MCP) joints.

Papilion* Hook of Hamate Position *(continued)*

IMAGE EVALUATION

The hook of the hamate should be seen in its broadest aspect, free of superimposition. The base of the hook should be well demonstrated. Correct degree of hand supination is essential and is evidenced by visualization of the fifth metacarpal just anterior to the second metacarpal. Sufficient radial deviation (radial flexion) has been achieved when the first and second metacarpal bases are *not* superimposed on the hamate hook.

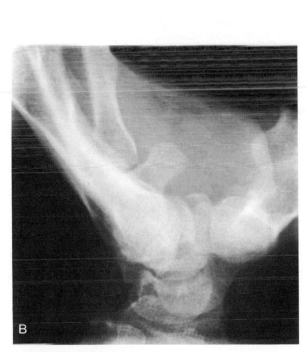

B

C

□ **FIGURE 3–18.** *(continued)*

---

*Papilion JD, DuPuy TE, Aulicino PL, et al. Radiographic evaluation of the hook of the hamate: a new technique. *J Hand Surg* 1988; 13Λ(3):437–439.

Radial Deviation (Flexion) PA Wrist Projection

RATIONALE FOR USE

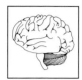

The radial deviation (radial flexion) projection *improves visualization of the carpal interspaces within the ulnar (medial) portion of the carpus* and places stress on the associated intercarpal ligaments.

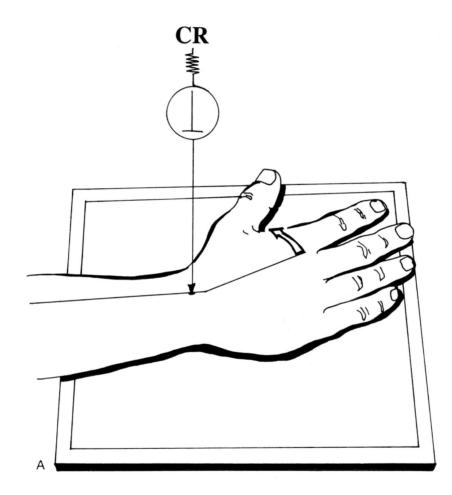

□ **FIGURE 3–19.**

POSITION DESCRIPTION

Part Position: The wrist is positioned as for a PA projection. The patient deviates the hand maximally toward the radial (lateral) side.

Central Ray: Perpendicular to the cassette, through the midcarpus.

Radial Deviation (Flexion) PA Wrist Projection *(continued)*

IMAGE EVALUATION

The wrist should be seen in PA projection, with the carpus in maximal radial deviation. The ulnar (medial) carpal interspaces should be open. The trapezium should appear in close proximity to the radial styloid.

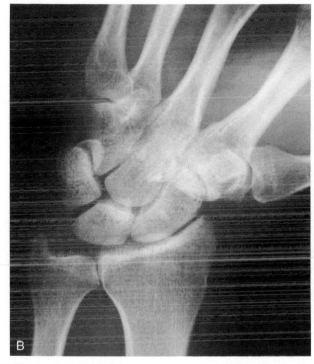

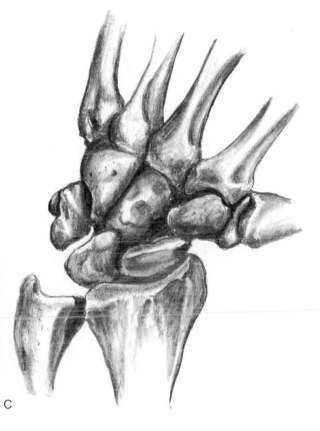

□ **FIGURE 3–19.** *(continued)*

Ulnar Deviation (Flexion) PA Wrist Projection

RATIONALE FOR USE

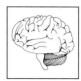

The ulnar deviation (ulnar flexion) PA wrist projection *improves visualization of the scaphoid articulations* and places stress on the associated intercarpal ligaments. The *scaphoid waist is more clearly demonstrated*, as a result of a reduction in foreshortening.

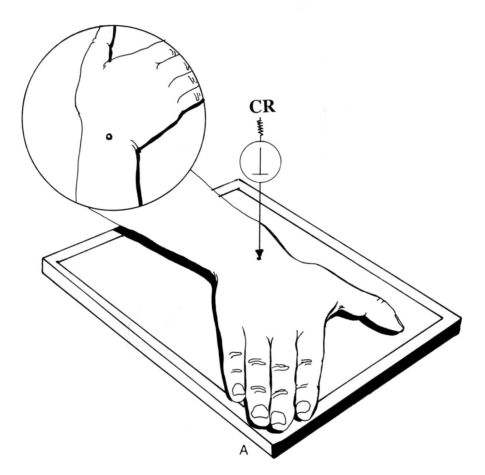

CR

A

□ **FIGURE 3–20.**

POSITION DESCRIPTION

Part Position: The wrist is positioned as for a PA projection. The patient deviates the hand maximally toward the ulnar (medial) side.

Central Ray: Perpendicular to the cassette, through the midcarpus.

Ulnar Deviation (Flexion) PA Wrist Projection *(continued)*

IMAGE EVALUATION

The wrist should be seen in PA projection, with the carpus in maximal ulnar deviation. All scaphoid articulations should be demonstrated without superimposition. The scaphoid waist should be well demonstrated. The entire lunate should be seen adjacent to the radial articular surface. The pisiform should appear in close proximity to the ulnar styloid.

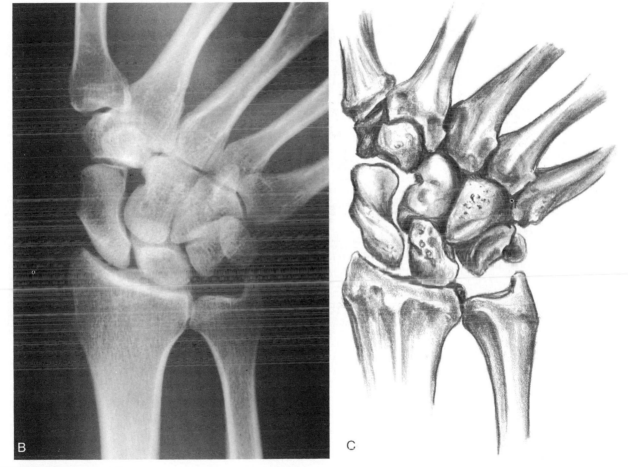

B   C

□ **FIGURE 3–20.** *(continued)*

Zero-Rotation* Lateral Wrist Position

RATIONALE FOR USE

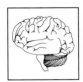

The zero-rotation lateral wrist position allows the *greatest degree of radius and ulna superimposition* by placing the forearm in neutral rotation.

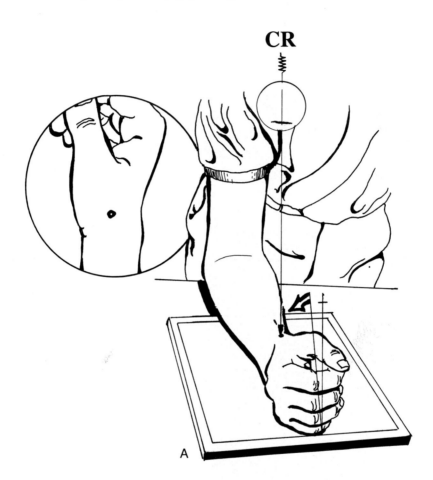

□ **FIGURE 3–21.**

POSITION DESCRIPTION

Part Position: The arm is placed against the side (0° of shoulder abduction), the elbow is flexed, and the wrist placed in an ulnar lateral position on the cassette. Forearm rotation is adjusted to neutral position, resulting in superimposition of the radius and ulna. The hand will be slightly supinated.

Central Ray: Perpendicular to the cassette, through the midcarpus.

Zero-Rotation* Lateral Wrist Position *(continued)*

IMAGE EVALUATION

The distal radius and ulna should be demonstrated in full superimposition, without radiocarpal flexion-extension or deviation. The carpals and proximal portions of the metacarpals should appear as they do in a routine lateral position.

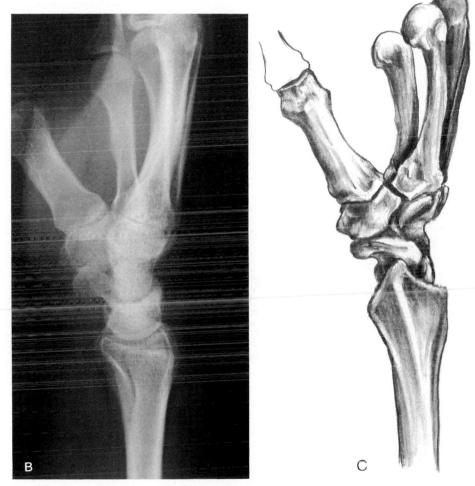

B

C

□ **FIGURE 3–21.** *(continued)*

*Epner RA, Bowers WH, Guilford WB. Ulnar variance—the effect of wrist positioning and roentgen filming technique. *J Hand Surg* 1982; 7:298–305.

Zero-Rotation* PA Wrist Projection

RATIONALE FOR USE

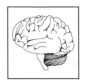

The zero-rotation PA wrist projection is used to *evaluate "ulnar variance," the relative lengths of the radius and ulna*. It has been determined that forearm rotation and radial wrist deviation adversely affect the radiographic appearance of ulnar variance. Changes in ulnar variance may be significant in the diagnosis of conditions such as repetitive motion disorders and Kienböck's disease.

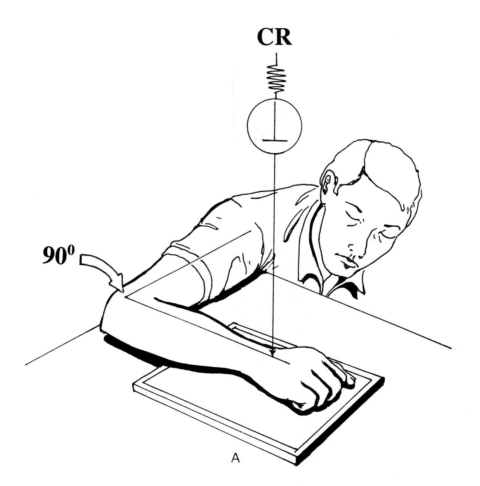

□ **FIGURE 3–22.**

POSITION DESCRIPTION

Part Position: The shoulder is abducted 90°, the elbow flexed 90°, and the wrist positioned on the cassette as for a routine PA projection.

Central Ray: Perpendicular to the cassette, through the midcarpus.

Zero-Rotation* PA Wrist Projection *(continued)*

IMAGE EVALUATION

The distal radius and ulna should be demonstrated in PA projection, without forearm rotation or wrist deviation. Neutral forearm rotation has been achieved when the ulnar and radial styloids are seen farthest apart, at the medial and lateral edges of the bones. Neutral wrist deviation results in approximately half the lunate positioned over the radius.

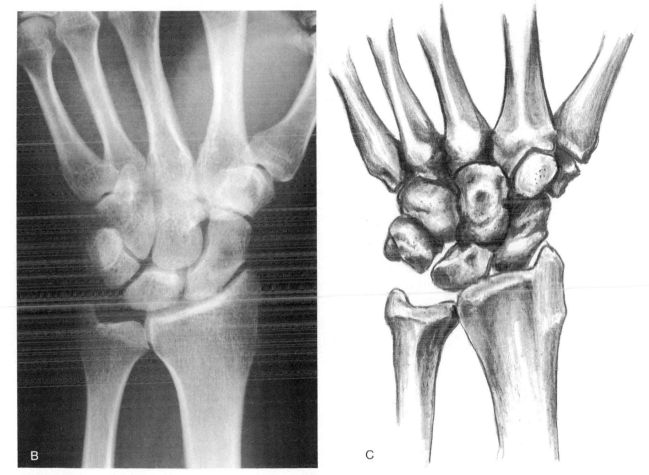

□ **FIGURE 3-22.** *(continued)*

*Epner RA, Bowers WH, Guilford WB. Ulnar variance—the effect of wrist positioning and roentgen filming technique. *J Hand Surg* 1982; 7:298–305.

Zero-Rotation–Ulnar Deviation* PA Wrist Projection

RATIONALE FOR USE

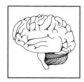

The zero-rotation–ulnar deviation wrist projection is used to *evaluate "ulnar variance," the relative lengths of the radius and ulna.* It has been determined that forearm rotation and radial wrist deviation adversely affect the radiographic appearance of ulnar variance. Changes in ulnar variance may be significant in the diagnosis of conditions such as repetitive motion disorders and Kienböck's disease. *The originators of this position recommended this ulnar deviated position over the neutral deviation.*

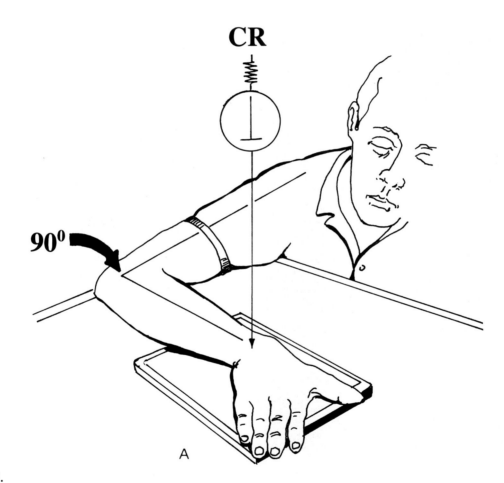

□ **FIGURE 3–23.**

POSITION DESCRIPTION

Part Position: The shoulder is abducted 90°, the elbow flexed 90°, and the wrist positioned on the cassette as for a routine PA projection. The hand is deviated toward the ulnar side of the wrist.

Central Ray: Perpendicular to the cassette, through the midcarpus.

Zero-Rotation–Ulnar Deviation* PA Wrist Projection *(continued)*

IMAGE EVALUATION

The distal radius and ulna should be demonstrated in PA projection, without forearm rotation. Neutral forearm rotation has been achieved when the ulnar and radial styloids are seen farthest apart, at the medial and lateral edges of the bones. The carpus should be seen in ulnar deviation as evidenced by the entire lunate adjacent to the radial articular surface and the trapezium in close proximity to the radial styloid.

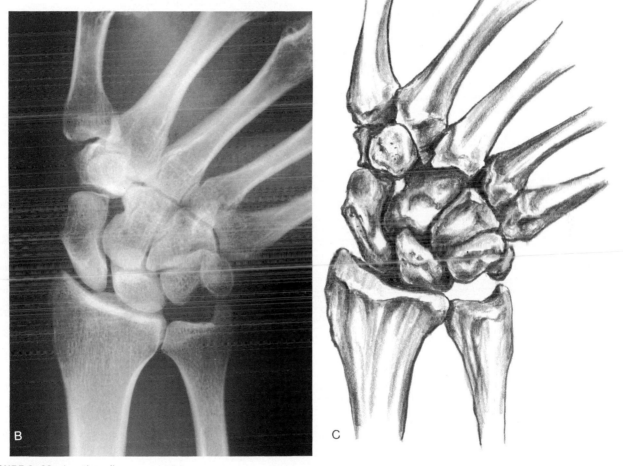

□ **FIGURE 3–23.** *(continued)*

*Epner RA, Bowers WH, Guilford WB. Ulnar variance—the effect of wrist positioning and roentgen filming technique. *J Hand Surg* 1982; 7:298–305.

References

1. Weber ER, Chao EY. An experimental approach to the mechanism of scaphoid waist fractures. *J Hand Surg* 1978; 3:142–148.
2. Rogers LF. *Radiology of Skeletal Trauma.* London: Churchill Livingstone; 1982:503.
3. Colles A. On fracture of the carpal extremity of the radius. *Edinb Med Surg* 1814; 10:182–186. (Abr. transl. *Clin Orthop* 1972; 83:3–5.)
4. Smith RW. *A Treatise on Fractures in the Vicinity of Joints, and on Certain Forms of Accidental and Congenital Dislocations.* Dublin: Hodges and Smith; 1854.
5. Louis DS. Barton's and Smith's fractures. *Hand Clin* 1988; 4:399–402.
6. Beekman F, Sullivan JE. Some observations on fractures of long bones in children. *Am J Surg* 1941; 51:722–738.
7. O'Brien ET. Fractures of the hand and wrist. *In* Rockwood CA, Wilkins KE, King RE (eds). *Fractures in Children,* 3rd ed. Philadelphia: JB Lippincott; 1991:319–413.
8. Barton JR. Views and treatment of an important injury to the wrist. *Med Exam* 1838; 1:365.
9. Wiot JF, Dorst JP. Less common fractures and dislocations of the wrist. *Radiol Clin North Am* 1966; 4:261.
10. Galeazzi R. Di una particulare sindrome, traumatica delle scheletro dell avambraccio. *Attie Mem Soc Lombardi di Chir* 1934; 2:12.
11. Thomas EM, Tuson KWR, Browne PSH. Fractures of the radius and ulna in children. *Injury* 1975; 7:120.
12. Rogers LF. The radiography of epiphyseal injuries. *Radiology* 1970; 96:289.
13. Johnson RP. The acutely injured wrist and its residuals. *Clin Orthop* 1980; 149:33.
14. Dunn AW. Fractures and dislocations of the carpus. *Surg Clin North Am* 1972; 52:1513.
15. Hanks GA, Kalenak A, Bowman LS, Sebastianelli WJ. Stress fractures of the carpal scaphoid. *J Bone Joint Surg* 1989; 71A:938–941.
16. Mayfield JK. Mechanism of carpal injuries. *Clin Orthop* 1980; 149:45–54.
17. Stecher W. Roentgenography of the carpal navicular bone. *AJR* 1937; 37:704.
18. Rafert JA, Long BW. Technique for diagnosis of scaphoid fractures. *Radiol Technol* 1991; 63(1):16–21.
19. Cooney WP, Linscheid RL, Dobyns JH. Fractures and dislocations of the wrist. *In* Rockwood CA, Green DP, Buckholz RW (eds). *Rockwood and Green's Fractures in Adults.* Philadelphia: JB Lippincott; 1991:563–678.
20. Kienböck R. Uber tramatische malazie des mondbiens und ihre folgezustände: entartungsformen und kompressionsfrakturen. *Fortschr Geb Roentgenstr Nuklearmed Erganzungsband* 1910–1911; 16:78–103. (Abr. transl. Kienböck R. Concerning traumatic malacia of the lunate and its consequences: degeneration and compression fractures. *Clin Orthop* 1980; 149:4–8.)
21. Gelberman RH, Salamon PB, Jurist JM, Posch JL. Ulnar variance in Kienböck's disease. *J Bone Joint Surg* 1975; 57:674–676.
22. Epner RA, Bowers WH. Ulnar variance—the effect of wrist positioning and roentgen filming technique. *J Hand Surg* 1982; 7:298–305.
23. Bryan RS, Dobyns JH. Fractures of the carpal bones other than the lunate and navicular. *Clin Orthop* 1980; 149:107–111.
24. Levy M, Fischel RE, Stern GM, Goldberg I. Chip fractures of the os triquetrum: the mechanism of injury. *J Bone Joint Surg* 1979; 61B:355–357.
25. Botte MJ, Gelberman RH. Fractures of the carpus, excluding the scaphoid. *Hand Clin* 1987; 3(1):149–161.
26. Rogers LF. *Radiology of Skeletal Trauma.* London: Churchill Livingstone; 1982:542–543.
27. Cordrey LJ, Ferrer-Torells M. Management of fractures of the greater multangular. *J Bone Joint Surg* 1960; 42A(7):1111–1118.
28. Holly EW. Radiography of the greater multangular bone. *Med Radiog Photog* 1948; 24(3):79.
29. Clements RW, Nakayama HK. Radiography of the polyarthritic hands and wrists. *Radiol Technol* 1981; 53(3):203–217.
30. Palmer AK. Trapezial ridge fractures. *J Hand Surg* 1981; 6:561–564.
31. Stark HH, Chao EK, Zemel NP, et al. Fracture of the hook of the hamate. *J Bone Joint Surg* 1989; 71A:1202–1207.
32. Vasilas A, Grieco RV, Bartone NF. Roentgen aspects of injuries to the pisiform bone and pisitriquetral joint. *J Bone Joint Surg* 1960; 42A:1317.
33. Holly EW. Radiography of the pisiform bone. *Radiogr Clin Photogr* 1945; 21(3):69–70.
34. Vance RM, Gelberman RH, Evans EF. Scaphocapitate fractures: patterns of dislocation, mechanisms of injury, and preliminary results of treatment. *J Bone Joint Surg* 1980; 62A:271–276.
35. Kuhlmann JN, Fournol S, Mimoun M, Baux S. Fracture of the lesser multangular (trapezoid) bone. *Ann Chir Main* 1986; 5:133–134.
36. Green DP, O'Brien ET. Classification and management of carpal dislocations. *Clin Orthop* 1980; 149:5–72.
37. Weissman BNW, Sledge CB. *Orthopedic Radiology.* Philadelphia: WB Saunders; 1986:147.
38. Sebald JR, Dobyns JH, Linscheid RL. The natural history of collapse deformities of the wrist. *Clin Orthop* 1974; 104:140.
39. Linscheid RL, Dobyns JH, Beabout JW, Bryan RS. Traumatic instability of the wrist: diagnosis, classification and pathomechanics. *J Bone Joint Surg* 1972; 54:1612–1632.
40. Landsmeer JMF. Studies in the anatomy of articulation. I. The equilibrium of the "intercalated" bone. *Acta Morph Neerl Scand* 1961; 3:287–303.
41. Dobyns JH, Linscheid RL, Chao EYS, et al. Traumatic instability of the wrist. *AAOS Instr Course Lectures* 1975; 24:182–199.
42. Cooney WP, Garcia-Elias M, Dobyns JH, Linscheid RL. Anatomy and mechanics of carpal instability. *Surg Rounds Orthop* 1989; 1:15–24.
43. Levinsohn EM. Imaging of the wrist. *Radiol Clin North Am* 1990; 28(5):905–921.
44. Viegas SF, Patterson RM, Peterson RD, et al. Ulnar-sided perilunate instability: an anatomic and biomechanic study. *J Hand Surg* 1990; 15A(2):268–278.
45. Rayhack JM, Linscheid RL, Dobyns JH, Smith JH. Posttraumatic ulnar translation of the carpus. *J Hand Surg* 1987; 12A:180–187.
46. Gilula LA, Weeks PM. Post-traumatic ligamentous instabilities of the wrist. *Radiology* 1978; 129:641–651.
47. Buckwalter KA, Swan JS, Braunstein EM. Evaluation of joint disease in the adult hand and wrist. *Hand Clin* 1991; 7(1):135–151.
48. Gold RH, Bassett LW, Seeger LL. Other arthritides: roentgenologic features of osteoarthritis, erosive osteoarthritis, ankylosing spondylitis, psoriatic arthritis, Reiter's disease, multicentric reticulohistiocytosis, and progressive systemic sclerosis. *Radiol Clin North Am* 1988; 26:1195.
49. Weston WJ. Soft tissue changes of rheumatoid arthritis at the wrist. *Aust Radiol* 1968; 12:384–392.
50. Renner WR, Weinstein AS. Early changes of rheumatoid arthritis in the hand and wrist. *Radiol Clin North Am* 1988; 26(6):1185–1193.
51. Chernin MM, Pitt MJ. Radiographic disease patterns at the carpus. *Clin Orthop* 1984; 187:72–80.
52. Collins LC, Lidsky MD, Sharp JT, Moreland J. Malposition of carpal bones in rheumatoid arthritis. *Radiology* 1972; 103:95–98.
53. Kaye JJ. Arthritis: roles of radiography and other imaging techniques in evaluation. *Radiology* 1990; 177:601–608.

FOUR

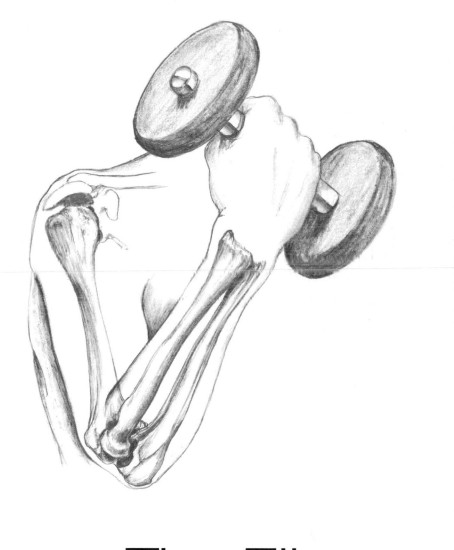

The Elbow

THE ELBOW: AN OVERVIEW

ROUTINE ELBOW RADIOGRAPHY

Routine AP Elbow Projection
Routine Lateral Elbow Position

SPECIALIZED ELBOW RADIOGRAPHY

AP Acute Flexion Elbow Projection (Distal Humerus)
AP Partial Flexion Elbow Projections (Distal Humerus)
AP Partial Flexion Elbow Projections (Proximal Forearm)
Axial Distal Humerus Projection
Axial Olecranon Process Projection
Coronoid-Trochlea Position (Coyle Trauma Elbow Position for Coronoid)
Cubital Tunnel Position
Gravity Stress Elbow Position
Gunsight Elbow Position
Lateral (External) Oblique Elbow Position
Lateral Radial Head Rotation Positions
Medial (Internal) Oblique Elbow Position
Radial Head–Capitellum Position (Coyle Trauma Elbow Position for Radial Head)

The Elbow: An Overview

Proper function of the elbow is crucial to effective use of the hand. The elbow functions to provide fine motor control over spatial placement of the hand through forearm rotation and flexion or extension at the elbow. An injury or a disease that results in decreased mobility or strength of the elbow may profoundly affect the ability of a patient to work or function normally. For this reason, prompt and accurate diagnosis is essential to prevent delayed or inappropriate treatment.

The elbow is the site of a variety of fractures. The type and location of the fracture are often age dependent. The most common elbow fracture in adults involves the radial head or neck. The next most common fracture is that of the olecranon process. A variety of fractures of the distal humerus are also seen. In children, the supracondylar fracture of the distal humerus is the most common. Next in frequency is fracture of the lateral condyle, followed by separation of the medial epicondylar apophysis and fracture of the radial head or neck.

Certain radiographic soft-tissue signs indicate the possibility of elbow injury. The supinator line is a radiolucent layer of fat anterior to the proximal radius. It is visible on a lateral radiograph of the elbow in flexion and is usually elevated or obliterated in the presence of radial head/neck fractures. Rogers and MacEwan[1] found this sign in 100% of radial head/neck fractures and 82% of other elbow fractures. Another soft-tissue sign involves the anterior and posterior fat pads. On a routine lateral elbow radiograph, the anterior fat pads are normally seen as a single triangular lucency contacting the anterior surface of the humerus. The posterior fat pad is not usually visible, because it is situated within the olecranon fossa.[2] However, the posterior fat pad is visible if the elbow is radiographed in extension. A positive fat pad sign consists of elevation of the anterior fat pads or visualization of the posterior fat pad.[3] The sign results from displacement of the fat pads as a result of elbow joint distention. The intrasynovial distention may result from either inflammation or hemorrhage caused by trauma. Lipohemarthrosis (the presence of fat and blood within the joint) is thought to indicate an intra-articular fracture or a significant capsular injury. This condition may be diagnosed by use of a horizontal beam–lateral elbow radiograph with the forearm held vertically.[4]

Fracture of the radial head accounts for about one third of all elbow fractures in adults.[5] If the fracture of the radial neck is included, the frequency is nearly one half.[6] The most common mechanism of injury is a fall on the outstretched arm with the forearm in pronation. This results in axial and valgus forces, causing the radial head to hit the capitellum.[7] Nearly half of radial head and neck fractures are nondisplaced,[8] making radiographic diagnosis more difficult. The fracture line in the radial head is most commonly anterolateral and oriented vertically. This explains the frequent inability to visualize the fracture line on routine anteroposterior (AP) and lateral radiographs. Special radiographs, such as the lateral (external) oblique or the radial head–capitellum[9] (Coyle[10] radial head trauma) positions, are useful when a radial head fracture is suspected.

Fracture of the olecranon process ranks second in frequency, accounting for approximately 20% of all adult elbow injuries.[11] The usual mechanisms of injury include direct falls on the elbow and falls on the outstretched hand with elbow flexion and triceps muscle contraction.[12] An olecranon fracture can also occur as a

115

result of hyperextension forces during elbow dislocation.[13] The fracture line is most commonly transverse, angled either proximal or distal, and located in the midportion of the trochlear notch.[14] Nondisplaced fractures present the greatest diagnostic challenge for the radiologist. The necessity of producing a true lateral elbow radiograph has been reported by Hotchkiss and Green[15] to allow accurate assessment of fracture extent, degree of comminution, amount of articular surface disruption in the semilunar notch, and any radial head displacement. Associated soft-tissue signs, such as a visible posterior fat pad or prominent olecranon bursa, can also be appraised. Inability of the patient to extend the elbow usually necessitates obtaining the AP projection radiograph in partial flexion. This radiograph is necessary in order to visualize the fracture line in the sagittal plane and should be obtained with the ulna parallel to the cassette, as described in the positioning guide of this chapter.

A variety of fractures involving the distal humerus may be seen in adults. Most of these (up to 95%[16]) are intra-articular. Almost half are bicondylar or intercondylar, T- or Y-shaped fractures.[17] In this type of fracture, a vertical fracture line involves the trochlea and branches to include both condyles. It most commonly results from a direct impact on the ulnar aspect of the flexed elbow.[18] Of the extra-articular fractures found in the elbow, the supracondylar fracture is most frequently seen. However, it is *not* a common elbow fracture in adults.[19] It consists of an oblique or transverse fracture just above the condyles. This injury most frequently occurs as the result of a fall on the outstretched arm with elbow hyperextension.[20] If the elbow is displaced, the lateral elbow radiograph will demonstrate the distal fragment distracted posteriorly and proximally. A supracondylar fracture can also result from a direct blow to the flexed elbow. A variation of the supracondylar fracture, seen more commonly in elderly osteoporotic adults,[15] is the transcondylar fracture. This fracture has the same mechanism of injury and similar radiographic features. However, the location of the fracture line is more distal and crosses both humeral condyles.

Isolated fracture of one condyle may result from a fall on the outstretched arm with the elbow in extension and varus or valgus stress added.[12] These fractures can also occur from a fall on the flexed elbow with the axial force concentrated over one condyle or from a direct blow to the posterior aspect of the condyle.[21] The lateral condyle is more frequently fractured. Other structures less commonly fractured in the adult elbow include the epicondyles (medial fractures are most common), the capitellum, and the trochlea.

The high activity level of children, coupled with immature balance and immature dexterity, results in frequent falls. The natural tendency for children is to protect themselves with outstretched arms. The result is a vulnerability of the upper extremity to injury. Large case analysis has demonstrated that the distal forearm is most frequently involved.[22] Fracture of the elbow accounts for 7%–9% of these upper extremity injuries.[23, 24] Elbow fractures in children differ from those in adults in frequency of both type and location. In an analysis of numerous studies, Wilkins[25] found that 86.4% were fractures of the distal humerus; 79.8% were of the supracondylar type, 16.9% involved the lateral condyle, and 12.5% consisted of avulsion of the medial epicondyle. Radial head and neck fractures are also relatively frequent. The commonly seen supracondylar fracture varies in severity. Over half are complete, with the distal fragment markedly displaced posteromedially. The remainder are divided approximately equally between moderately and minimally displaced complete or incomplete fractures.[26]

The minimally displaced fractures present the greatest challenge to radiological diagnosis. *True* AP and lateral elbow radiographs must be obtained because the signs are often subtle. Baumann's angle[27] is commonly used to assess varus-valgus alignment of the humeral shaft with the distal humeral metaphysis on the AP radiograph. The need to accurately image the elbow in AP projection has resulted in development of radiographic procedures enabling evaluation when the elbow is held in varying degrees of flexion. These positions and projections are described in this chapter. The lateral elbow radiograph enables evaluation of the fat pads for elevation and/or displacement. The relationship between the anterior humeral shaft and the capitellum, the anteversion angle, may also be demonstrated. The need to evaluate the elbow for these signs underscores the importance of obtaining a true lateral radiograph. The importance of accurate frontal and lateral positioning holds true for all other fractures involving a child's elbow. As in adults, radiographs in oblique positions in children may be necessary. In addition, comparison radiographs of the other elbow may be needed in order to rule out normal variants that may mimic injury.

The elbow is also susceptible to dislocation and fracture-dislocation. In adults, the elbow ranks third in frequency of dislocation, behind the shoulder (most common) and finger interphalangeal joints.[11] The elbow is the most common site of dislocation in children.[28, 29] Most elbow dislocations are posterior, resulting from hyperextension forces caused by a fall on the hand with the arm extended.[30] There is often an associated valgus force that may result in a variety of fractures. The most common are fracture of the medial condyle and avulsion of the medial epicondyle; these are followed in frequency by fracture of the radial head and neck.[11] Fracture of the coronoid process is also common in adults with a posterior dislocation.[31] Fractures in these locations are found to occur with the same relative frequency in children.[32]

Postreduction radiographs are important, not only for demonstrating reduction of the dislocation, but also for demonstrating associated fractures. These fractures are occasionally missed on the initial radiographs because of positioning difficulties or obscured anatomy. Only after re-establishing the normal anatomical relationships are some of these fractures seen.

Isolated dislocation of the radial head may also occur, although it is more frequently associated with fracture of the proximal ulna. This fracture-dislocation is termed **Monteggia's fracture**.[33] Bado[34] applied the term **Monteggia lesion** to any fracture of the ulna with associated dislocation of the radial head. Most cases of isolated traumatic radial head dislocation have been found in young children. It is thought to be due to the greater ligamentous laxity and the elasticity of immature bone.[35]

Several sports-related and overuse injuries are found in the elbow. They are primarily related to throwing and to racket sports but may be seen in occupations requiring stressful forearm use. Tendinitis of the elbow, or "tennis elbow," may involve either the lateral or medial aspect. The soft-tissue injuries and inflammatory process are not visible on radiographs.

On occasion, associated bony spurs, cortical hypertrophy, and loose bodies within the joint may be seen.[36] These radiographic findings are more commonly demonstrated in baseball pitchers and other athletes participating in throwing sports.[37]

Throwing stress injuries in children manifest somewhat differently. The so-called "Little League elbow" results from injury to the medial epicondylar apophysis. The radiographic manifestation of the injury ranges from widening of the epiphysis to complete avulsion of the medial epicondyle.[38] If there is question of medial elbow instability resulting from this condition, the instability can be radiographically assessed with the use of the gravity stress elbow position described in this chapter. Another condition associated with Little League elbow is osteochondritis dissecans. Found most commonly in boys 10 to 15 years old, the injury is believed to be caused by microtrauma to the capitellar articular cartilage, resulting in fragmentation and eventual loose body formation.[39]

A number of nontraumatic conditions afflict the elbow. A variety of arthritides manifest with elbow involvement. These include rheumatoid, crystalline-induced (gout, crystal pyrophosphate dihydrate deposition disease [CPPD], hydroxyapatite), spondyloarthropathic, degenerative, septic, hematologic (hemophilia, sickle cell disease), and neurotrophic disorders. The elbow may be involved in 40%–50% of patients with long-term rheumatoid arthritis.[40, 41] Early involvement is manifested as soft-tissue signs. The associated joint effusion and synovial hypertrophy may be demonstrated on lateral elbow radiographs as displacement of the anterior fat pads and the supinator fat line.[42] Soft-tissue nodules or olecranon bursitis may be evident. Bony and cartilaginous changes are identical to those found in other joints. Gout in the elbow often manifests as acute olecranon bursitis.[43] Degenerative arthritis is uncommon and is usually post-traumatic.

Nerve entrapment or compression syndromes occur, involving all major nerves around the elbow. Their diagnosis is primarily based on symptoms, physical examination, and electromyographic evaluation. Radiography is limited to demonstration of soft-tissue swelling and bony changes in the area adjacent to the suspected lesion.

Congenital anomalies of bone and soft tissue may be seen in the elbow. Both benign and malignant tumors of bone or soft tissue can occur in this area. For the sake of brevity, these less commonly seen entities are not discussed.

Routine Elbow Radiography

Routine AP Elbow Projection

CR

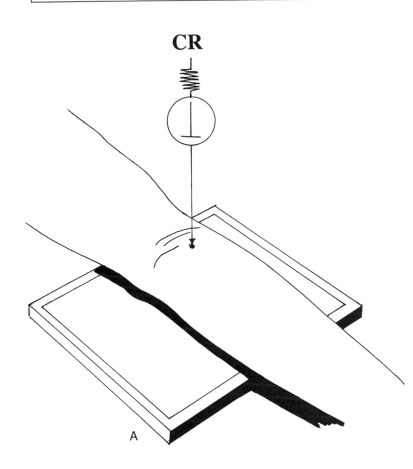

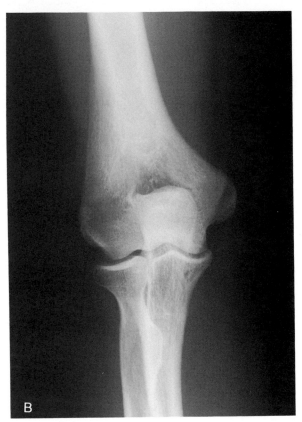

□ **FIGURE 4–1.**

POSITION DESCRIPTION

Part Position: The elbow is extended and the hand supinated. Rotation of the arm is adjusted to place the coronal plane of the epicondyles parallel to the cassette surface.

Central Ray: Perpendicular to the cassette, through the midpoint of the elbow joint.

IMAGE EVALUATION

The humeral epicondyles should be demonstrated without rotation. The olecranon process of the ulna should be seen in its broadest aspect, within the olecranon fossa of the distal humerus. The radial head, neck, and tuberosity should be slightly superimposed over the proximal ulna.

Routine Lateral Elbow Position

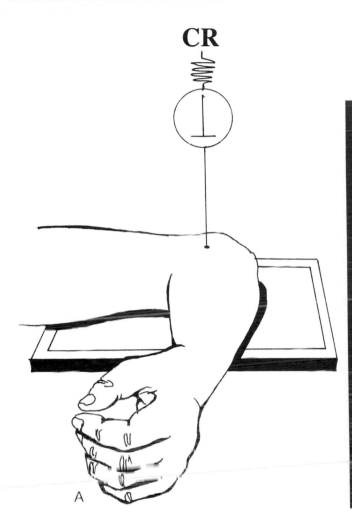

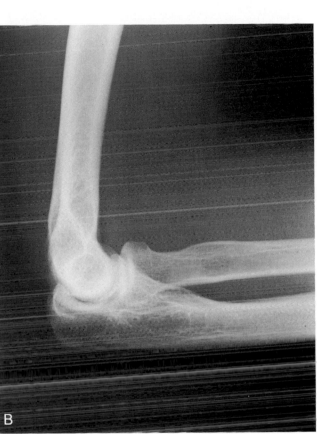

□ **FIGURE 4–2.**

POSITION DESCRIPTION

Part Position: The arm is abducted so that the humerus and forearm are in the same horizontal plane. The elbow is flexed 90°, and the hand is placed in ulnar lateral position.

Central Ray: Perpendicular to the cassette, through the midpoint of the elbow joint.

IMAGE EVALUATION

The long axes of the humerus and ulna should form a 90° angle. Correct arm position will be evidenced by superimposition of the humeral epicondyles and open ulnohumeral joint space. The olecranon process and radial tuberosity should be seen in profile. A portion of the radial head will be superimposed over the coronoid process.

Specialized Elbow Radiography

AP Acute Flexion Elbow Projection (Distal Humerus)

RATIONALE FOR USE

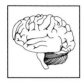

This projection, also called the **Jones position**, is used to achieve an *AP projection radiograph of the distal humerus, with the elbow in acute flexion.* This acutely flexed position may be used for closed reduction treatment of moderately displaced, incomplete supracondylar fractures in children.

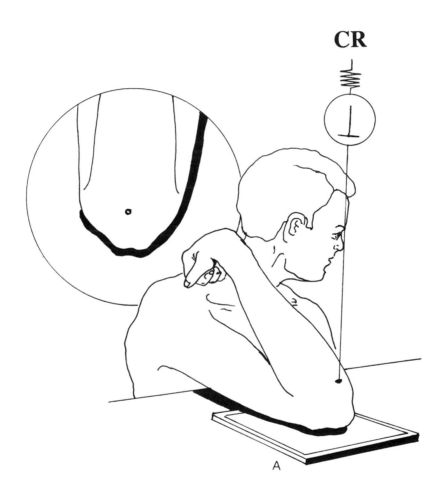

□ **FIGURE 4–3.**

POSITION DESCRIPTION

Part Position: The distal humerus is placed in contact with the cassette and rotated so that the coronal plane of the humeral epicondyles is parallel to the plane of the cassette.

Central Ray: Perpendicular to the cassette, entering the forearm 2 inches distal to the olecranon process.

AP Acute Flexion Elbow Projection (Distal Humerus) *(continued)*

IMAGE EVALUATION

The proximal forearm and distal humerus will be superimposed. An AP projection of the distal humerus should be demonstrated. The proximal radius and ulna will be seen with shape distortion.

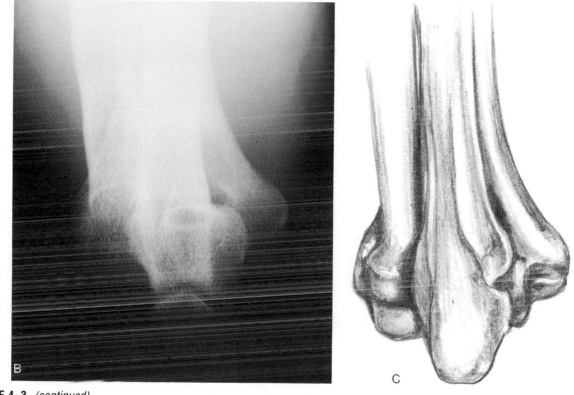

□ **FIGURE 4–3.** *(continued)*

AP Partial Flexion Elbow Projections (Distal Humerus)

RATIONALE FOR USE

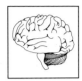

These projections are used to achieve *AP projection radiographs of the proximal radius and ulna or the distal humerus, when the patient's condition limits elbow extension.*

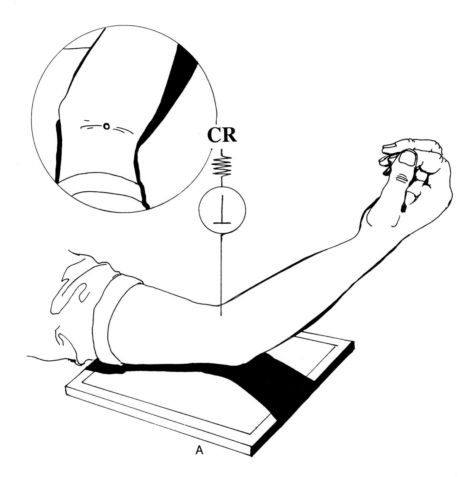

CR

A

☐ **FIGURE 4–4.**

POSITION DESCRIPTION

Part Position: The distal humerus is placed in contact with the cassette and rotated so that the coronal plane of the humeral epicondyles is parallel to the plane of the cassette. The elbow is extended as much as the patient's condition allows, and the forearm is supported for the patient's comfort.

Central Ray: Perpendicular to the cassette, through the midpoint of the elbow joint.

AP Partial Flexion Elbow Projections (Distal Humerus) *(continued)*

IMAGE EVALUATION

An AP projection of the distal humerus should be demonstrated. The proximal radius and ulna will be seen with some degree of shape distortion and humeral superimposition, depending on the amount of elbow extension achieved.

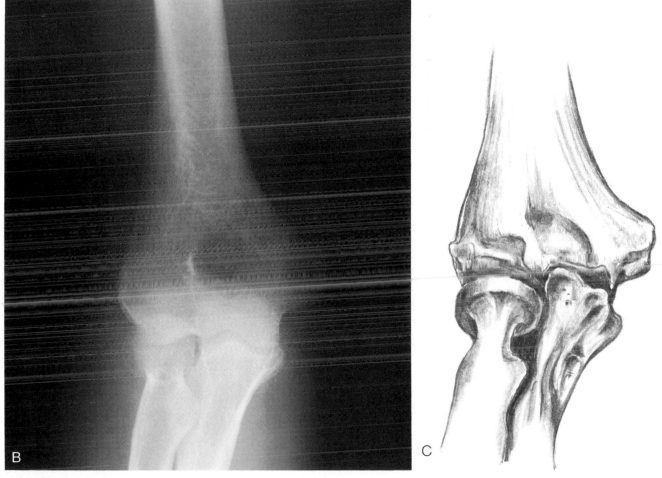

□ **FIGURE 4–4.** *(continued)*

AP Partial Flexion Elbow Projections (Proximal Forearm)

RATIONALE FOR USE

These projections are used to achieve *AP projection radiographs of the proximal radius and ulna or the distal humerus, when the patient's condition limits elbow extension.*

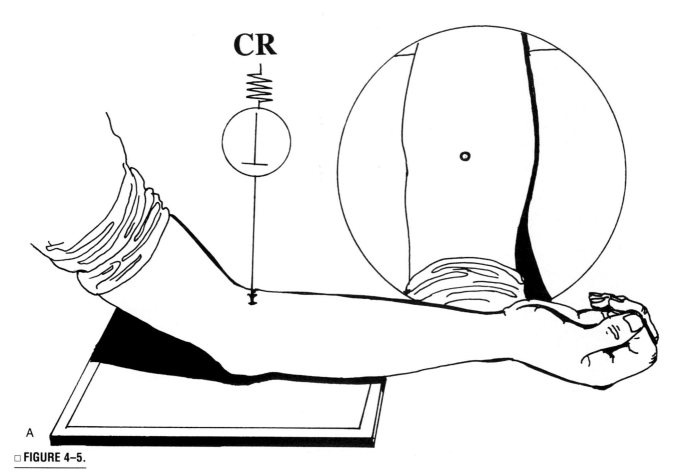

□ **FIGURE 4–5.**

POSITION DESCRIPTION

Part Position: The dorsum of the proximal forearm is placed in contact with the cassette and the elbow is extended as much as the patient's condition allows. The hand is supinated as much as possible, and the arm is adjusted, by the patient's lateral leaning, so that a line through the humeral epicondyles is parallel to the plane of the cassette.

Central Ray: Perpendicular to the cassette, through the midpoint of the elbow joint.

AP Partial Flexion Elbow Projections (Proximal Forearm) *(continued)*

IMAGE EVALUATION

An AP projection of the proximal radius and ulna should be demonstrated. The distal humerus will be seen with some degree of shape distortion and radial head superimposition, depending on the amount of elbow extension achieved.

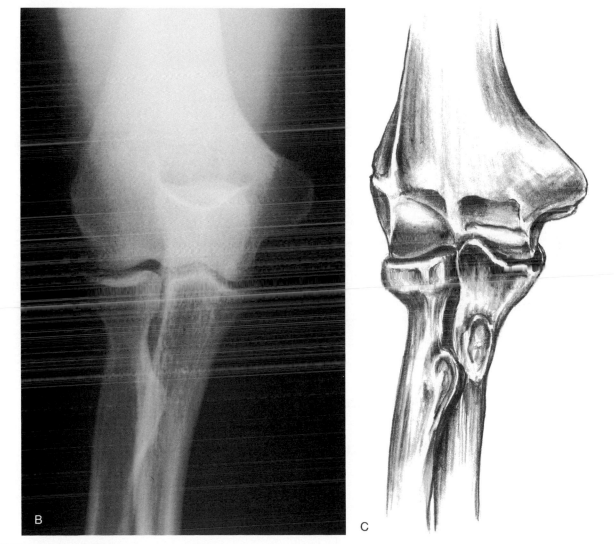

B

C

□ **FIGURE 4–5.** *(continued)*

Axial Distal Humerus Projection*

RATIONALE FOR USE

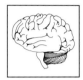

The axial distal humerus projection allows evaluation of *abnormalities of the humeral epicondyles, trochlea, ulnar sulcus, or olecranon fossa*. It may be used to evaluate distal humeral trauma, tennis elbow, or ulnar neuropathy. The projection was originally developed to document avulsion of the apophysis of the medial humeral epicondyle.

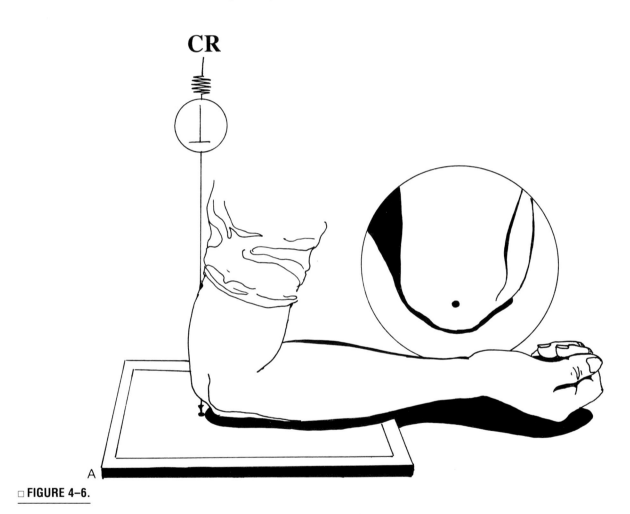

□ **FIGURE 4–6.**

POSITION DESCRIPTION

Part Position: The dorsum of the distal forearm is placed on the cassette with the hand supinated and directed anteriorly. The elbow is flexed to form an ulnohumeral angle of 75°–80°. Arm position is adjusted so that there is no abduction of the humerus.

Central Ray: Perpendicular to the cassette, through the olecranon process.

Axial Distal Humerus Projection* *(continued)*

IMAGE EVALUATION

An axial projection of the distal humerus should be demonstrated. The humeral epicondyles, trochlea, ulnar sulcus, and olecranon fossa should be seen. A portion of the radial head may be visible, but the remainder of the elbow anatomy will be obscured by superimposition.

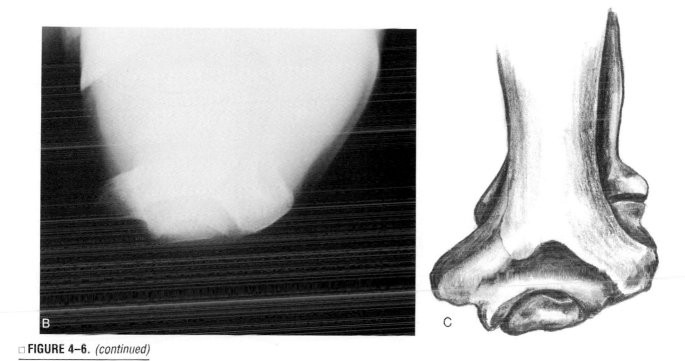

□ **FIGURE 4–6.** *(continued)*

---

*Viehweger G. Zum problem der deutung der knöchernen gebilde distal des epikondylus medialis humeri. *Fortschr Roentgenstr* 1957; 86:643–652.

Axial Olecranon Process Projection*

RATIONALE FOR USE

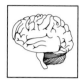

This axial projection allows evaluation of *abnormalities of the olecranon process.* The projection provides a second radiograph of the olecranon process without superimposition, in addition to the lateral position.

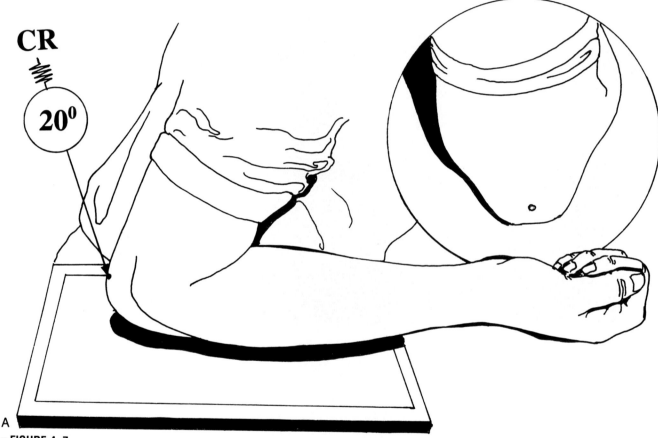

CR

20⁰

□ **FIGURE 4–7.**

POSITION DESCRIPTION

Part Position: The dorsum of the distal forearm is placed on the cassette with the hand supinated and directed anteriorly. The elbow is flexed maximally. Arm position is adjusted so that there is no abduction of the humerus.

Central Ray: Angled 20° distally (toward the hand), along the long axis of the forearm, through the olecranon process.

Note: The central ray may be directed perpendicular to the cassette to demonstrate the more distal portion of the olecranon process.

Axial Olecranon Process Projection* *(continued)*

IMAGE EVALUATION

An axial projection of the olecranon process should be demonstrated. The tip of the olecranon process and its distal articular margin should be seen without superimposition. The capitellum, trochlea, ulnar sulcus, and medial epicondyle should be seen. The remainder of the elbow anatomy will be obscured by superimposition.

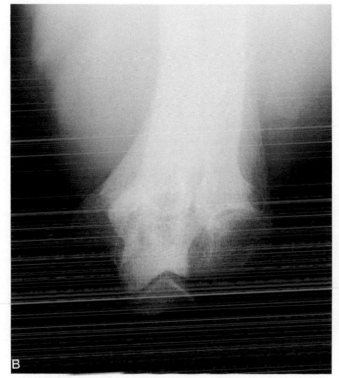

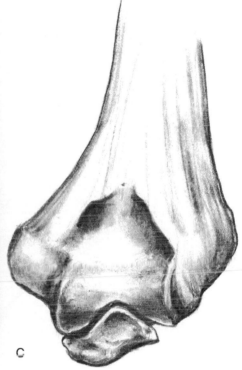

□ **FIGURE 4–7.** *(continued)*

*Laquerriére and Pierquin. De la nécessité d'employer une technique radiographique spéciale pour obtenir certains détails squelettiques. *J Radiol Electr* 1918; 3(4):145–148.

Coronoid-Trochlea Position*
(Coyle† Trauma Elbow Position for Coronoid)

RATIONALE FOR USE

The coronoid-trochlea position (also called the Coyle trauma elbow position for the coronoid) demonstrates *fractures of the coronoid process and trochlea*. Separating the coronoid process from the radial head and the trochlea from the capitellum eliminates much of the bone superimposition seen on the standard lateral position of the elbow.

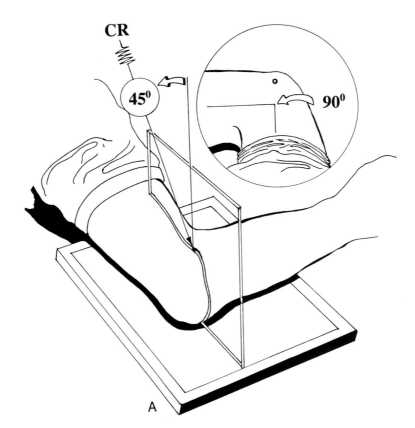

□ FIGURE 4–8.

POSITION DESCRIPTION

Part Position: The elbow is placed in the standard lateral position (elbow in 90° flexion, humerus and forearm parallel to plane of cassette).

Central Ray: The central ray is angled 45° from the shoulder toward the elbow, oriented parallel to the long axis of the humerus and passing through the midpoint of the elbow joint.

Note: If the elbow cannot be flexed 90°, the central ray should be oriented perpendicular to the long axis of the proximal forearm when the coronoid process is of primary interest.

Coronoid-Trochlea Position*
(Coyle† Trauma Elbow Position for Coronoid) *(continued)*

IMAGE EVALUATION

The coronoid process should be seen free of superimposition by the radial head. The trochlea should be separated from the capitellum and the trochlear articular surface well demonstrated. The radial head will be obscured by the ulna. Angulation distortion will be evident.

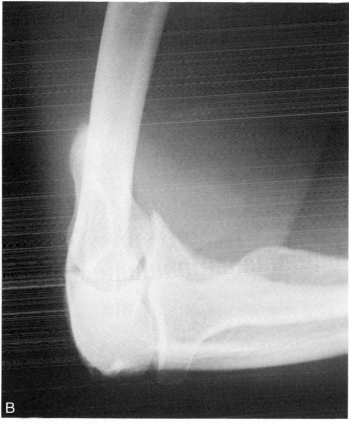

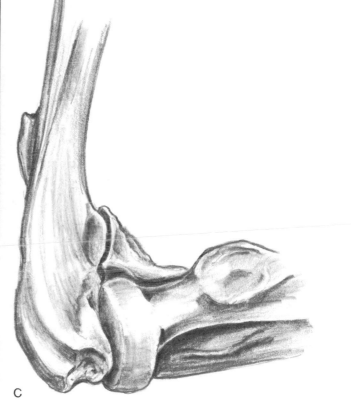

□ **FIGURE 4–8.** *(continued)*

---

*Guilbeau JC, Mouelhi MM, Nahum H. Les profils modifiés du coude en traumatologie: intérêt de l'incidence tête radiale–capitellum et d'une nouvelle incidence coronoïde-trochlée. *J Radiol* 1986; 67(5):439–444.
†Coyle GF. Unit 7, Special angled views of joints—elbow, knee, ankle. *Radiographing Immobile Trauma Patients.* Denver: Multi-Media Publishing; 1980.

Cubital Tunnel Position*†

RATIONALE FOR USE

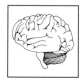

The cubital tunnel position demonstrates the bony portions of the cubital tunnel through which the ulnar nerve passes. Cubital tunnel syndrome, or ulnar neuritis, may be caused by bone irregularities impinging on the cubital tunnel.

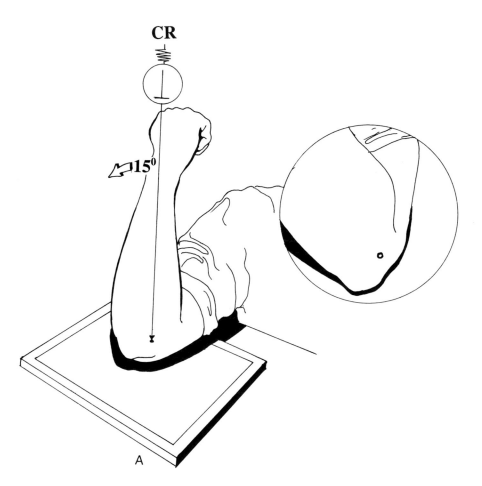

□ **FIGURE 4–9.**

POSITION DESCRIPTION

Part Position: The dorsal aspect of the distal humerus is placed on the cassette with the elbow in full flexion. The arm is adjusted in 15° of external rotation.

Central Ray: Perpendicular to the cassette, through the midpoint of the elbow joint.

Cubital Tunnel Position*† *(continued)*

IMAGE EVALUATION

An AP projection of the entire cubital tunnel should be demonstrated. The cubital tunnel includes both the bony notch between the medial epicondyle and medial aspect of the trochlea and the area between the medial aspect of the trochlea and the medial aspect of the olecranon process.

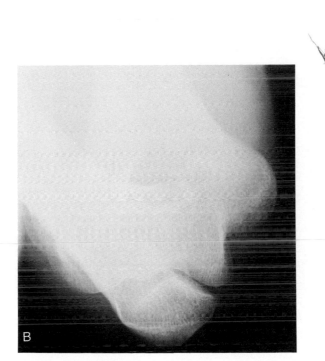

□ **FIGURE 4–9.** *(continued)*

---

*St. John JN, Palmaz JC. The cubital tunnel in ulnar entrapment neuropathy. *Radiology* 1986; 158:119–123.
†Wadsworth TG, Williams JR. Cubital tunnel external compression syndrome. *Br J Med* 1973; 1:662–666.

Cubital Tunnel Position *(continued)*

CASE STUDY

The patient presented with numbness in the fourth and fifth digits of the right hand.

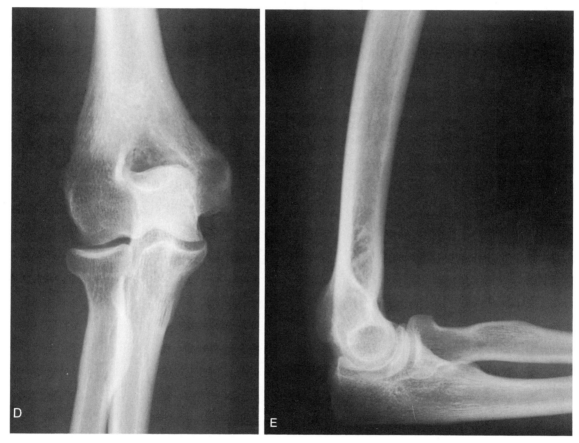

☐ **FIGURE 4–9.** *(continued)*

Routine AP and lateral elbow radiographs were taken. The AP radiograph revealed degenerative changes medially, but the extent of cubital tunnel involvement could not be assessed.

Cubital Tunnel Position *(continued)*

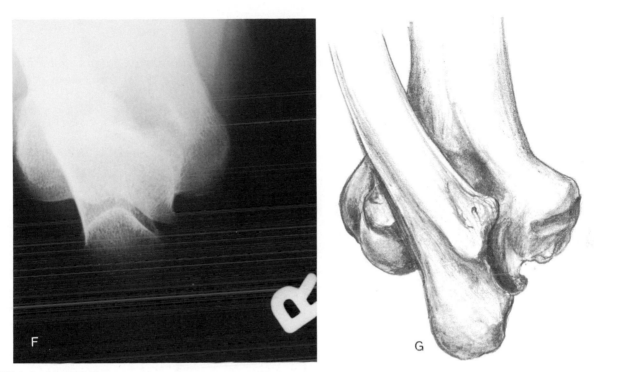

□ **FIGURE 4–9.** *(continued)*

The cubital tunnel elbow radiograph demonstrated bone spurs projecting into the area of the cubital tunnel.

Gravity Stress Elbow Position*

RATIONALE FOR USE

The gravity stress elbow position allows *evaluation of valgus instability of the elbow*. The degree of instability may be assessed by AP projection of the elbow during gravity-induced valgus stress.

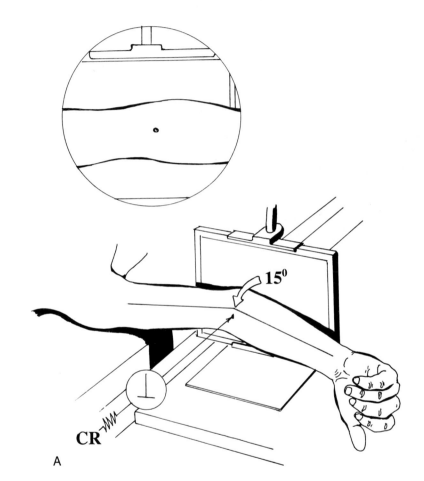

A

☐ **FIGURE 4–10.**

POSITION DESCRIPTION

Part Position: The patient is supine on the radiographic table with the arm abducted 90° from the body. The arm, excluding the shoulder, is extended over the side of the table and is in external rotation with the thumb pointing toward the floor. The elbow is flexed 15°. The cassette is oriented vertically and placed against the dorsal aspect of the elbow.

Central Ray: Perpendicular to the cassette, through the midpoint of the elbow joint.

Gravity Stress Elbow Position* *(continued)*

IMAGE EVALUATION

The elbow should be seen in AP projection, with slight angulation distortion as a result of elbow flexion. Valgus instability will be evident as a widening of the medial aspect of the joint space.

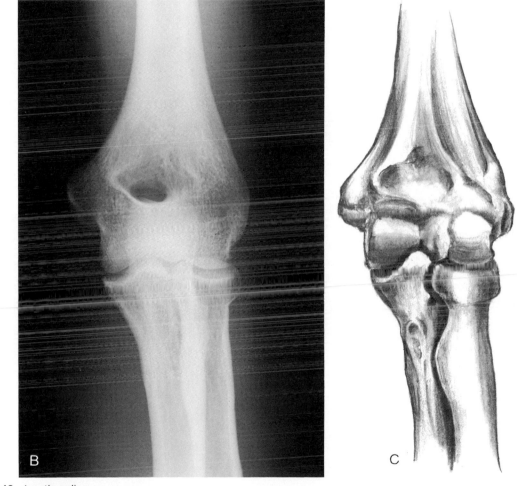

□ **FIGURE 4–10.** *(continued)*

---

*Schwab GH, Bennett JB, Woods GW, Tullos HS. Biomechanics of elbow instability: the role of the medial collateral ligament. *Clin Orthop* 1980; 146:42–52.

Gunsight Elbow Position*

RATIONALE FOR USE

The gunsight elbow position may demonstrate the presence of an *osteophyte (spur) on the lateral humeral epicondyle*. Such osteophytes are often associated with epicondylitis, or tennis elbow. This position provides excellent visualization of the epicondylar osteophyte, which is easily missed on routine projections.

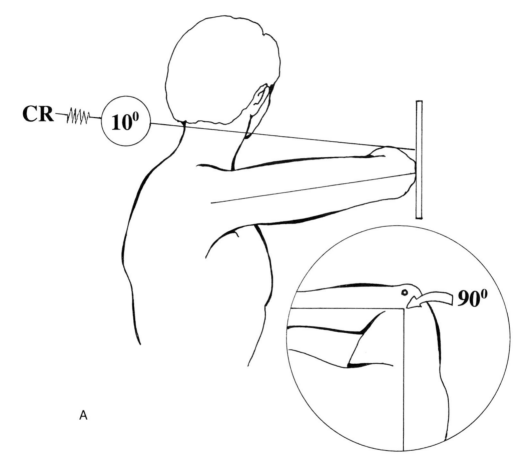

A

□ **FIGURE 4–11.**

POSITION DESCRIPTION

Part Position: The patient stands or sits facing the vertically oriented cassette, with the entire arm raised slightly above horizontal and in front of the body. The elbow is flexed 90°, and the dorsal surface of the distal ulna is in contact with the cassette.

Central Ray: The tube is positioned behind the shoulder with the central ray directed along the long axis of the humerus, angled 10° caudad (down) from horizontal and entering the elbow at the lateral epicondyle.

Gunsight Elbow Position* *(continued)*

IMAGE EVALUATION

A tangential image of the lateral humeral epicondyle should be demonstrated. A portion of the radial head may be visible.

Note: Overexposure of the lateral epicondyle could mask the presence of an osteophyte.

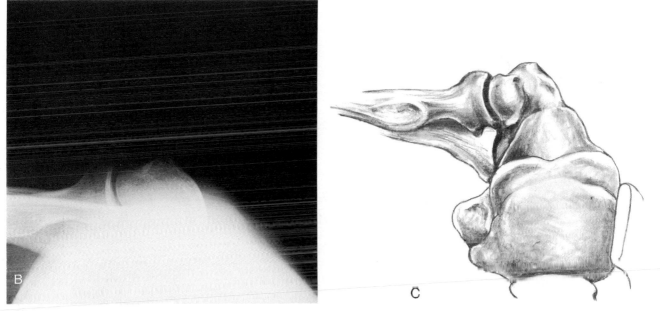

□ **FIGURE 4–11.** *(continued)*

---

*Begg RE. Epicondylitis or tennis elbow: frequent findings of gunsight type spur in lateral epicondyle of distal humerus. *Ortho Review* 1980; 9(8):33–42.

Gunsight Elbow Position *(continued)*

CASE STUDY

The patient presented with pain in the elbow. The pain extended distally, and the patient had difficulty moving the hand.

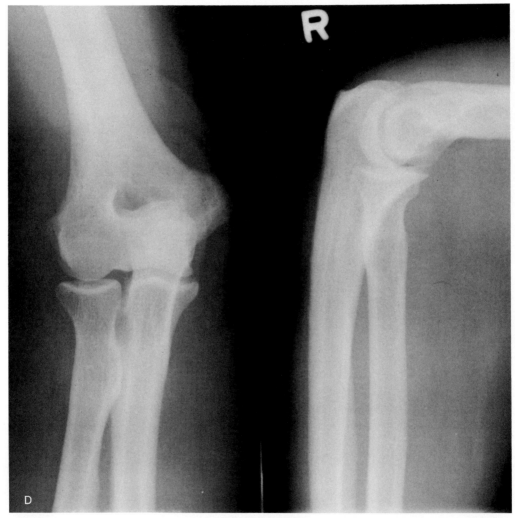

□ **FIGURE 4–11.** *(continued)*

(Courtesy of Larry Robinson, RT[R].)

Routine AP and lateral radiographs were taken. There appeared to be an added bony density at the lateral epicondyle, but this was considered inconclusive.

Gunsight Elbow Position *(continued)*

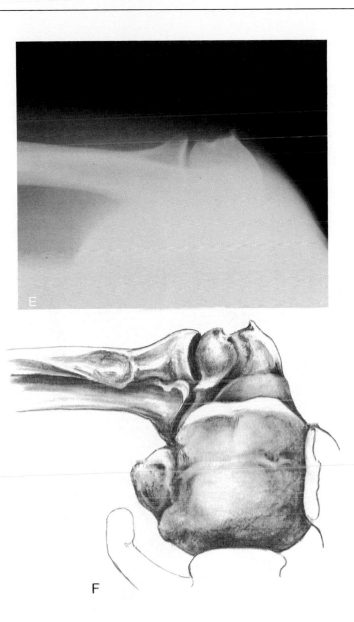

□ **FIGURE 4–11.** *(continued)*

(*E,* courtesy of Larry Robinson, RT[R].)

The gunsight elbow projection clearly demonstrated the presence of the epicondylar osteophyte.

Note: The terms *tennis elbow* and *epicondylitis* are often used interchangeably. However, *tennis elbow* may also refer to radial head capsulitis and radiohumeral bursitis.

Lateral (External) Oblique Elbow Position

RATIONALE FOR USE

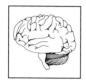

The lateral (external) oblique elbow position enables visualization of the *radial head, neck, and tuberosity without bone superimposition.* Fractures of the radial head are often not well demonstrated on routine elbow radiographs. The position also enables evaluation of the elbow for other fractures not demonstrated on the routine radiographs.

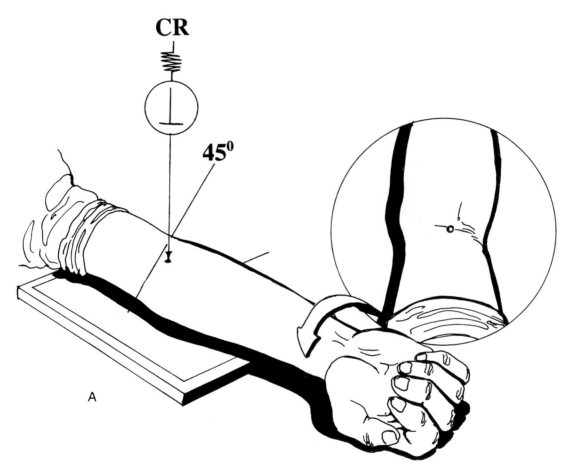

□ **FIGURE 4–12.**

POSITION DESCRIPTION

Part Position: The elbow is first positioned as for a routine AP projection. The entire arm is then rotated laterally (externally) so that the coronal plane of the humeral epicondyles is at a 45° angle to the cassette.

Note: External rotation of the arm is easier if the patient leans slightly laterally.

Central Ray: Perpendicular to the cassette, through the midpoint of the elbow joint.

Lateral (External) Oblique Elbow Position *(continued)*

IMAGE EVALUATION

The radial head, neck, and tuberosity should be seen without bone superimposition. The capitellum of the humerus should be well demonstrated. The medial humeral epicondyle will be superimposed over the olecranon process of the ulna.

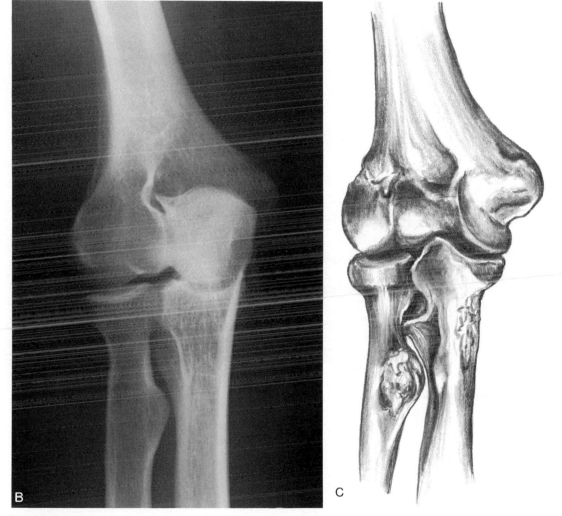

□ **FIGURE 4–12.** *(continued)*

Lateral Radial Head Rotation Positions

RATIONALE FOR USE

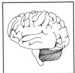

The lateral radial head rotation positions enable *demonstration of the entire profile of the radial head* for evaluation of occult fractures not visible on other positions or projections.

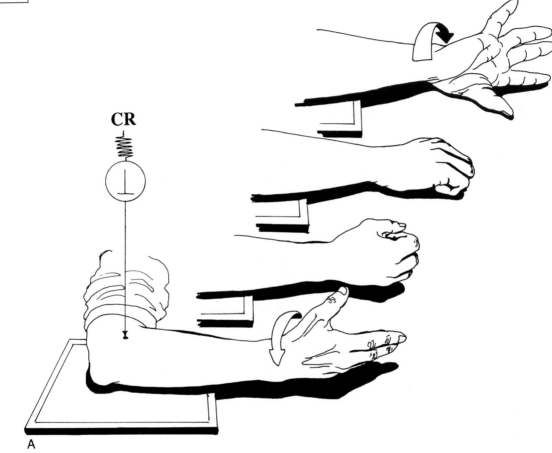

□ **FIGURE 4–13.**

POSITION DESCRIPTION

Part Position: The elbow is positioned as for a routine lateral radiograph. Four exposures of the hand are made: maximal supination, ulnar lateral, pronation, and maximal hyperpronation (internal rotation with radial side down).

Central Ray: Perpendicular to the cassette, through midpoint of the elbow joint.

Lateral Radial Head Rotation Positions *(continued)*

IMAGE EVALUATION

The elbow should be seen in lateral position. A different portion of the radial head profile is demonstrated on each image. The change in position of the radial tuberosity is the most apparent indicator of radial head rotation. In supination, the radial tuberosity is oriented away from the ulna. In ulnar lateral position, it is obscured by the radius. In pronation, it is oriented toward the ulna. In hyperpronation, it is again obscured by the radius.

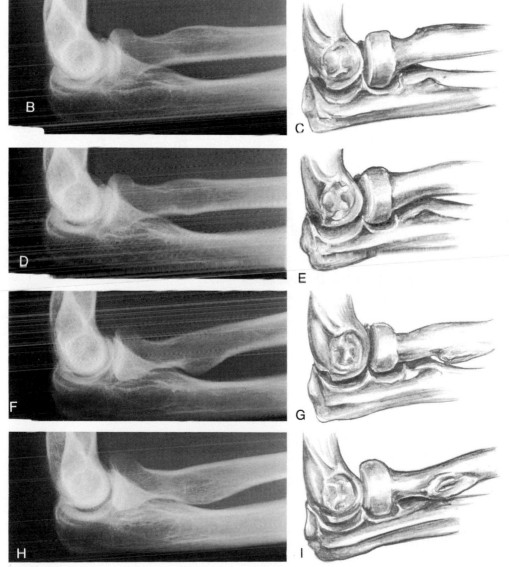

□ **FIGURE 4–13.** *(continued)*

(B, supination; *D,* ulnar lateral; *F,* pronation; *H,* hyperpronation.)

Medial (Internal) Oblique Elbow Position

RATIONALE FOR USE

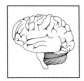

The medial (internal) oblique elbow position enables visualization of the *coronoid process without bone superimposition.* Fractures of the coronoid are not well demonstrated on routine elbow radiographs. The position also allows evaluation of the elbow for other fractures not demonstrated on the routine radiographs.

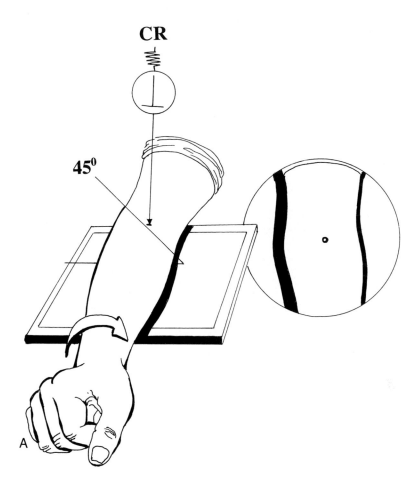

□ **FIGURE 4–14.**

POSITION DESCRIPTION

Part Position: The elbow is first positioned as for a routine AP projection. The entire arm is then rotated medially (internally) so that the coronal plane of the humeral epicondyles is at a 45° angle to the cassette.

Central Ray: Perpendicular to the cassette, through the midpoint of the elbow joint.

Medial (Internal) Oblique Elbow Position *(continued)*

IMAGE EVALUATION

The coronoid process should be seen without bone superimposition, distal to the elongated medial humeral epicondyle. The trochlea should be well demonstrated. The radial head, neck, and tuberosity will be superimposed over the proximal ulna.

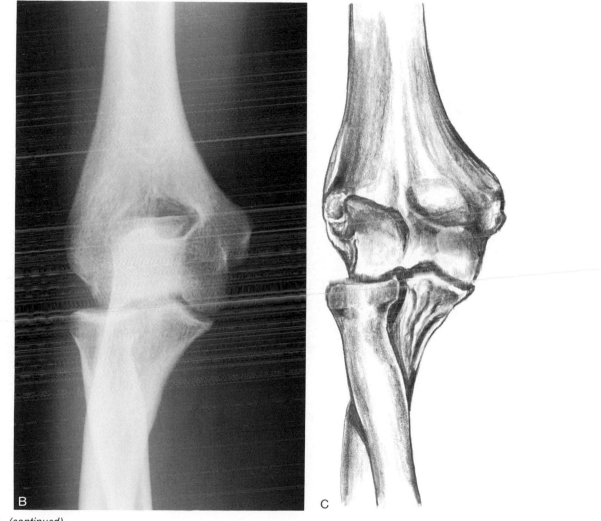

B

C

□ **FIGURE 4–14.** *(continued)*

Radial Head–Capitellum Position*
(Coyle† Trauma Elbow Position for Radial Head)

RATIONALE FOR USE

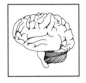

The radial head–capitellum position (also called the Coyle trauma elbow position for the radial head) demonstrates *fractures of the radial head, coronoid process, and capitellum*. By separating the radial head from the coronoid process and the capitellum from the trochlea, it eliminates much of the bone superimposition seen on the standard lateral position of the elbow.

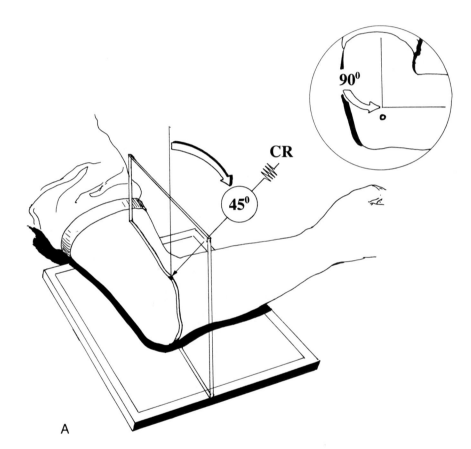

A

□ **FIGURE 4–15.**

POSITION DESCRIPTION

Part Position: The elbow is placed in the standard lateral position (elbow in 90° flexion, humerus and forearm parallel to plane of cassette).

Central Ray: The central ray is angled 45° toward the shoulder, oriented parallel to the long axis of the humerus and passing through the midpoint of the elbow joint.

Note: If the elbow cannot be flexed 90°, the central ray should be oriented perpendicular to the long axis of the proximal forearm when the radial head is of primary interest.

Radial Head–Capitellum Position*
(Coyle† Trauma Elbow Position for Radial Head) *(continued)*

IMAGE EVALUATION

The radial head and coronoid process should be minimally overlapped. The capitellum should be separated from the trochlea and the capitellar articular surface well demonstrated. Angulation distortion will be evident.

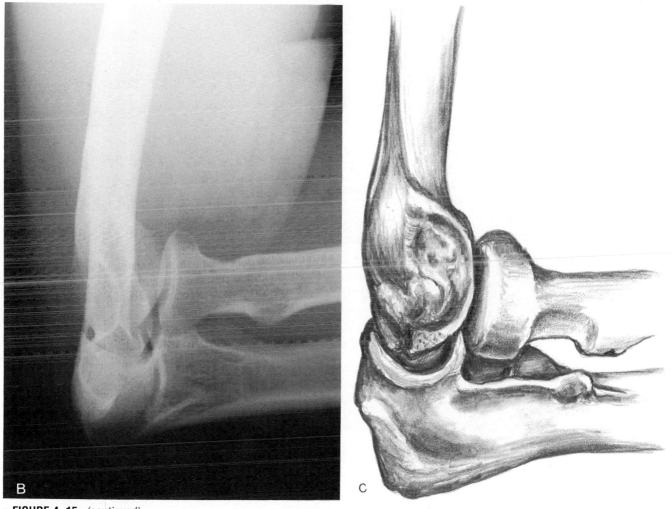

B

C

☐ **FIGURE 4–15.** *(continued)*

*Greenspan A, Norman A. The radial head–capitellum view: useful technique in elbow trauma. *AJR* 1982; 138:1186–1188.
†Coyle GF. Unit 7, Special angled views of joints—elbow, knee, ankle. *Radiographing Immobile Trauma Patients.* Denver: Multi-Media Publishing; 1980.

Radial Head–Capitellum Position
(Coyle Trauma Elbow Position for Radial Head) *(continued)*

CASE STUDY

The patient fell on her outstretched hand. She complained of pain in the elbow.

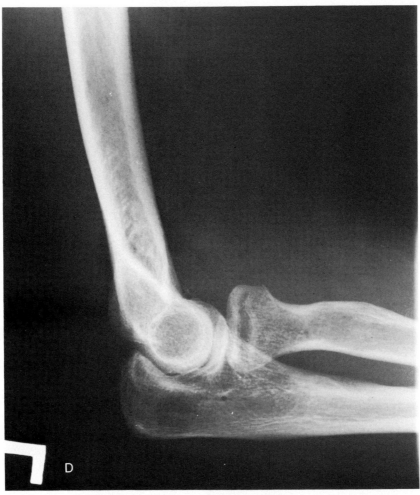

□ **FIGURE 4–15.** *(continued)*

Routine AP and lateral radiographs were taken. The lateral radiograph showed a barely visible radiolucent line, which is suggestive of a fracture of the radial neck.

Radial Head–Capitellum Position
(Coyle Trauma Elbow Position for Radial Head) *(continued)*

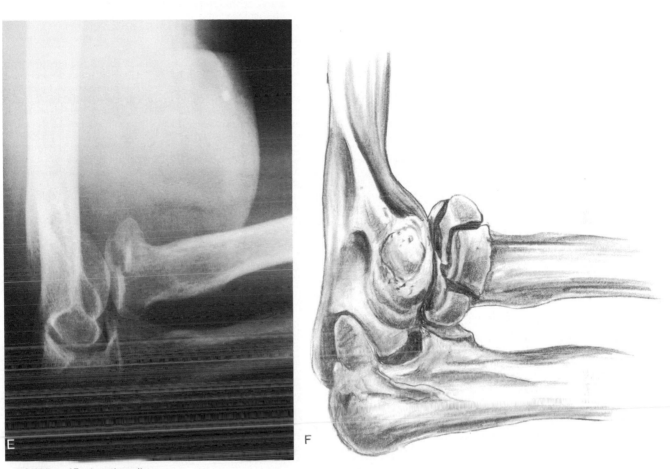

E   F

□ **FIGURE 4–15.** *(continued)*

The radial head–capitellum radiograph demonstrated an angular deformity and an impacted radial head and neck fracture.

References

1. Rogers SL, MacEwan DW. Changes due to trauma in the fat plane overlying the supinator muscle. *Radiology* 1969; 92:954.
2. Norell HG. Roentgenologic visualization of the extracapsular fat. Its importance in the diagnosis of traumatic injuries to the elbow. *Acta Radiol* 1954; 42:205.
3. Bledsoe RC, Izenstark JL. Displacement of fat pads in disease and injury of the elbow. A new radiographic sign. *Radiology* 1959; 73:717.
4. Yousefzadeh DK, Jackson JH. Lipohemarthrosis of the elbow joint. *Radiology* 1978; 128:643–645.
5. Mason MB. Some observations on fractures of the head of the radius with a review of one hundred cases. *Br J Surg* 1954; 42:123.
6. Conn J, Wade PA. Injuries of the elbow: a ten year review. *J Trauma* 1961; 1:248–268.
7. Morrey BF. Radial head fracture. *In* Morrey BF (ed). *The Elbow and Its Disorders.* Philadelphia: WB Saunders; 1985:355.
8. Radin EL, Riseborough EJ. Fractures of the radial head. *J Bone Joint Surg* 1966; 48A:1055.
9. Greenspan A, Norman A. The radial head–capitellum view: useful technique in elbow trauma. *AJR* 1982; 138:1186–1188.
10. Coyle GF. Unit 7, Special angled views of joints—elbow, knee, ankle. *Radiographing Immobile Trauma Patients.* Denver: Multi-Media Publishing; 1980.
11. Rogers LF. *Radiology of Skeletal Trauma,* 2nd ed. London: Churchill Livingstone; 1992.
12. Horne JG, Tanzer TL. Olecranon fractures: a review of 100 cases. *J Trauma* 1981; 21:469.
13. Watson JT. Fractures of the forearm and elbow. *Clin Sports Med* 1990; 9:59–83.
14. Pitt MJ, Speer DP. Imaging of the elbow with an emphasis on trauma. *Radiol Clin North Am* 1990; 28(2):293–305.
15. Hotchkiss RN, Green DP. Fractures and dislocation of the elbow. *In* Rockwood CA, Green DP, Bucholz RW (eds). *Fractures in Adults,* 3rd ed. Philadelphia: JB Lippincott; 1991:739–841.
16. Aitken GK, Rorabeck CH. Distal humeral fractures in the adult. *Clin Orthop* 1986; 207:191.
17. Knight RA. Fractures of the humeral condyles in adults. *South Med J* 1955; 48:1165.
18. Miller WE. Comminuted fractures of the distal end of the humerus in adults. *J Bone Joint Surg* 1964; 46A:644.
19. Wade FV, Batdorf J. Supracondylar fractures of the humerus: a twelve year review with follow-up. *J Trauma* 1961; 1:269.
20. Bryan RS, Morrey BF. Fractures of the distal humerus. *In* Morrey BF (ed). *The Elbow and Its Disorders.* Philadelphia: WB Saunders; 1985:304.
21. Milch H. Fractures and fracture-dislocations of the humeral condyles. *J Trauma* 1964; 4:592.
22. Lichtenberg RP. A study of 2532 fractures in children. *Am J Surg* 1954; 87:330–338.
23. Landin LA. Fracture patterns in children. Analysis of 8,682 fractures with special reference to incidence, etiology, and secular changes in a Swedish urban population 1950–1979. *Acta Orthop Scand (Suppl)* 1983; 54(202):1–109.
24. Reed MH. Fractures and dislocations of the extremities in children. *J Trauma* 1977; 17:351–354.
25. Wilkins KE. Fractures and dislocations of the elbow region. *In* Rockwood CA, Wilkins KE, King RE (eds). *Fractures in Children,* 3rd ed. Philadelphia: JB Lippincott; 1991:509–828.
26. Rogers LF, Malave S, White H, Tachdijian MO. Plastic bowing, torus, and greenstick supracondylar fractures of the humerus: radiographic clues to obscure fractures of the elbow in children. *Radiology* 1978; 128:145.
27. Baumann E. Beitrage zur kenntnis dur frackturen am ellbogengelenk. *Bruns Beitr F Klin Chir* 1929; 146:1–50.
28. Asher MA. Dislocations of the upper extremity in children. *Orthop Clin North Am* 1976; 7:583.
29. Blount WP. *Fractures in Children.* Baltimore: Williams & Wilkins; 1955:26–75.
30. Josefsson PO, Nilsson BE. Incidence of elbow dislocation. *Acta Orthop Scand* 1986; 57:537.
31. Linscheid RL. Elbow dislocation. *In* Morrey BF (ed). *The Elbow and Its Disorders.* Philadelphia: WB Saunders; 1985:422.
32. Carlioz H, Abols Y. Posterior dislocation of the elbow in children. *J Pediatr Orthop* 1984; 4:8–12.
33. Monteggia GB. *Instituzioni Chirurgiche,* vol 5. Milan: Maspero; 1814.
34. Bado JL. The Monteggia lesion. *Clin Orthop* 1967; 50:71.
35. Hudson DA, DeBeer JD. Isolated traumatic dislocation of the radial head in children. *J Boint Joint Surg* 1986; 68B:378–381.
36. Priest JD, Jones HH, Nagel DA. Elbow injuries in highly skilled tennis players. *J Sports Med* 1974; 2:137.
37. Gore RM, Rogers LF, Bowerman J, et al. Osseous manifestations of elbow stress associated with sports activities. *AJR* 1980; 134:971–977.
38. Bennett JB, Tullos HS. Ligamentous and articular injuries in the athlete. *In* Morrey BF (ed). *The Elbow and Its Disorders.* Philadelphia: WB Saunders; 1985:505–507.
39. Karasick D, Burk DL, Gross GW. Trauma to the elbow and forearm. *Semin Roentgenol* 1991; 25(4):318–330.
40. Berens DL, Lin RK. *Roentgen Diagnosis of Rheumatoid Arthritis.* Springfield, IL: Charles C Thomas; 1969.
41. Porter BB, Park N, Richardson C, et al. Rheumatoid arthritis of the elbow. The results of synovectomy. *J Bone Joint Surg* 1974; 56B:427.
42. Weissman BNW, Sledge CB. *Orthopedic Radiology.* Philadelphia: WB Saunders; 1986:181.
43. Tompkins RB. Nonrheumatoid inflammatory arthritis. *In* Morrey BF (ed). *The Elbow and Its Disorders.* Philadelphia: WB Saunders; 1985:657.

FIVE

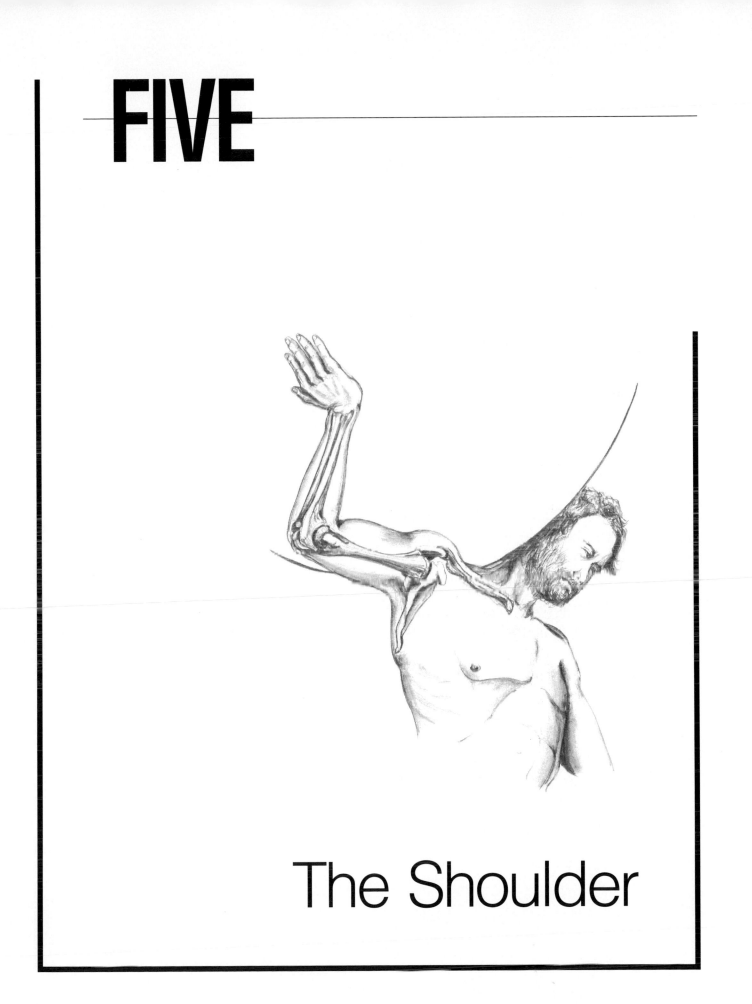

The Shoulder

THE SHOULDER: AN OVERVIEW

ROUTINE SHOULDER RADIOGRAPHY

Routine AP Internal Rotation Shoulder Projection
Routine AP External Rotation Shoulder Projection

SPECIALIZED SHOULDER RADIOGRAPHY

Apical AP Shoulder Projection
Coracoid Process Position
Didiee Shoulder Position
Exaggerated External Rotation Axillary Shoulder Position
Fisk Bicipital Groove Position
Garth Apical Oblique Shoulder Position
Lawrence Axillary Shoulder Position
Stryker Notch Shoulder Position
Superoinferior Axillary Shoulder Position
Supraspinatus Outlet Shoulder Position
True AP (Grashey) Shoulder Position
True Lateral (Scapular "Y") Shoulder Position
Westpoint Axillary Shoulder Position

ACROMIOCLAVICULAR AND STERNOCLAVICULAR JOINT RADIOGRAPHY

AP Acromioclavicular Joint Projections (No Weights)
AP Acromioclavicular Joint Projections (With Weights)
PA Oblique Sternoclavicular Joint Position
PA Sternoclavicular Joints Projection
Serendipity Axial Sternoclavicular Joint Projection

The Shoulder: An Overview

The shoulder girdle is primarily responsible for the infinite variety of arm positions used by humans to manipulate their environment. The shoulder is the most mobile joint in the body. The complex shoulder motions result from the combined movements of the glenohumeral, acromioclavicular, and sternoclavicular joints, as well as the scapulothoracic articulation. The greatest amount of movement occurs at the glenohumeral joint.

Pathology of the shoulder girdle may be acute or chronic, and traumatic, degenerative, or destructive. Patients usually present with pain, joint instability, or decreased mobility as a result of pain, stiffness, or muscle weakness. Prompt and definitive diagnosis of fracture, dislocation, or other pathology involving the shoulder girdle is of paramount importance, because any disruption in the balance of forces across the shoulder will interfere with proper function.

Fractures occur, to varying degrees, in each of the three bones constituting the shoulder girdle. The clavicle is commonly fractured both in children and in adults. Clavicular fracture is believed to be the most common fracture in children.[1] Such fractures usually involve the midshaft, followed in frequency by the distal third. The common mechanisms of injury, both in children and in adults, are falls on the outstretched hand and direct impacts or falls on the superolateral aspect of the shoulder.[2, 3] In addition, clavicular fracture is recognized as the most common birth injury.[4] Radiographic evaluation consists of anteroposterior/posteroanterior (AP/PA) and axial radiographs. The radiographic findings are easily demonstrated in adults, but the frequency of greenstick and plastic deformity injuries in children complicates diagnosis.

Fractures of the proximal humerus are common in older adults, whereas distal humeral fractures are common in children. The usual mechanism of injury is a fall on the outstretched hand. The prevalence of proximal humeral fractures in the elderly is believed to be related to osteoporosis.[5] The amount of force involved in many of these injuries is moderate, and the majority of these fractures are nondisplaced or minimally displaced with one fracture line. The more complex fractures and fracture-dislocations are more often seen in younger patients and are associated with severe trauma. Radiographic evaluation of proximal humeral fractures is best accomplished with the use of the "trauma series" recommended by Neer.[6] The series consists of a true AP (Grashey[7]), a true lateral (scapular "Y"[8]), and a Lawrence[9] axillary radiograph, if possible. These positions and projections are described in this chapter.

Fractures of the scapula are relatively uncommon in adults and even less common in children. The body of the scapula is most often fractured; the scapular neck is second in frequency of involvement.[10] The scapular body is usually fractured by a direct blow or fall. Fractures involving the scapular neck result from indirect forces generated from a fall on the outstretched arm, a direct blow, or a direct fall on the point of the shoulder.[11] Intra-articular fractures of the glenoid process may occur, usually in association with humeral dislocation or with the mechanisms of scapular neck fracture.[12] The acromion process is occasionally fractured by a direct superior blow, but acromioclavicular joint separation is much more common with this event.[11] Acromion fracture is also associated with superior displacement of the humeral head. Fracture of the coracoid process may occur from a direct blow, from a fall on the point of the shoulder, or as an avulsion associated with acromioclavicular joint separation.[13] Radiographic evaluation of the scapula should include true AP (Grashey[7]) and either true lateral (scapular "Y"[8]) or axillary (Lawrence[9] or Westpoint[14]) radiographs. The coracoid and acromion processes are best visualized with the Stryker Notch[15] or coracoid process[16] positions.

The shoulder is believed to be the most commonly dislocated major joint in adults.[17] Shoulder dislocations are considered very rare in children; the incidence increases with age. In a large study of shoulder injuries, Cave[18] reported that the majority (84%) were anterior glenohumeral dislocations. Other reported dislocations were acromioclavicular (12%), sternoclavicular (2.5%), and posterior glenohumeral (1.5%). Inferior and superior glenohumeral dislocations have been found to occur less frequently than the posterior type.

Radiographic evaluation of shoulder dislocations or subluxations necessitates imaging in planes parallel, perpendicular, or tangential to the joint surfaces. Glenohumeral dislocations are best evaluated in the scapular planes with the true AP (Grashey)[7] and either the true lateral (scapular "Y"[8]) or Lawrence[9] axillary positions. The classic radiographic signs of anterior glenohumeral dislocation—the Hill-Sachs[19] defect of the superolateral humeral head and the Bankart[20] lesion of the anteroinferior glenoid rim—may be further evaluated through a number of accessory positions, including special axillary positions (Westpoint,[14] exaggerated external rotation[21]), the Stryker Notch[15] position, the Didiee[22] position, and the Garth[23] apical oblique position.

Dislocation of the acromioclavicular joint is most commonly caused by a fall or a direct blow on the point of the shoulder.[24] The distal clavicle is usually seen to be displaced superiorly, but posterior and inferior dislocations may occur. The dislocation is best demonstrated with bilateral AP upright radiographs. Bilateral examination enables comparison of the affected joint with the normal joint to assess widening (or, occasionally, narrowing) of the joint space. The upright position allows gravity to displace the scapula and humerus downward when the integrity of the acromioclavicular joint has been disrupted by fracture or ligamentous rupture. AP radiographs, with weights attached to the wrists, may be used when a dislocation is suspected but not revealed by gravity alone.

In sternoclavicular joint dislocation, the medial end of the clavicle may be displaced anteriorly or posteriorly. The anterior dislocation is most common.[25] Most of these dislocations result from indirect forces generated during compression to the lateral shoulder. Rockwood[26] explained that if the shoulder is rolled forward during compression, a posterior dislocation results, whereas if the shoulder is rolled backward during the compression incident, an anterior dislocation results. Dislocation may also result from a direct blow to the chest or clavicle. Findings of several studies[27, 28] indicate that the most common cause of sternoclavicular joint dislocation is a vehicular accident. This is followed in frequency by sports-related injury. Sternoclavicular dislocation is often difficult to diagnose radiographically. AP radiographs demonstrate inferosuperior displacement of the medial clavicle but not anterior or posterior displacement. The Serendipity[29] axial sternoclavicular joint projection, described in this chapter, effectively demonstrates anterior or posterior dislocations.

The shoulder is subject to a number of conditions that Rowe[30] termed "subacromial syndromes." He included tendinitis, bursitis, impingement, snapping scapula, calcific tendinitis, rotator cuff tears, and idiopathic chronic adhesive capsulitis (frozen shoulder). Only shoulder impingement syndrome and calcific tendinitis produce significant signs that are readily apparent on radiographs. According to Neer,[31] the shoulder impingement syndrome is caused by impingement of the supraspinatus tendon on the anterior acromion when the arm is abducted or forward flexed. It is thought that impingement is more likely when the anterior portion of the acromion is abnormally long or when a subacromial spur is present.[32] The axial

AP shoulder projection (30° caudad angle) demonstrates the extent of anterior acromial projection. The supraspinatus outlet shoulder position[33] may demonstrate the presence of a subacromial spur. Both of these positions or projections are described in this chapter. Calcific tendinitis manifests radiographically as calcium deposits within the supraspinatus (most common), infraspinatus, teres minor, and, occasionally, subscapularis tendons. These calcium deposits can be localized on routine AP internal and external rotation shoulder radiographs.

The shoulder is involved in most forms of arthritis. Mills[34] stated that the rheumatic diseases commonly encountered in the shoulder include seronegative spondyloarthropathies (i.e., psoriatic arthritis, ankylosing spondylitis, Reiter's syndrome), seropositive rheumatoid arthritis, pseudogout, gout, juvenile rheumatoid arthritis, and hemochromatosis. Osteoarthritis in the shoulder is rarely of the primary type. It is usually associated with previous trauma. Radiographic findings of these arthritides are similar to those seen in other involved joints.

Many additional conditions affect the shoulder, including infection, tumors, neurological problems, and congenital abnormalities. For the sake of brevity and because their radiographic evaluation usually requires no special techniques, these abnormalities are not covered.

Routine Shoulder Radiography

Routine AP Internal Rotation Shoulder Projection

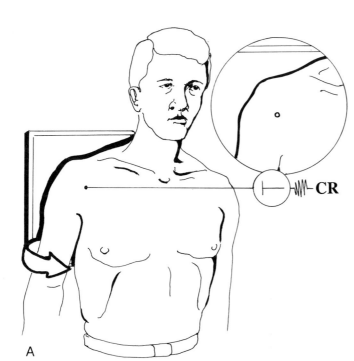

A

□ **FIGURE 5-1.**

POSITION DESCRIPTION

Part Position: Patient faces the tube with the dorsal aspect of the shoulder against the table or upright bucky/cassette holder. The body and cassette are adjusted to place the center of the cassette slightly below the coracoid process. The humerus is placed in internal rotation, by adjusting the coronal plane of the distal humeral epicondyles perpendicular to the plane of the cassette.

Central Ray: Perpendicular to the cassette, entering slightly inferior to the coracoid process.

IMAGE EVALUATION

An AP projection of the shoulder girdle, in anatomical position, should be demonstrated. The lesser tuberosity should be profiled on the medial aspect of the proximal humerus, with the greater tuberosity seen en face and superimposed over the middle of the humeral head.

Routine AP External Rotation Shoulder Projection

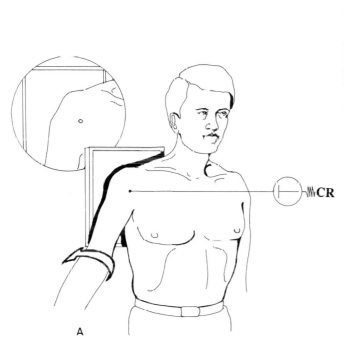

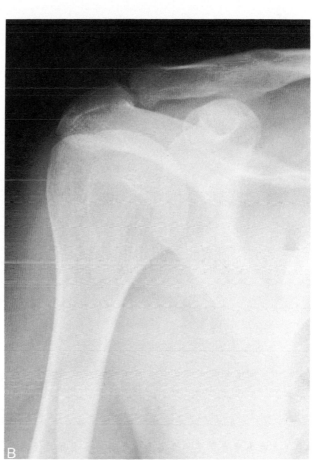

□ **FIGURE 5–2.**

POSITION DESCRIPTION

Part Position: Patient faces the tube with the dorsal aspect of the shoulder against the table or upright bucky/cassette holder. The body and cassette are adjusted to place the center of the cassette slightly below the coracoid process. The humerus is placed in external rotation by adjusting the coronal plane of the distal humeral epicondyles parallel to the plane of the cassette.

Central Ray: Perpendicular to the cassette, entering slightly inferior to the coracoid process.

IMAGE EVALUATION

An AP projection of the shoulder girdle, in anatomical position, should be demonstrated. The articular surface of the humeral head should be seen in profile. The greater tuberosity should be profiled on the lateral aspect of the proximal humerus, with the lesser tuberosity seen en face and medial to the greater tuberosity.

Specialized Shoulder Radiography

Apical AP Shoulder Projection

RATIONALE FOR USE

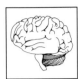

The apical AP shoulder projection may demonstrate *overgrowth or spurs of the anterior/inferior aspects of the acromion process and narrowing of the acromiohumeral space,* which have been found to be associated with the shoulder "impingement syndrome."

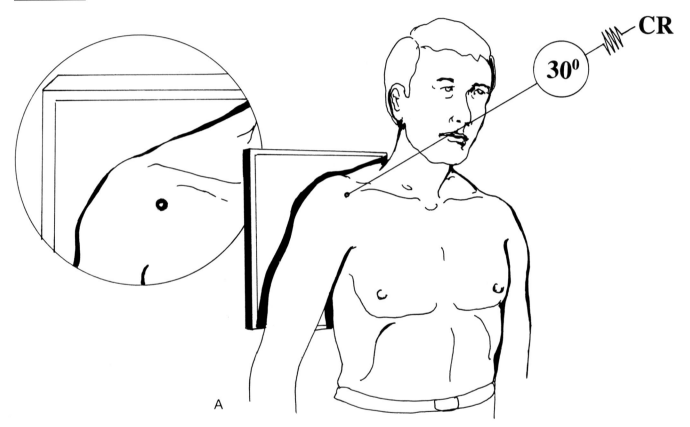

A

□ **FIGURE 5–3.**

POSITION DESCRIPTION

Part Position: Patient and part are positioned as for a routine AP shoulder projection. The humerus is placed in neutral rotation.

Central Ray: Angled 30° caudad, through the coracoid process.

Apical AP Shoulder Projection *(continued)*

IMAGE EVALUATION

The anteroinferior aspect of the acromion process should be demonstrated. The acromiohumeral space will appear wider than on the routine AP projection. The shoulder girdle will exhibit angulation distortion.

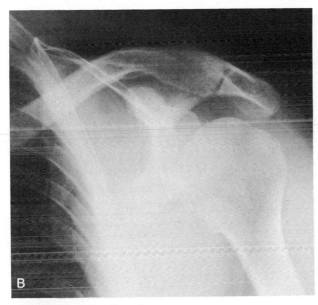

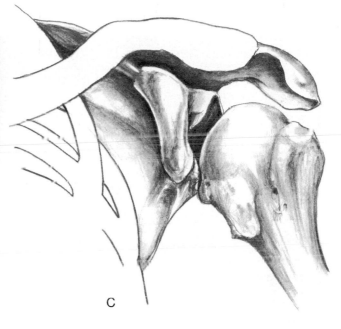

⊔ **FIGURE 5–3.** *(continued)*

Apical AP Shoulder Projection *(continued)*

CASE STUDY

The patient presented with pain on shoulder abduction or anterior flexion.

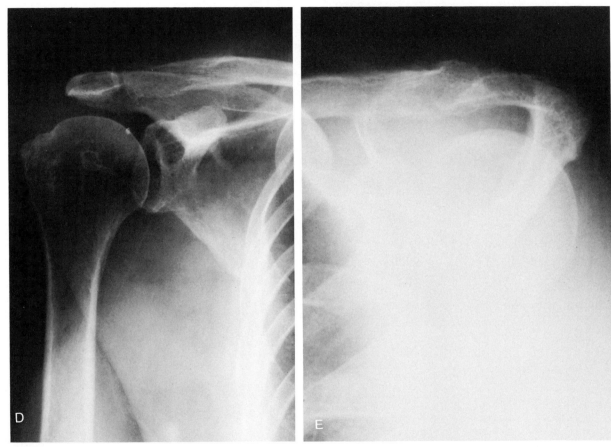

□ **FIGURE 5–3.** *(continued)*

True AP (Grashey) and supraspinatus outlet shoulder radiographs were taken. Degenerative changes of the greater tuberosity were evident, and the presence of acromial abnormality could not be ruled out.

Apical AP Shoulder Projection *(continued)*

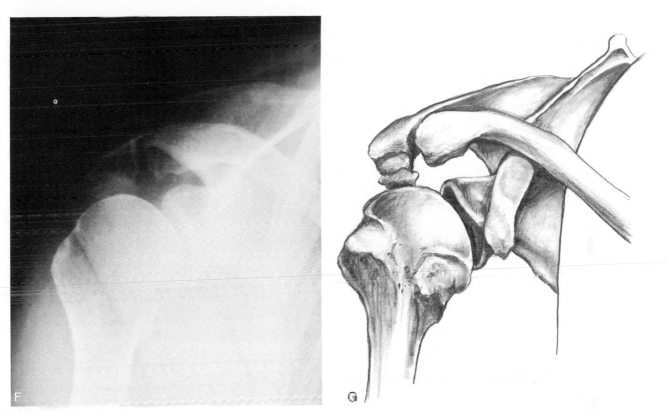

□ **FIGURE 5–3.** *(continued)*

An apical AP radiograph demonstrated an outgrowth of the anterior acromion.

Coracoid Process Position*

RATIONALE FOR USE

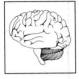

This position *alleviates the usual foreshortening and overlap of the coracoid process,* allowing evaluation for fractures or other pathology. The position also demonstrates the acromioclavicular joint without superimposition.

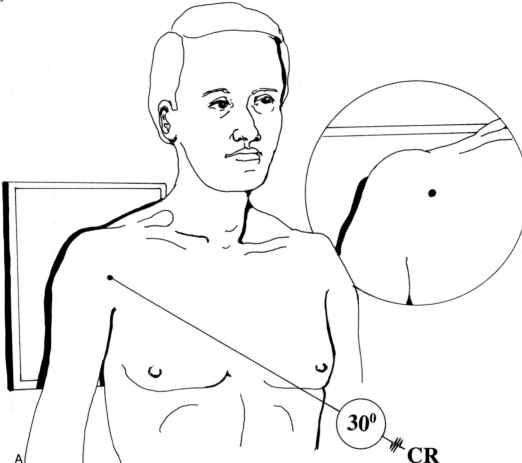

□ **FIGURE 5–4.**

POSITION DESCRIPTION

Part Position: Patient and part are positioned as for a routine AP shoulder projection. The humerus is placed in neutral rotation.

Central Ray: Angled 20°–30° cephalad, through the coracoid process.

Note: Amount of central ray angulation depends on the degree of dorsal kyphosis. The greater the kyphosis, the greater the angle needed.

Coracoid Process Position* *(continued)*

IMAGE EVALUATION

The coracoid process should be demonstrated with minimal foreshortening, inferior to the distal clavicle. The acromioclavicular joint should be well demonstrated. The shoulder girdle will exhibit angulation distortion.

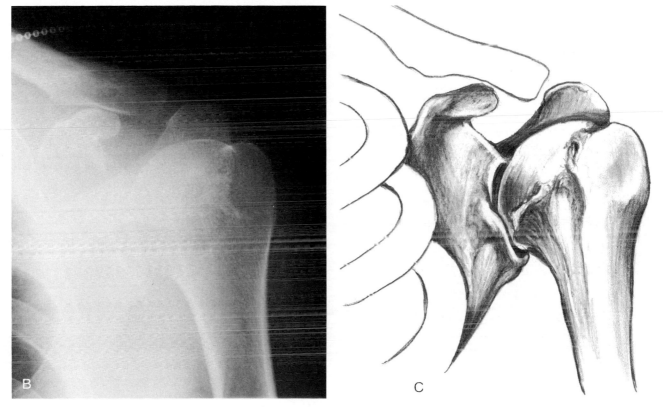

□ **FIGURE 5–4.** *(continued)*

---

*Fengler K. Special projections for the coracoid process and clavicle. *AJR* 1948; 59:435–438.

Didiee* Shoulder Position

RATIONALE FOR USE

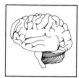

The Didiee shoulder position may be *used in cases of suspected anterior dislocation or subluxation of the shoulder to demonstrate the classic Hill-Sachs compression fracture* on the posterolateral aspect of the humeral head *and/or a Bankart lesion* of the anteroinferior glenoid rim.

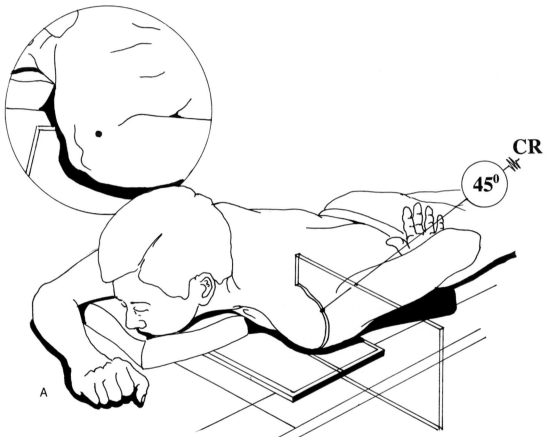

□ **FIGURE 5–5.**

POSITION DESCRIPTION

Part Position: The patient is prone with the cassette under the shoulder. The arm is abducted, and the back of the hand placed on the posterior iliac crest. The elbow is elevated to place the humeral shaft horizontal.

Central Ray: Angled 45° lateromedially, through the glenohumeral joint.

Note: This is a modification of the original Didiee‡ position, in which the central ray was directed from the elbow toward the shoulder along the long axis of the humerus.

Didiee* Shoulder Position *(continued)*

IMAGE EVALUATION

An elongated projection of the humeral head and neck should be demonstrated. The posterolateral aspect of the humeral head should be well seen. The glenoid rim will be elongated but should be well demonstrated.

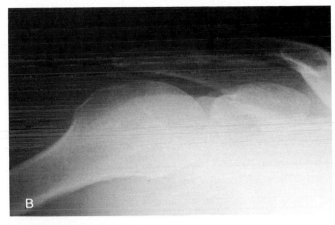

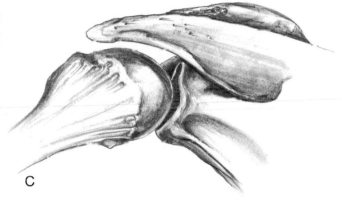

□ **FIGURE 5–5.** *(continued)*

*Didiee J. Le radiodiagnostic dans la luxation récidivante de l'épaule. *J Radiol Electrologic* 1930; 14(4):209–218.

Exaggerated External Rotation Axillary Shoulder Position*

RATIONALE FOR USE

The exaggerated external rotation axillary shoulder position may be used *in cases of suspected anterior dislocation or subluxation of the shoulder to demonstrate the classic Hill-Sachs compression fracture* on the posterolateral aspect of the humeral head *and/or a Bankart lesion* of the anterior-inferior glenoid rim.

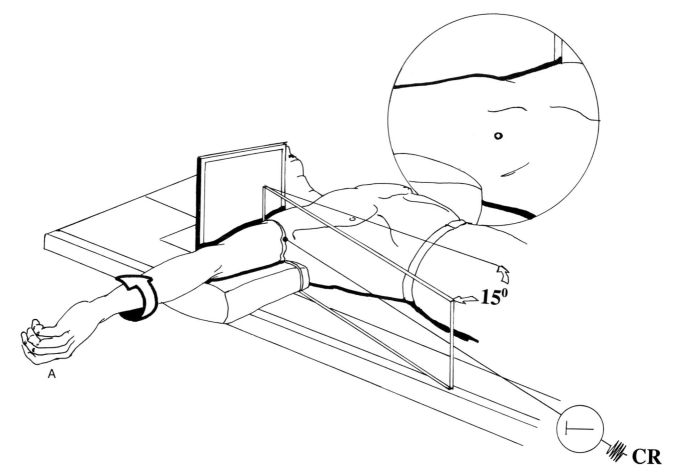

□ **FIGURE 5–6.**

POSITION DESCRIPTION

Part Position: The patient is supine with the shoulder slightly elevated and the arm is abducted to 90°. The vertically oriented cassette is placed against the superior surface of the shoulder and in contact with the side of the neck. The arm is then adjusted in maximal external rotation with the thumb pointing down.

Central Ray: Horizontal and angled approximately 15° medially, entering the axilla and passing through the acromioclavicular joint.

Exaggerated External Rotation Axillary Shoulder Position* *(continued)*

IMAGE EVALUATION

The shoulder girdle is demonstrated in axial projection. The glenohumeral joint should be well demonstrated. The greater tuberosity of the humerus will be in partial profile and oriented dorsally. The area of the acromioclavicular joint will be superimposed on the humerus. The coracoid process, if included, will be pointed ventrally.

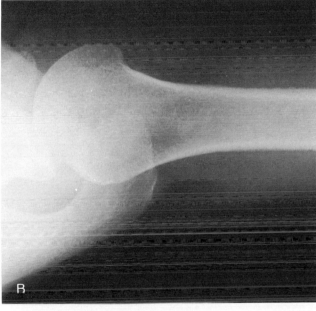

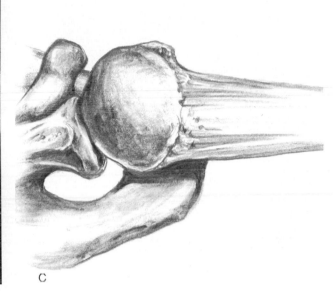

□ **FIGURE 5–6.** *(continued)*

---

*Rafert JA, Long BW, Hernandez EM, Kreipke DL. Axillary shoulder with exaggerated rotation: the Hill-Sachs defect. *Radiol Technol* 1990; 62(1):18–23.

Exaggerated External Rotation Axillary Shoulder Position *(continued)*

CASE STUDY

The patient presented with a history of recurrent anterior shoulder dislocation.

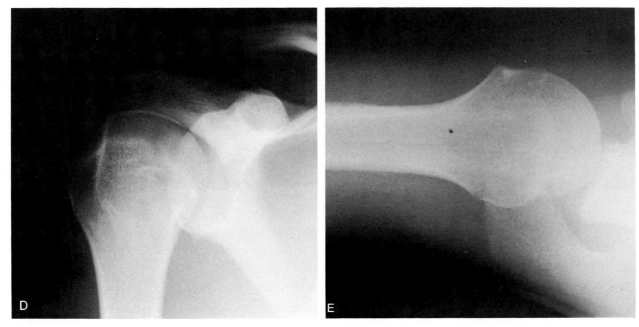

□ **FIGURE 5–6.** *(continued)*

Routine AP and axillary shoulder radiographs were taken. The neutral rotation AP demonstrated a vertically oriented "condensation line" on the superolateral humeral head. The Lawrence axillary also demonstrated a possible defect in this area but was thought to be inconclusive.

Exaggerated External Rotation Axillary Shoulder Position *(continued)*

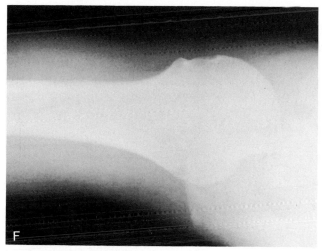

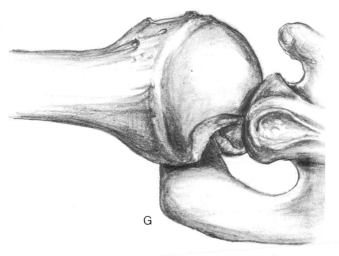

□ **FIGURE 5–6.** *(continued)*

The exaggerated external rotation axillary shoulder radiograph demonstrates a Hill-Sachs defect on the superolateral aspect of the humeral head. This depressed fracture occurs during anterior dislocation, as the humeral head impinges on the glenoid rim.

Fisk* Bicipital Groove Position

RATIONALE FOR USE

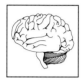

The Fisk bicipital groove position results in an axial projection of the proximal humeral tuberosities and the bicipital groove between them. This allows *evaluation of the humeral tuberosities for bony overgrowth projecting into the bicipital groove.*

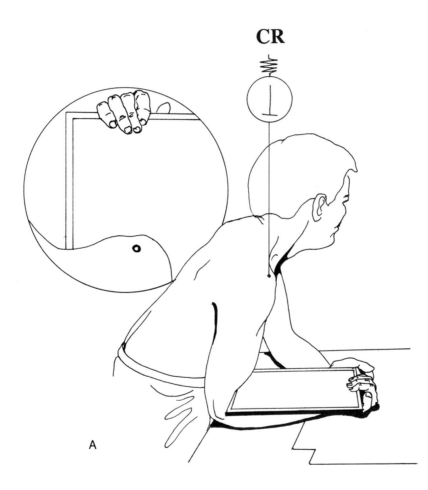

CR

A

□ FIGURE 5–7.

POSITION DESCRIPTION

Part Position: The patient leans forward over the cassette, which rests on the forearm and is held by the supinated hand. The forward leaning is adjusted so as to place the shoulder joint slightly anterior to the elbow.

Central Ray: Vertical and perpendicular to the cassette, through the humeral head.

Fisk* Bicipital Groove Position *(continued)*

IMAGE EVALUATION

An axial projection of the humeral tuberosities and the bicipital groove should be demonstrated. The acromion process will be superimposed over the bicipital groove but should not appreciably obscure it.

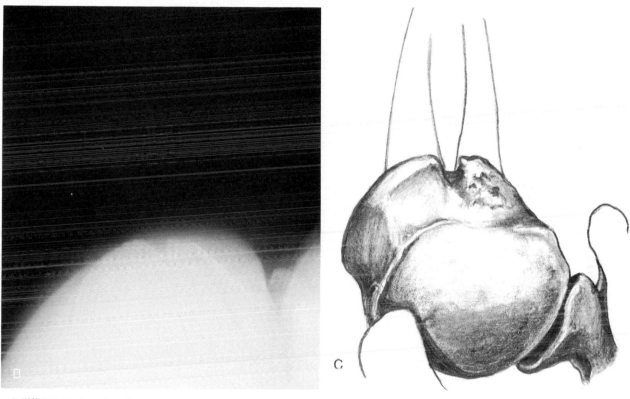

□ **FIGURE 5–7.** *(continued)*

---

*Fisk C. Adaptation of the technique for radiography of the bicipital groove. *Radiol Technol* 1965; 37:47–50.

Garth* Apical Oblique Shoulder Position

RATIONALE FOR USE

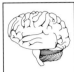

The Garth apical oblique shoulder position demonstrates a *coronal profile of the glenohumeral joint, allowing evaluation for instability, dislocations, or intra-articular fractures.*

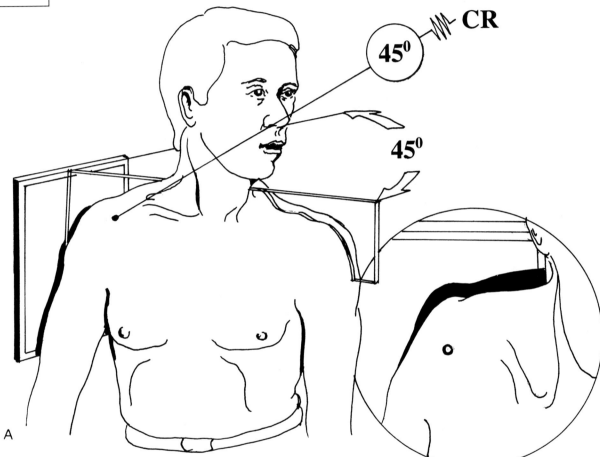

□ **FIGURE 5–8.**

POSITION DESCRIPTION

Part Position: Patient and part are positioned as for a true AP or Grashey shoulder (45° posterior oblique) position. The humerus is usually in neutral or slight internal rotation.

Note: When the patient is supine, a greater degree of obliquity may be required. Medial beam angulation may replace obliquity in severely injured patients.

Central Ray: Angled 45° caudad, entering slightly superior to the coracoid process.

Garth* Apical Oblique Shoulder Position *(continued)*

IMAGE EVALUATION

A coronal projection of the glenohumeral joint should be demonstrated. The coracoid process will be superimposed over the glenoid. The humeral head will appear elongated.

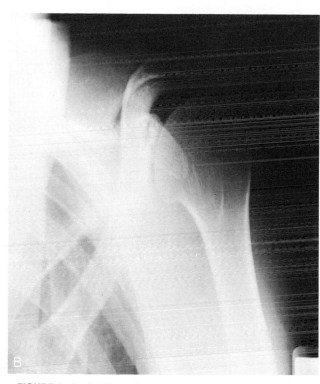

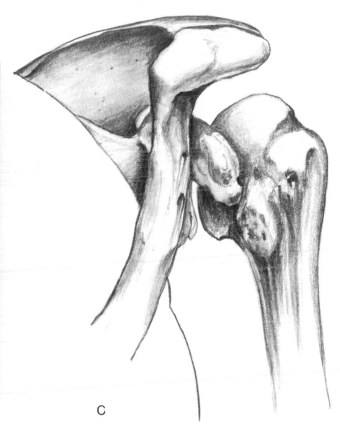

□ **FIGURE 5–8.** *(continued)*

---

*Garth WP, Slappey CE, Ochs CW. Roentgenographic demonstration of instability of the shoulder: the apical oblique projection—a technical note. *J Bone Joint Surg* 1984; 66A(9):1450–1453.

Garth Apical Oblique Shoulder Position *(continued)*

CASE STUDY

The patient presented with signs of anterior shoulder dislocation.

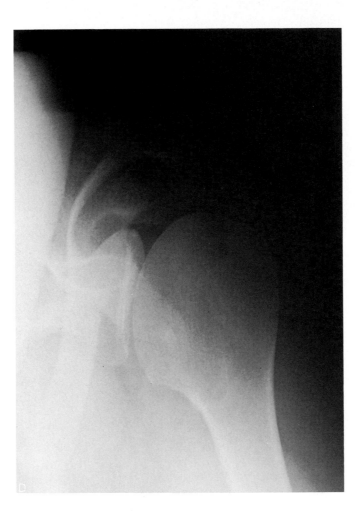

□ **FIGURE 5–8.** *(continued)*

The routine radiographs from this case were unavailable. A "normal" apical oblique shoulder radiograph is included for comparison with the following radiograph.

Garth Apical Oblique Shoulder Position *(continued)*

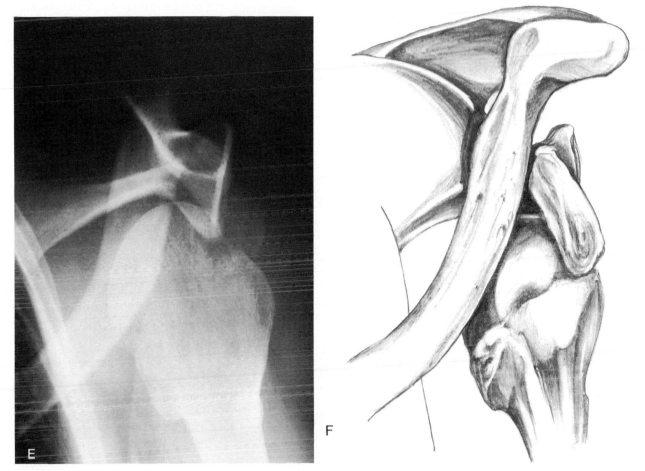

□ **FIGURE 5–8.** *(continued)*

(*E*, Courtesy of Vickie Byers, RT[R].)

The Garth apical oblique shoulder radiograph demonstrates an anterior dislocation of the proximal humerus. The humeral head is seen to lie beneath the coracoid process; this juxtaposition is common with anterior dislocation.

Lawrence* Axillary Shoulder Position

RATIONALE FOR USE

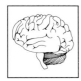

The Lawrence axillary shoulder position is *the most commonly performed axillary shoulder position*. It demonstrates the glenoid, proximal humerus, and glenohumeral joint integrity. The acromioclavicular joint and coracoid process may also be evaluated.

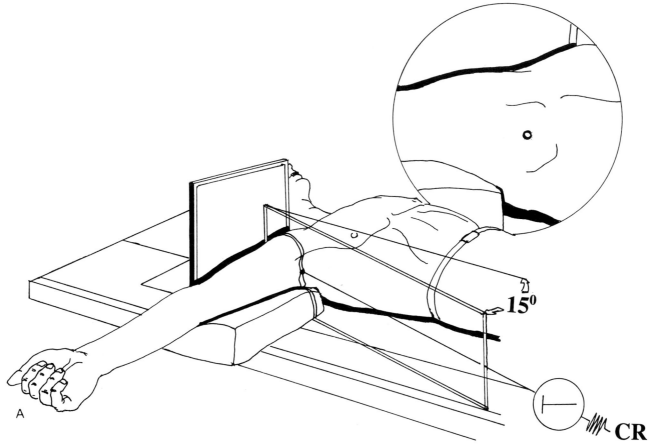

□ **FIGURE 5–9.**

POSITION DESCRIPTION

Part Position: The patient is supine with the affected shoulder slightly elevated and the arm abducted to 90°. The vertically oriented cassette is placed against the superior surface of the shoulder and in contact with the side of the neck. The arm is then adjusted in external rotation with the hand supinated.

Note: This position can be performed with as little as 30° of arm abduction if the tube can be brought close enough to the patient's body.

Central Ray: Horizontal and angled approximately 15° medially, entering the axilla and passing through the acromioclavicular joint.

Lawrence* Axillary Shoulder Position *(continued)*

IMAGE EVALUATION

The shoulder girdle is demonstrated in axial projection. The glenohumeral joint should be well demonstrated. The lesser tuberosity of the humerus should be in profile and oriented ventrally. The area of the acromioclavicular joint will be superimposed on the humerus. If included, the coracoid process will be pointed ventrally.

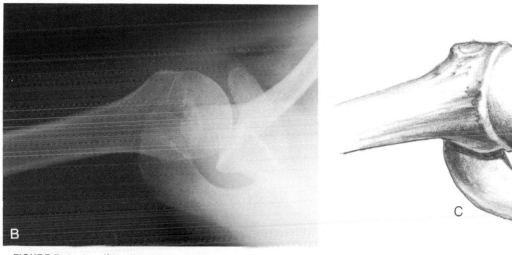

☐ **FIGURE 5-9.** *(continued)*

---

*Lawrence WS. New position in radiographing the shoulder joint. *AJR* 1915; 2:728–730.

Lawrence Axillary Shoulder Position *(continued)*

CASE STUDY

The patient presented with signs of anterior shoulder dislocation.

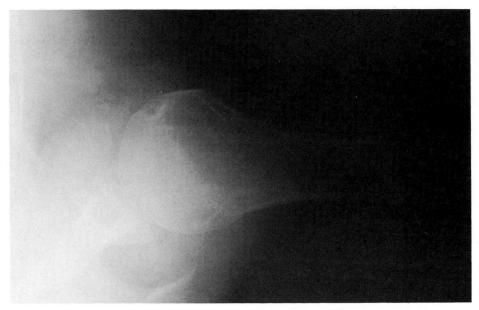

□ **FIGURE 5–9.** *(continued)*

The routine radiographs from this case were unavailable. A "normal" Lawrence axillary shoulder radiograph is included for comparison with the following radiograph.

Lawrence Axillary Shoulder Position *(continued)*

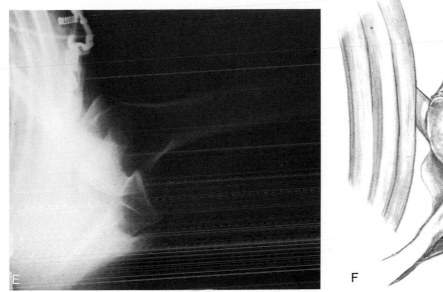

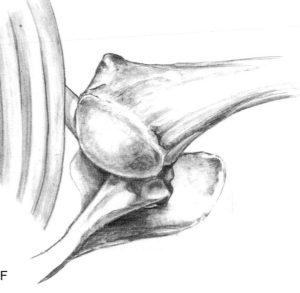

☐ **FIGURE 5–9.** *(continued)*

The Lawrence axillary shoulder radiograph demonstrates an anterior dislocation of the proximal humerus. The humeral head is seen to lie medial to the glenoid fossa and, from this inferior perspective, beneath the coracoid process.

Stryker Notch Shoulder Position*,†

RATIONALE FOR USE

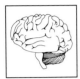

The Stryker Notch shoulder position may be *used in cases of suspected anterior dislocation or subluxation of the shoulder to demonstrate the classic Hill-Sachs compression fracture* on the posterolateral aspect of the humeral head *and/or a Bankart lesion* of the anterior-inferior glenoid rim.

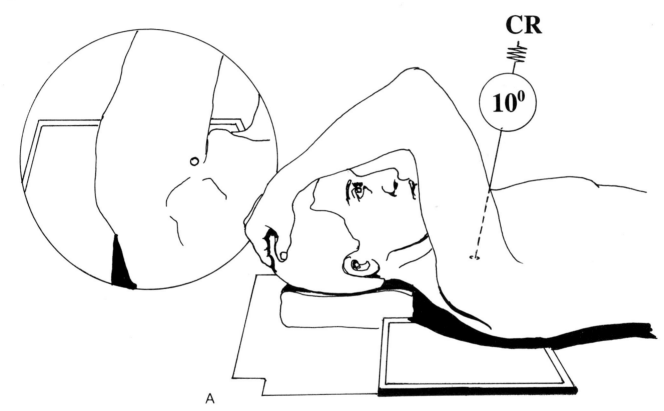

A

□ **FIGURE 5–10.**

POSITION DESCRIPTION

Part Position: The patient is supine with the affected arm raised in forward flexion, the elbow flexed, and the palm resting on top of the head. The cassette is placed beneath the affected shoulder.

Central Ray: Angled 10° cephalad, entering at the coracoid process.

Stryker Notch Shoulder Position*,† *(continued)*

IMAGE EVALUATION

A semi-axial projection of the shoulder girdle should be demonstrated. The gleno-humeral joint will be seen with the humeral shaft directed anteriorly. The postero-lateral aspect of the humerus and the anteroinferior glenoid rim should be well visualized.

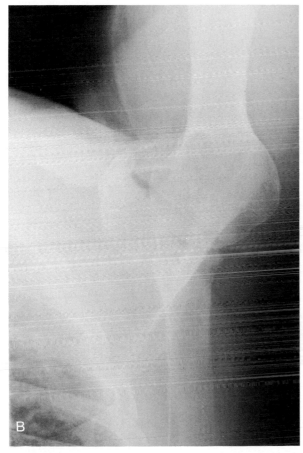

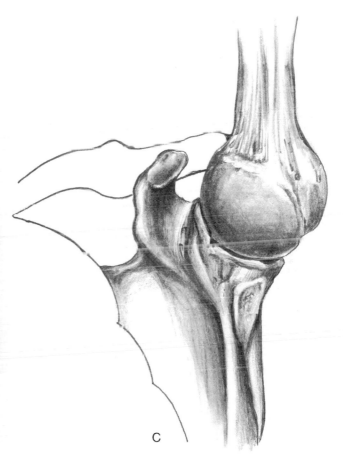

□ **FIGURE 5–10.** *(continued)*

---

*Hall RH, Isaac F, Booth CR. Dislocations of the shoulder with special reference to accompanying small fractures. *J Bone Joint Surg* 1959; 41A(3):489–494.
†In their article, R. H. Hall and associates gave credit for this position to W. S. Stryker. It was originally called the "Notch" view but was later termed the "Stryker Notch" view by CA Rockwood, as stated in Rockwood CA, Szalay EA, Curtis RJ, et al. X-ray evaluation of shoulder problems. *In* Rockwood CA, Matsen FA (eds). *The Shoulder*. Philadelphia: WB Saunders; 1990:178–200.

Superoinferior Axillary Shoulder Position

RATIONALE FOR USE

The superoinferior axillary shoulder position is commonly used as an *alternative to the Lawrence axillary shoulder position* when the patient's condition permits. The position is customarily used *to assess nontraumatic conditions of the shoulder girdle.*

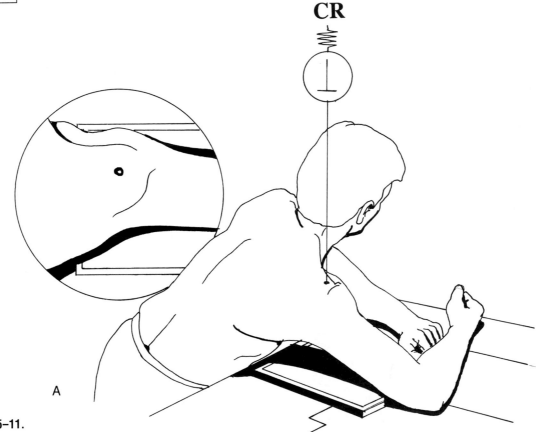

CR

A

□ **FIGURE 5–11.**

POSITION DESCRIPTION

Part Position: The patient is seated with the affected shoulder adjacent to the end of the table. The arm is abducted, and the elbow is flexed 90° and rests on the table. The cassette is placed on the table beneath the arm, and the patient leans laterally over the cassette until the axilla is centered. The arm is abducted as much as the patient's condition allows (up to 90°). The cassette should be as close as possible to the axilla. If possible, the humerus is adjusted in external rotation with the coronal plane of the humeral epicondyles perpendicular to the plane of the cassette. The patient's head and neck are tilted away from the affected side.

Central Ray: Angled 5°–15° toward the elbow, through the glenohumeral joint.

Note: The more the patient is able to lean over the cassette, the less angulation is required.

Superoinferior Axillary Shoulder Position *(continued)*

IMAGE EVALUATION

The shoulder girdle is demonstrated in axial projection. The glenohumeral joint is demonstrated but usually not as well as in the Lawrence position. The lesser tuberosity of the humerus will be in profile and oriented ventrally if the humerus has been placed in external rotation. The area of the acromioclavicular joint will be superimposed on the humerus. The coracoid process, if included, will be pointed ventrally and partially superimposed over the distal clavicle.

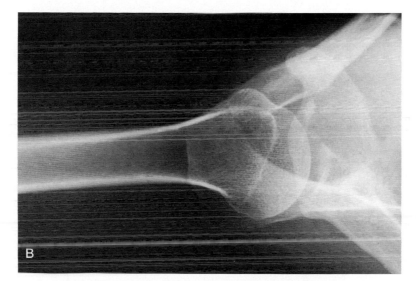

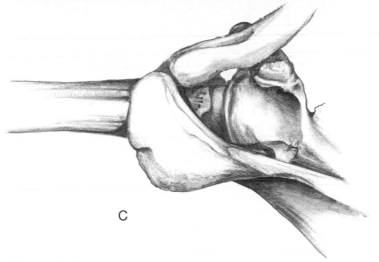

C

□ **FIGURE 5–11.**
(continued)

Supraspinatus Outlet Shoulder Position*

RATIONALE FOR USE

The supraspinatus outlet shoulder position may be used in cases of *suspected* *"impingement syndrome,"* to demonstrate acromial abnormalities such as *a subacromial spur.*

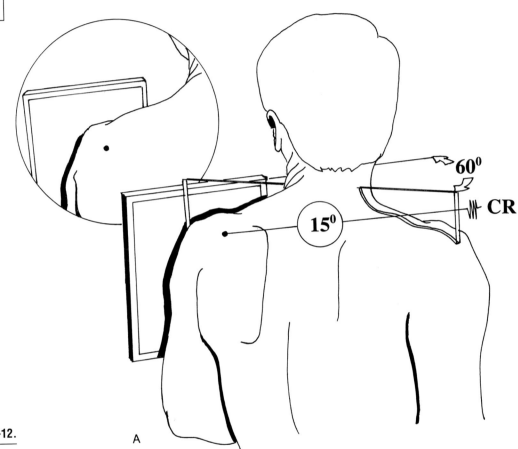

□ **FIGURE 5–12.**

A

POSITION DESCRIPTION

Part Position: The patient is erect, facing the vertical bucky/cassette holder. The body is adjusted in an approximately 60° anterior oblique position with the affected shoulder against and centered to the bucky/cassette holder. Also, the shoulder is adjusted, by forward or backward leaning, in order to place the long axis of the scapular spine perpendicular to the plane of the cassette. The arm should be adducted at the patient's side.

Note: The degree of the patient's obliquity is adjusted to place the plane of the scapula perpendicular to the plane of the cassette. Scapular orientation may be approximated by palpation of the scapular spine.

Central Ray: Angled approximately 10°–15° down from horizontal, entering 1 inch superior to the medial end of the scapular spine.

Supraspinatus Outlet Shoulder Position* *(continued)*

IMAGE EVALUATION

The scapula should be seen in lateral position. In this orientation the scapula appears as a "Y"; the scapular body forms the vertical portion, and the acromion and coracoid processes represent the upper limbs. The glenoid process is seen en face at the junction of the three "Y" limbs. In the normal shoulder, the humeral head will be superimposed on the glenoid process. The acromiohumeral space will appear wider than in the non-angled true lateral radiograph.

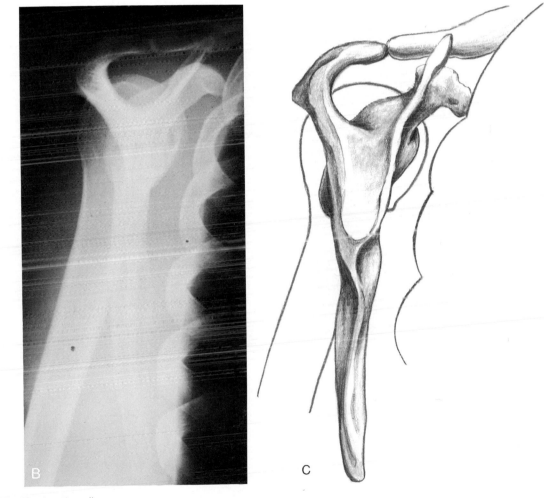

□ **FIGURE 5–12.** *(continued)*

(*B,* courtesy of Paula Shyko, RT[R].)

*Neer CS. Supraspinatus outlet. *Orthop Trans* 1987; 11:234.

Supraspinatus Outlet Shoulder Position *(continued)*

CASE STUDY

The patient presented with pain on shoulder abduction or anterior flexion.

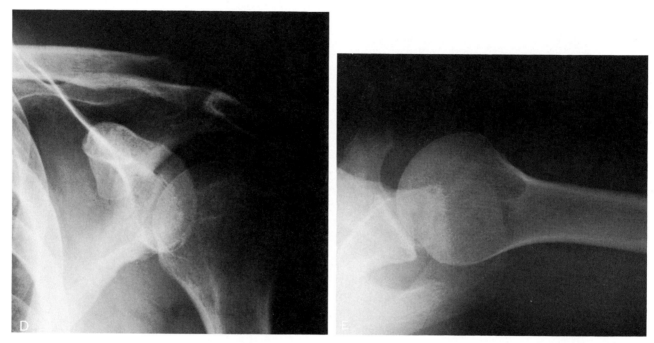

□ **FIGURE 5–12.** *(continued)*

Routine AP internal rotation and axillary shoulder radiographs reveal mild degenerative changes of the acromioclavicular joint, but the extent of inferior spurring could not be assessed.

Supraspinatus Outlet Shoulder Position *(continued)*

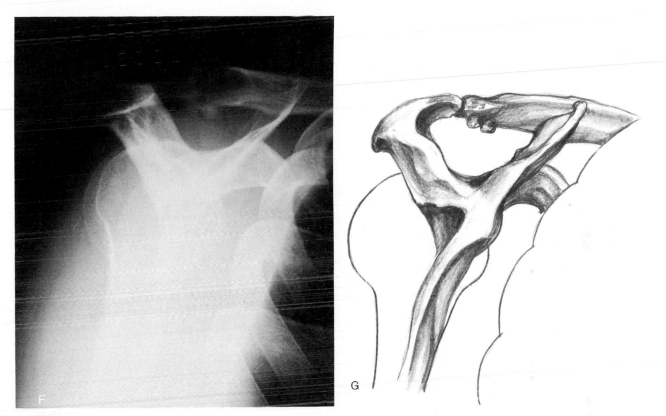

□ **FIGURE 5–12.** *(continued)*

The supraspinatus outlet shoulder radiograph demonstrated spurring of the lateral end of the clavicle, projecting inferiorly into the area of the supraspinatus outlet.

True AP (Grashey*) Shoulder Position

RATIONALE FOR USE

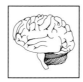

The true AP or Grashey shoulder position places the plane of the scapula parallel to the cassette. The resulting radiograph demonstrates a *"true" AP projection of the shoulder girdle, with the glenoid labrum seen in profile and the glenohumeral joint space open.* The routine AP shoulder position places the shoulder girdle in an oblique orientation to the cassette and obscures the glenohumeral joint space.

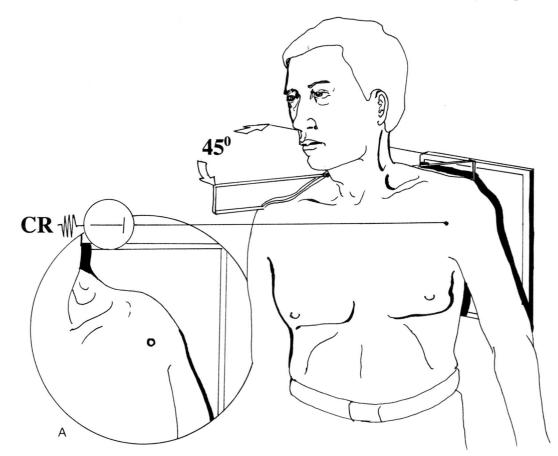

□ **FIGURE 5–13.**

POSITION DESCRIPTION

Part Position: The patient is positioned as for a routine AP shoulder. The body is then obliqued approximately 45° to place the plane of the scapula of the affected shoulder parallel to the plane of the cassette and against the table or upright bucky/cassette holder. The humerus is adjusted in internal rotation by placing the distal forearm on the abdomen.

Note: When the patient is supine, a greater degree of obliquity may be required. Scapular orientation may be approximated by palpation of the scapular spine. This position may also be performed with the humerus in external rotation.

Central Ray: Perpendicular to the cassette, entering slightly medial and inferior to the coracoid process.

True AP (Grashey*) Shoulder Position *(continued)*

IMAGE EVALUATION

A true AP projection of the shoulder girdle should be demonstrated. The glenoid labrum should be seen in profile, and glenohumeral joint space should be open.

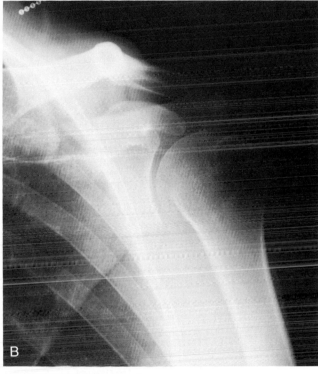

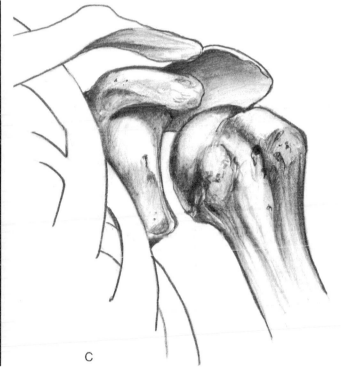

□ **FIGURE 5–13.** *(continued)*

*Grashey R. *Allgemeine aufnahme Technik und Deutung der Rontgenbilder.* Berlin & Wein: Urban & Schwarzenberg; 1926.

True Lateral (Scapular "Y") Shoulder Position*

RATIONALE FOR USE

The true lateral or scapular "Y" shoulder position may be used in cases of suspected shoulder dislocation or other injury. The position results in a *true lateral orientation of the shoulder girdle, allowing assessment of fractures or glenohumeral dislocation.*

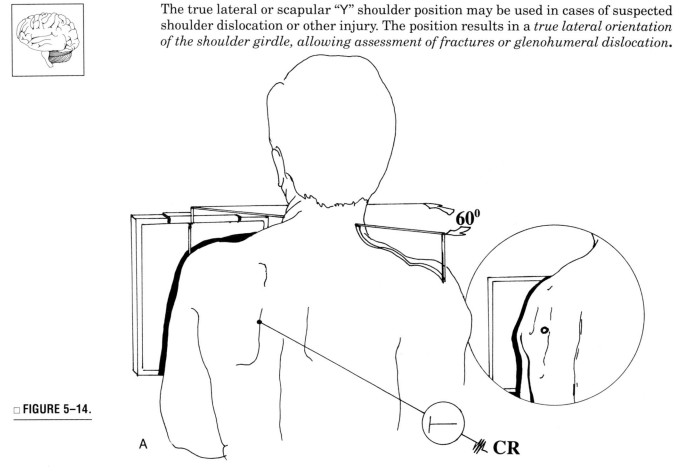

□ **FIGURE 5–14.**

POSITION DESCRIPTION

Part Position: The patient is erect, facing the vertical bucky/cassette holder. The body is adjusted in an approximately 60° anterior oblique position with the affected shoulder against and centered on the bucky/cassette holder. Also, the shoulder is adjusted, by forward or backward leaning, to place the long axis of the scapular spine perpendicular to the plane of the cassette. The arm is adducted along the patient's side.

Note: The degree of the patient's obliquity is adjusted so as to place the plane of the scapula perpendicular to the plane of the cassette. Scapular orientation may be approximated by palpation of the scapular spine.

Alternative position: When trauma necessitates a recumbent position, a 60° posterior oblique position is used. The affected shoulder is elevated, and the central ray is directed vertically to enter just distal to the humeral head.

Central Ray: Horizontal and perpendicular to the cassette, entering 1 inch inferior to the medial end of the scapular spine and passing through the glenohumeral joint.

True Lateral (Scapular "Y") Shoulder Position* *(continued)*

IMAGE EVALUATION

The scapula should be seen in lateral position. In this orientation the scapula appears as a "Y"; the scapular body forms the vertical portion, and the acromion and coracoid processes represent the upper limbs. The glenoid process is seen en face at the junction of the three "Y" limbs. The humeral head will be superimposed on the glenoid process in the normal shoulder, under the coracoid process when anteriorly dislocated, and under the acromion process when posteriorly dislocated.

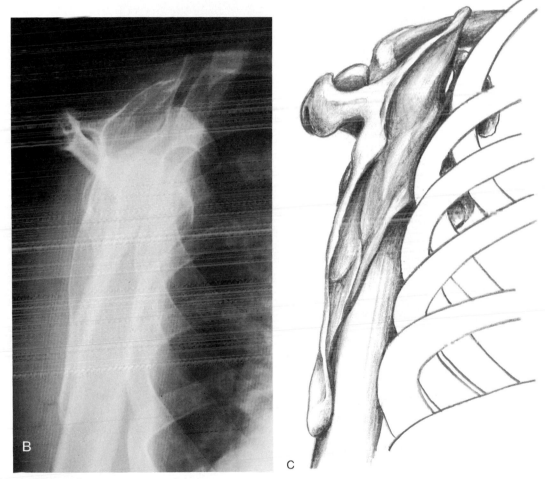

□ **FIGURE 5–14.** *(continued)*

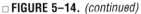

*Rubin SA, Gray RL, Green WR. The scapular "Y": a diagnostic aid in shoulder trauma. *Radiology* 1974; 110:725–726.

True Lateral (Scapular "Y") Shoulder Position *(continued)*

CASE STUDY

The patient presented on a stretcher with a diagnosis of acute shoulder dislocation.

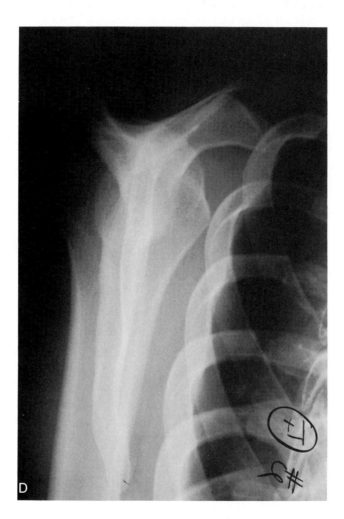

□ **FIGURE 5–14.** *(continued)*

The routine radiographs from this case were unavailable. This "normal" true lateral (scapular "Y") shoulder radiograph is included for comparison with the radiograph on the facing page. This comparison radiograph was taken with the patient in the recumbent, posterior oblique position.

True Lateral (Scapular "Y") Shoulder Position *(continued)*

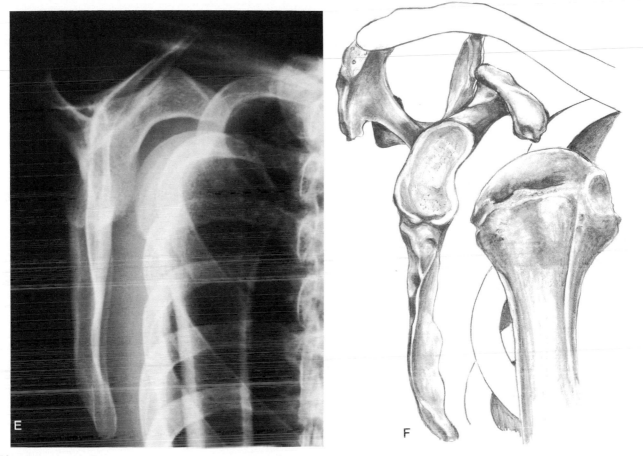

□ **FIGURE 5–14.** *(continued)*

The true lateral (scapular "Y") shoulder radiograph demonstrates anterior dislocation of the proximal humerus. The humeral head is seen to lie beneath the coracoid process. Because of the patient's condition, this radiograph was taken with the patient in the recumbent, posterior oblique position.

Westpoint Axillary Shoulder Position*,†

RATIONALE FOR USE

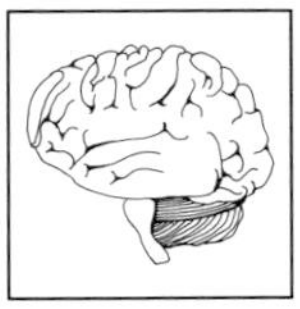

The Westpoint axillary shoulder position may be *used in cases of suspected anterior dislocation or subluxation of the shoulder to demonstrate the classic Hill-Sachs compression fracture* on the posterolateral aspect of the humeral head *and/or a Bankart lesion* of the anteroinferior glenoid rim.

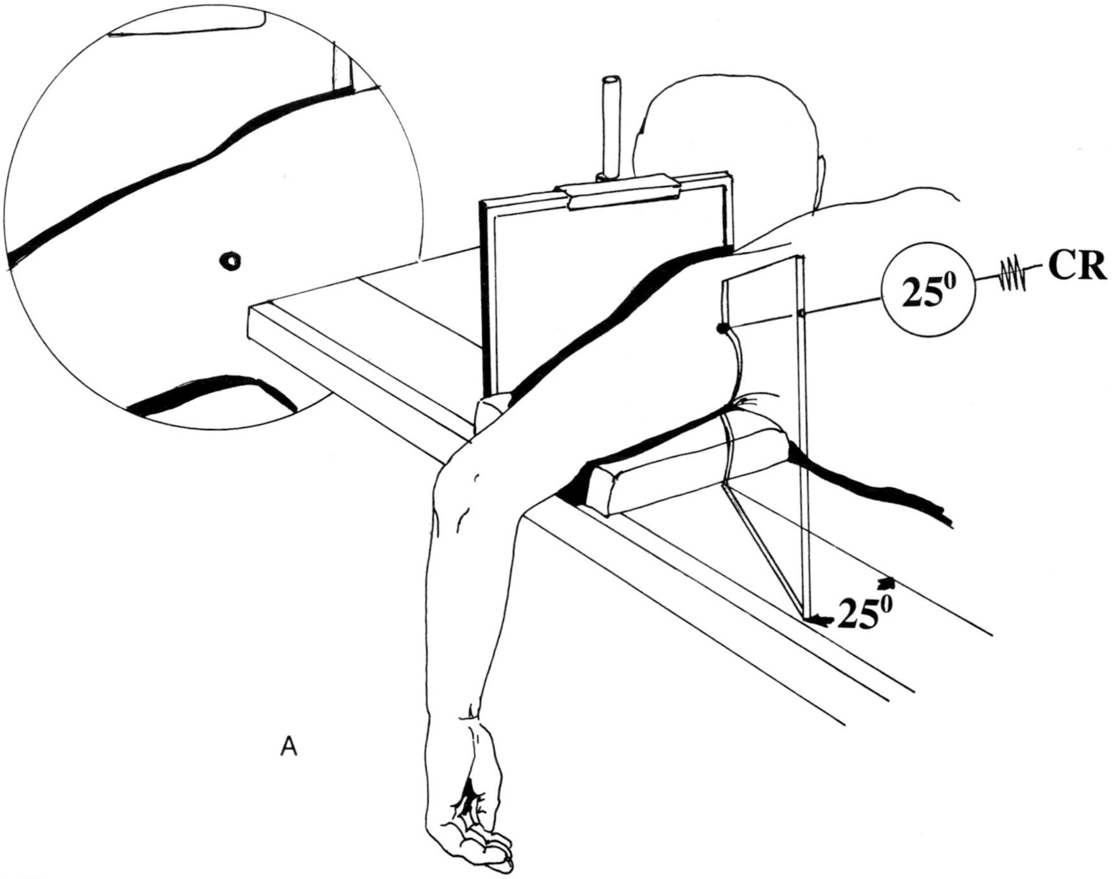

25° ⊪─ **CR**

25°

A

□ **FIGURE 5–15.**

POSITION DESCRIPTION

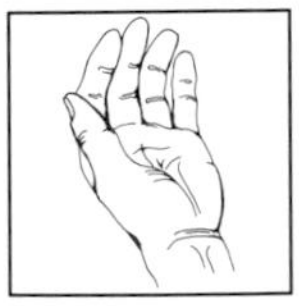

Part Position: The patient is prone on the table with the affected shoulder elevated approximately 3 inches. The arm is abducted 90°, and the elbow is flexed to allow the forearm to hang down over the side of the table. The vertically oriented cassette is placed against the superior surface of the shoulder and in contact with the side of the neck.

Central Ray: Angled 25° down from horizontal and 25° medially, entering the dorsal surface of the shoulder 3 inches above the axilla and passing through the glenohumeral joint.

Westpoint Axillary Shoulder Position*,† *(continued)*

IMAGE EVALUATION

The shoulder girdle is demonstrated in axial projection. The anteroinferior glenoid rim should be well demonstrated with minimal superimposition by the coracoid process or distal clavicle. The lesser tuberosity of the humerus will be in profile and oriented ventrally.

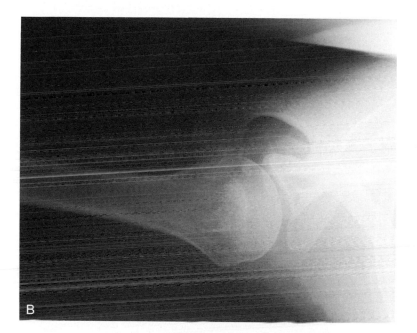

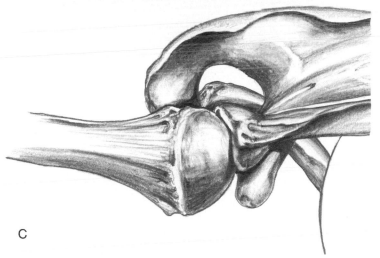

□ **FIGURE 5–15.** *(continued)*

---

*Rokous JR, Feagin JA, Abbott HG. Modified axillary roentgenogram. *Clin Orthop* 1972; 82:84–86.
†C. A. Rockwood stated that he had referred to this position as the "Westpoint view" since 1975, as stated in Rockwood CA, Szalay EA, Curtis RJ, et al. X-ray evaluation of shoulder problems. *In* Rockwood CA, Matsen FA (eds). *The Shoulder*. Philadelphia: WB Saunders; 1990:178–200.

Acromioclavicular and Sternoclavicular Joint Radiography

AP Acromioclavicular Joint Projections (No Weights)

RATIONALE FOR USE

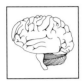

The AP acromioclavicular joint projections are used in cases of suspected dislocation of an acromioclavicular joint. This upright, bilateral radiograph allows evaluation of joint space widening by comparison of the normal with the injured joint. *This non–weight-bearing radiograph allows diagnosis of displaced, complete acromioclavicular joint dislocations (types III to VI).*

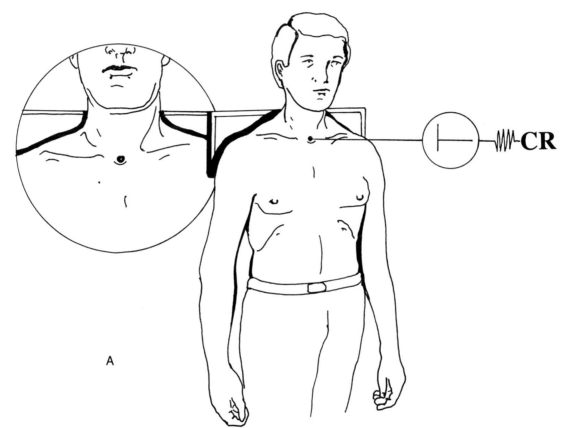

A

□ **FIGURE 5–16.**

POSITION DESCRIPTION

Part Position: The patient is standing or sitting with the back against an upright bucky/cassette holder. A cassette of sufficient width to include both joints is used (7 × 17 inch, 14 × 17 inch, or two 8 × 10 inch cassettes). The upright bucky/cassette holder is adjusted vertically to place the center of the cassette at the level of the acromioclavicular joints. Both arms must hang freely, without support.

Central Ray: Perpendicular to the cassette, directed to the midline and at the level of the acromioclavicular joints.

Note: A 72-inch source-to-image receptor distance (SID) should be used.

AP Acromioclavicular Joint Projections (No Weights) *(continued)*

IMAGE EVALUATION

A bilateral AP projection of the acromioclavicular joints should be demonstrated. Widening of the injured acromioclavicular joint will be demonstrated with complete dislocation.

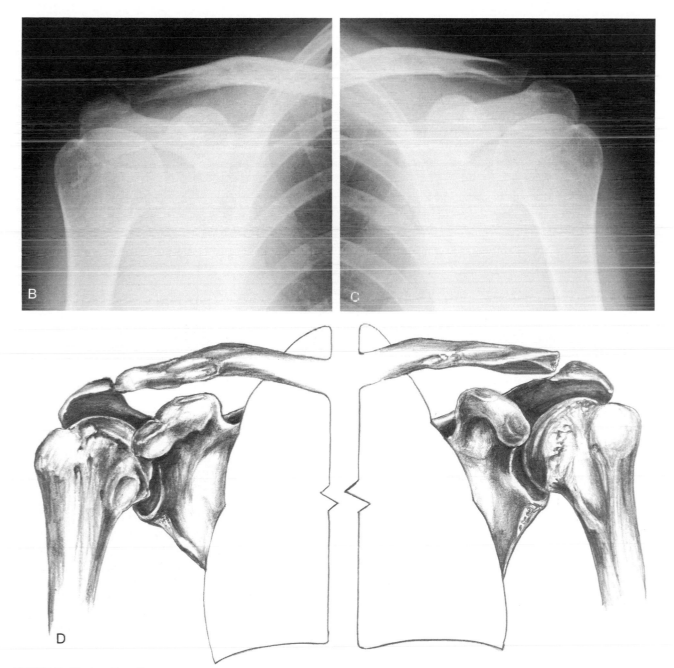

□ **FIGURE 5–16.** *(continued)*

AP Acromioclavicular Joint Projections (With Weights)

RATIONALE FOR USE

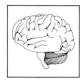

The AP acromioclavicular joint projections are used in cases of suspected dislocation of an acromioclavicular joint. This upright, bilateral radiograph enables evaluation of joint space widening by comparison of the normal with the injured joint. *This weight-bearing radiograph enables diagnosis of minimally displaced or non-displaced complete (type III) acromioclavicular joint dislocations.*

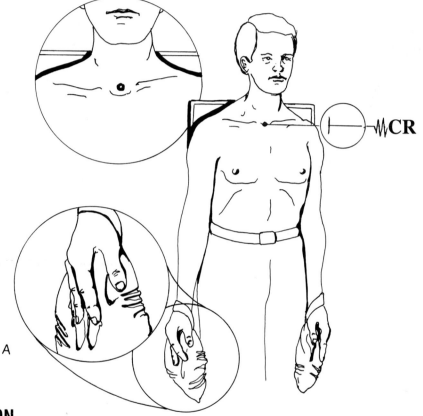

□ **FIGURE 5–17.**   A

POSITION DESCRIPTION

Part Position: The patient is standing or sitting with the back against an upright bucky/cassette holder. A cassette of sufficient width to include both joints is used (7 × 17 inch, 14 × 17 inch, or two 8 × 10 inch cassettes). The upright bucky/cassette holder is adjusted vertically to place the center of the cassette at the level of the acromioclavicular joints. Ten- to fifteen-pound weights are strapped to each wrist. The patient is instructed to relax the shoulders and allow the weights to pull the arms down.

Note: Patients should *not* hold the weights in their hands because they will be inclined to pull up on the weights, thus reducing the acromioclavicular joint space widening.

Central Ray: Perpendicular to the cassette, directed to the midline and at the level of the acromioclavicular joints.

Note: A 72-inch SID should be used.

AP Acromioclavicular Joint Projections (With Weights) *(continued)*

IMAGE EVALUATION

A bilateral AP projection of the acromioclavicular joints should be demonstrated. With complete dislocation, widening of the injured acromioclavicular joint space will be demonstrated.

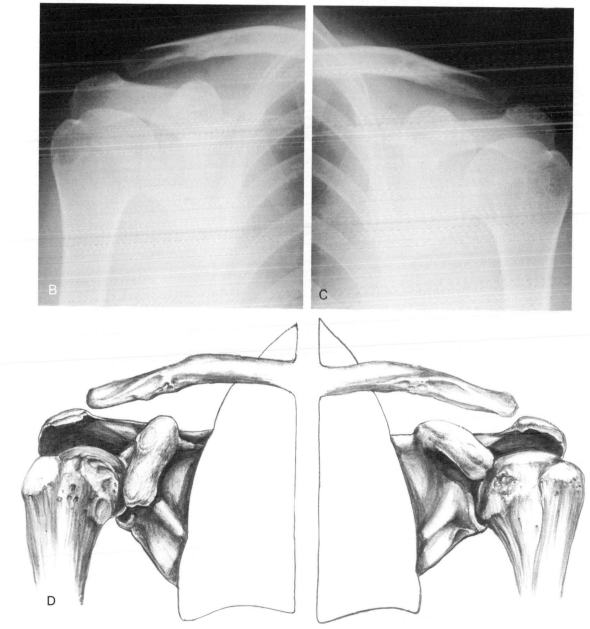

□ **FIGURE 5–17.** *(continued)*

PA Oblique Sternoclavicular Joint Position

RATIONALE FOR USE

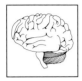

The PA oblique sternoclavicular joint position may be used to evaluate pathology of the sternoclavicular joint. This position *relieves superimposition of the sternoclavicular joint over the spine while minimizing image distortion*. Because this position does not result in axial presentation (as in the Serendipity position), evaluation of anteroposterior dislocation is very difficult. However, image detail is greater than in the Serendipity position, allowing more accurate assessment of fractures, arthritis, or other pathology.

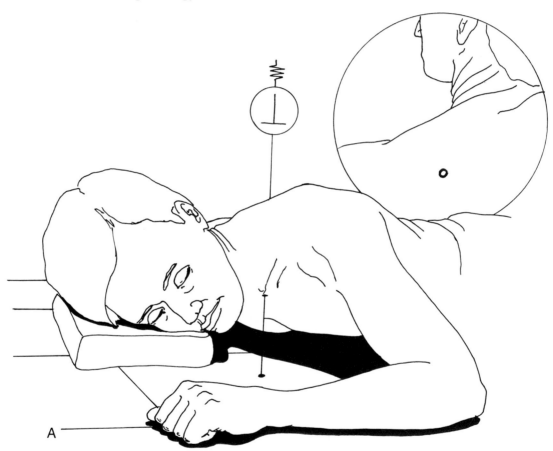

A

☐ **FIGURE 5–18.**

POSITION DESCRIPTION

Part Position: The patient is prone on the table with the head turned toward the side of interest. The arm on the affected side is abducted, and the forearm rests on the table, while the opposite arm is placed along the side. This should place the body in a shallow oblique position (approximately 10°). The affected sternoclavicular joint will be elevated approximately 2 inches from the tabletop.

Central Ray: Perpendicular to the cassette, entering the affected side 3 inches inferior and 2 inches lateral to the C7 spinous process and passing through the sternoclavicular joint of interest.

PA Oblique Sternoclavicular Joint Position *(continued)*

IMAGE EVALUATION

The affected sternoclavicular joint should be demonstrated just lateral to the T2 or T3 vertebra. The medial end of the clavicle should be well seen.

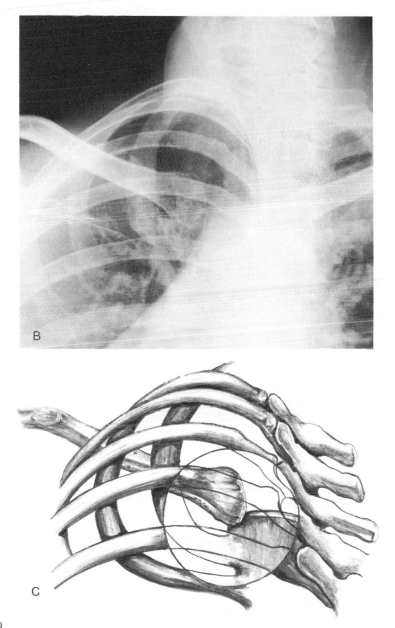

□ **FIGURE 5–18.** *(continued)*

PA Sternoclavicular Joints Projection

RATIONALE FOR USE

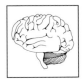

The PA sternoclavicular joints projection may be used to *evaluate pathology of the sternoclavicular joint*. Because this position does not result in axial presentation (as in the Serendipity position), evaluation of anteroposterior dislocation is very difficult. However, image detail is greater than in the Serendipity position, allowing more accurate assessment of fractures, arthritis, or other pathology.

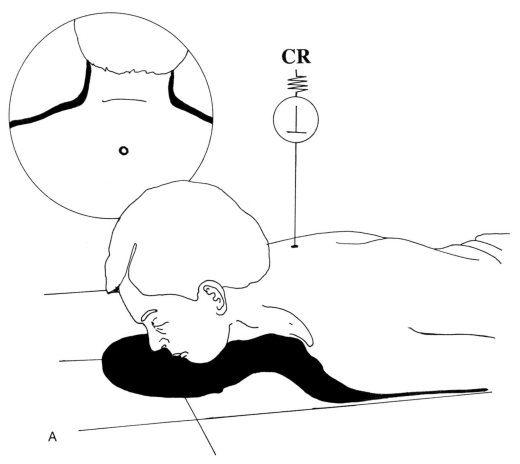

CR

A

□ **FIGURE 5–19.**

POSITION DESCRIPTION

Part Position: The patient is prone, with the chin resting on the table, or upright, facing the bucky/cassette holder. Both arms are placed along the sides. The sternoclavicular joints are centered to the cassette.

Central Ray: Perpendicular to the cassette, entering 3 inches inferior to the C7 spinous process and passing through the manubrium.

PA Sternoclavicular Joints Projection *(continued)*

IMAGE EVALUATION

The medial end of the clavicles and the sternoclavicular joints should be well demonstrated. There should be no body rotation, as evidenced by visualization of both joints. Body rotation will obscure one joint by superimposition over the spine.

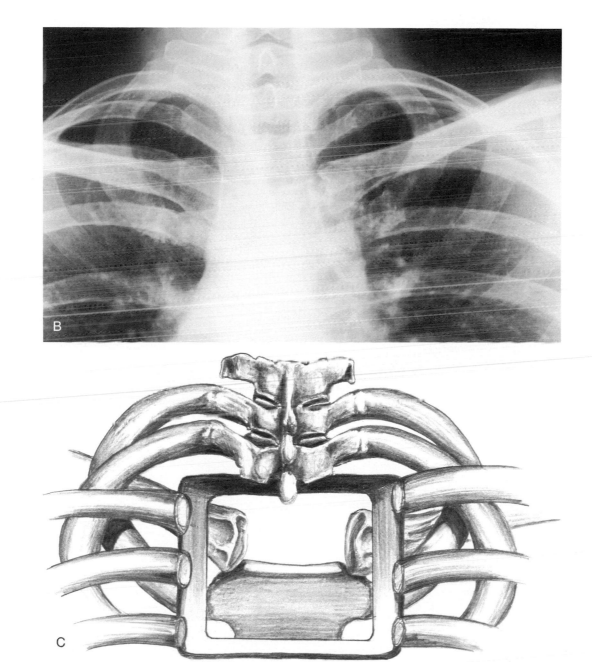

□ **FIGURE 5–19.** *(continued)*

Serendipity Axial Sternoclavicular Joint Projection*

RATIONALE FOR USE

The Serendipity axial sternoclavicular joint projection may be used in cases of suspected dislocation of the sternoclavicular joints. Projection of the medial end of the clavicles above the first ribs allows *assessment of anterior or posterior displacement.*

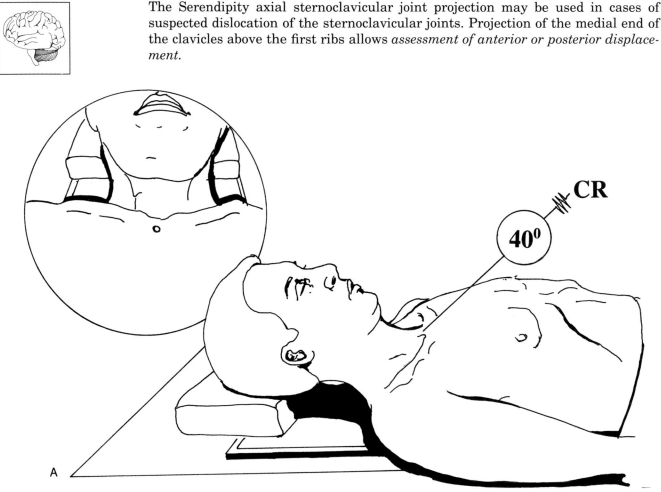

□ **FIGURE 5–20.**

POSITION DESCRIPTION

Part Position: The patient is supine on the table with the cassette under the head and neck.

Central Ray: Angled 40° cephalad, entering at the sternal angle.

Note: SID should be increased to minimize magnification. Rockwood* recommended 60 inches for thicker-chested adults and 45 inches for children and small adults.

Serendipity Axial Sternoclavicular Joint Projection* *(continued)*

IMAGE EVALUATION

An axial projection of the sternoclavicular joints should be demonstrated. The medial end of the clavicles should be projected superior to the first rib but will be superimposed over the cervical spine. The medial end of the clavicle will be superiorly displaced with anterior dislocation and inferiorly displaced with posterior dislocation.

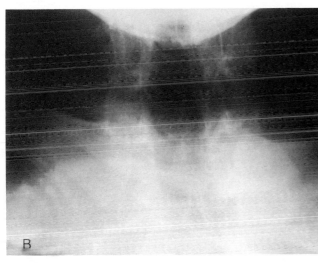

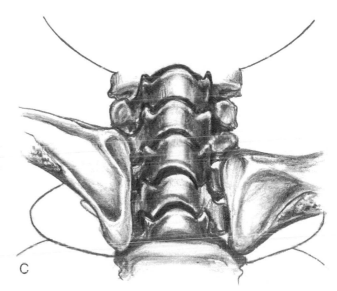

□ **FIGURE 5–20.** *(continued)*

*Rockwood CA. Injuries to the sternoclavicular joint. *In* Rockwood CA, Green DP, Bucholz RW (eds). *Fractures in Adults,* 3rd ed. Philadelphia: JB Lippincott; 1991:1269–1273.

References

1. Rang M. Clavicle. *In Children's Fractures,* 2nd ed. Philadelphia: JB Lippincott; 1983:84–86.
2. Tachdijian MO. *Paediatric Orthopaedics.* Philadelphia: WB Saunders; 1972.
3. Stanley D, Trowbridge EA, Norris SH. The mechanism of clavicular fracture. *J Bone Joint Surg* 1988; 70B:461–464.
4. Rubin A. Birth injuries: incidents, mechanisms, and end results. *Obstet Gynecol* 1964; 23:218–221.
5. Rose SH, Melton LJ, Morrey BF, et al. Epidemiologic features of humeral fractures. *Clin Orthop* 1982; 168:24–30.
6. Neer CS. Displaced proximal humeral fractures. Part I. Classification and evaluation. *J Bone Joint Surg* 1970; 52A:1077–1089.
7. Grashey R. *Allgemeine aufnahme Technik und Deutung der Rontgenbilder.* Berlin & Wein: Urban & Schwarzenberg; 1926.
8. Rubin SA, Gray RL, Green WR. The scapular "Y": a diagnostic aid in shoulder trauma. *Radiology* 1974; 110:725–726.
9. Lawrence WS. New position in radiographing the shoulder joint. *AJR* 1915; 2:728–730.
10. McGahan JP, Rab GT, Dublin A. Fractures of the scapula. *J Trauma* 1980; 20:880–883.
11. Butters KP. The scapula. *In* Rockwood CA, Matsen FA (eds). *The Shoulder.* Philadelphia: WB Saunders; 1990:335–361.
12. Ideberg R. Fractures of the scapula involving the glenoid fossa. *In* Bateman JE, Welsh RP. *Surgery of the Shoulder.* Toronto: BC Decker; 1984:63–66.
13. Bernard TN, Brunet ME, Haddad RJ. Fractured coracoid process in acromioclavicular dislocations. *Clin Orthop* 1983; 175:227–231.
14. Rokous JR, Feagin JA, Abbott HG. Modified axillary roentgenogram. *Clin Orthop* 1972; 82:84–86.
15. Hall RH, Isaac F, Booth CR. Dislocations of the shoulder with special reference to accompanying small fractures. *J Bone Joint Surg* 1959; 41A(3):489–494.
16. Fengler K. Special projections for the coracoid process and clavicle. *AJR* 1948; 59:435–438.
17. Rockwood CA, Thomas SC, Matsen FA. Subluxations and dislocations about the glenohumeral joint. *In* Rockwood CA, Green DP, Bucholz RW (eds). *Fractures in Adults,* 3rd ed. Philadelphia: JB Lippincott; 1991:1021–1179.
18. Cave ER, Burke JF, Boyd RJ. *Trauma Management.* Chicago: Year Book Medical; 1974:409–411.
19. Hill HA, Sachs MD. The grooved defect of the humeral head: a frequently unrecognized complication of dislocations of the shoulder joint. *Radiology* 1940; 35:690–700.
20. Bankart ASB. Recurrent or habitual dislocation of the shoulder joint. *B Med J* 1923; 2:1132–1133.
21. Rafert JA, Long BW, Hernandez EM, Kreipke DL. Axillary shoulder with exaggerated rotation: the Hill-Sachs defect. *Radiol Technol* 1990; 62(1):18–23.
22. Didiee J. Le radiodiagnostic dans la luxation récidivante de l'épaule. *J Radiol Electrologie* 1930; 14(4):209–218.
23. Garth WP, Slappey CE, Ochs CW. Roentgenographic demonstration of instability of the shoulder: the apical oblique projection—a technical note. *J Bone Joint Surg* 1984; 66A(9):1450–1453.
24. Rockwood CA. Injuries to the acromioclavicular joint. *In* Rockwood CA, Green DP, Bucholz RW (eds). *Fractures in Adults,* 3rd ed. Philadelphia: JB Lippincott; 1991.
25. Rockwood CA. Disorders of the sternoclavicular joint. *In* Rockwood CA, Matsen FA (eds). *The Shoulder.* Philadelphia: WB Saunders; 1990:486.
26. Rockwood CA. Injuries to the sternoclavicular joint. *Orthop Trans* 1977; 1:96.
27. Nettles JL, Linscheid R. Sternoclavicular dislocations. *J Trauma* 1968; 8(2):158–164.
28. Omer GE. Osteotomy of the clavicle in surgical reduction of anterior sternoclavicular dislocation. *J Trauma* 1967; 7(4):584–590.
29. Rockwood CA. Injuries to the sternoclavicular joint. *In* Rockwood CA, Green DP, Bucholz RW (eds). *Fractures in Adults,* 3rd ed. Philadelphia: JB Lippincott; 1991:1269–1273.
30. Rowe CR (ed). *The Shoulder.* New York: Churchill Livingstone; 1988.
31. Neer CS. Anterior acromioplasty for the chronic impingement syndrome in the shoulder. *J Bone Joint Surg* 1972; 54A:41–50.
32. Kilcoyne RF, Reddy PK, Lyons F, Rockwood CA. Optimal plain film imaging of the shoulder impingement syndrome. *AJR* 1989; 153:795–797.
33. Neer CS, Poppen NK. Supraspinatus outlet. *Orthop Trans* 1987; 11:234.
34. Mills JA. Arthritis of the shoulder. *In* Rowe CR (ed). *The Shoulder.* New York: Churchill Livingstone; 1988:471.

SIX

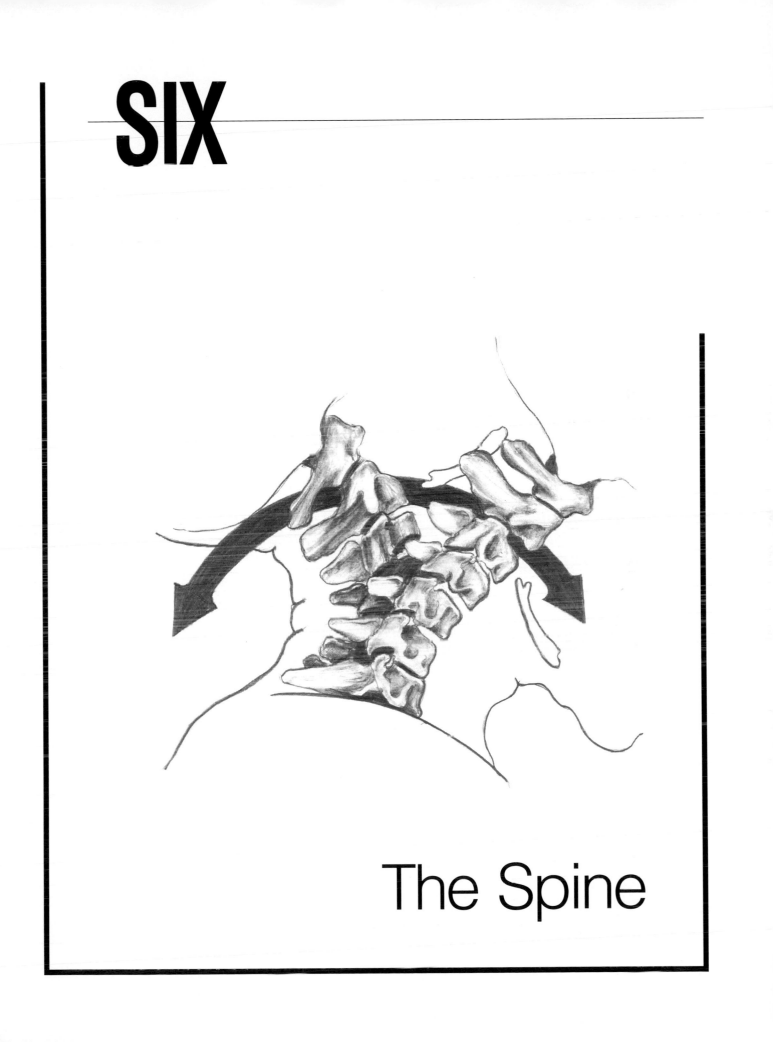

The Spine

THE SPINE: AN OVERVIEW

ROUTINE SPINE RADIOGRAPHY

Cervical Spine
Routine AP Cervical Spine Projection
Routine AP Open-Mouth Cervical Spine Projection
Routine AP Oblique Cervical Spine Position
Routine PA Oblique Cervical Spine Position
Routine Lateral Cervical Spine Position
Thoracic Spine
Routine AP Thoracic Spine Projection
Routine Lateral Thoracic Spine Position
Lumbar Spine
Routine AP Lumbar Spine Projection
Routine AP Oblique Lumbar Spine Position
Routine Lateral Lumbar Spine Position
Routine Lateral Lumbosacral Joint (L5 to S1) Position
Sacrum
Routine AP Sacrum Projection
Routine Lateral Sacrum Position
Coccyx
Routine AP Coccyx Projection
Routine Lateral Coccyx Position

SPECIALIZED CERVICAL SPINE RADIOGRAPHY

AP Axial Oblique (Pillars) Cervical Spine Position
Exaggerated Supine Oblique Cervical Spine Position
Extension Lateral Cervical Spine Position
Flexion Lateral Cervical Spine Position
Fuchs Odontoid Process Position
Lateral Cervicothoracic (Swimmer's) Position
Trauma Oblique Cervical Spine Position

SPECIALIZED LUMBAR SPINE RADIOGRAPHY

AP Axial (Ferguson) Lumbosacral Projection
AP Axial Oblique Lumbar Spine Position
Extension Lateral Lumbar Spine Position
Flexion Lateral Lumbar Spine Position
Lateral-Bending AP Lumbar Spine Projections
Vertebral Arch Lumbar Spine Position

RADIOGRAPHY OF ABNORMAL SPINAL CURVATURE

AP Scoliosis Projection
Lateral-Bending AP/PA Scoliosis Projections
Lateral Kyphosis-Lordosis Position
PA Scoliosis Projection

SACROILIAC JOINT RADIOGRAPHY

AP Axial Sacroiliac Joints Projection
AP Oblique Sacroiliac Joint Position
AP Sacroiliac Joints Projection

The Spine: An Overview

The spine provides support and mobility for the axial portion of the human body, as well as a protective pathway for the spinal cord and nerves. Conditions that affect the integrity, mobility, or interrelationships of the spinal segments often adversely affect the quality of the patient's life. The spine may be affected by trauma, degenerative and inflammatory conditions, metabolic disorders, congenital and developmental anomalies, a variety of infections, and benign and malignant tumors. Diagnostic imaging has an important role in the diagnosis of these spinal conditions, and radiography is very often the initial imaging modality utilized.

The spine is susceptible to a variety of fractures, dislocations, and fracture-dislocations. These injuries are usually the result of a combination of indirect forces, including flexion, extension, compression, distraction, rotation, and shearing. Although these forces often act in combination, the predominant force results in a characteristic radiographic appearance to the injured spinal component.[1] Flexion is characterized by anterior wedging of the vertebral body, whereas extension may result in small avulsion fractures of the anteroinferior or anterosuperior margin of the vertebral body. Severe compression forces result in burst fractures of the vertebral body, often with displacement of fragments. Distraction (pulling apart) may result in horizontally oriented fractures through the neural arch and posterior aspect of the vertebral body. Translation or dislocation injuries result in segmental malalignment, caused by subluxation, dislocation, or fracture-dislocation.

The incidence of vertebral column fracture is low: this type of fracture involves only 3% to 6% of all skeletal injuries.[2] Most of these injuries occur in young and middle-aged adults; only a small percentage involves children. The frequency of injury to spinal segments is not uniform, and three peaks of incidence have been identified at C1 to C2, C5 to C7, and T12 to L2.[3] The upper cervical spine injuries are more common in very young children,[4] although the overall incidence of cervical spine trauma is low in this population. Injuries to the lower cervical spine and thoracolumbar area are found most often in adolescents and adults.[5] The highest percentage (40%) of spinal cord injury is associated with trauma to the lower cervical spine.[6] Fracture of the thoracolumbar area, although common, has a low rate (4%) of association with spinal cord trauma.[3]

Radiographic examination of spinal injuries is used to assess the presence and relative stability of a fracture or dislocation. This is most often accomplished with routine anteroposterior (AP) and lateral radiographs. Additional oblique, axial, and motion-study radiographs are utilized when further information is required to clarify the initial findings. Bone involvement is often evident directly on the radiograph. However, injury to the equally important soft-tissue structures of the spinal column is more difficult to assess because these structures are radiolucent. Variations in distance or alignment between vertebral elements may be the only radiographic indicators of destabilizing soft-tissue injury. In 10% of patients with spinal cord injury from trauma, there is no radiographic evidence of fracture or dislocation.[7] Radiographers should continue to minimize movement of patients with suspected spinal injuries, even after the initial cross-table lateral and AP radiographs have demonstrated no abnormalities. Rogers[8] believed that the 5% to 10% of spinal cord injuries occurring in the immediate postoperative period are quite likely caused by mishandling of the patient.

A variety of fractures and dislocations may occur in the cervical spine. A large number of these injuries are the result of the accelerating head and body striking a stationary object.[9] These are usually classified into upper and lower cervical injuries. The upper cervical elements, the atlas (C1) and axis (C2), are best evaluated with AP open-mouth and lateral radiographs. The most common fractures of the atlas are hyperextension fractures of the anterior or posterior arch and **Jefferson's fracture**,[10] a burst (compression) fracture involving both anterior and posterior arches. Both in adults and in children, the odontoid process is most frequently involved in fractures of the axis, and such a fracture may be associated with atlanto-axial dislocation.[11, 12] This fracture is most often transverse and found at the base of the odontoid process. The other common fracture of the adult axis is the **hangman's fracture** or traumatic spondylolisthesis of C2, consisting of a bilateral avulsion fracture through the pedicles, with or without anterior subluxation of C2 on C3.[13] The usual mechanism of injury is impact of the forehead or face against the windshield during sudden deceleration, forcing neck hyperextension.[14]

As with lesions in the upper cervical spine, the extent and location of a lower cervical lesion is related to the mechanism of injury. A comminuted burst fracture of a lower cervical vertebral body results from the same axial compression mechanism that causes the Jefferson fracture of C1. Vertebral body wedge fractures may result from hyperflexion. The most serious hyperflexion injury to the lower cervical spine is the **teardrop fracture**. The injury consists of a fracture-dislocation with a characteristic "teardrop" fragment of the anteroinferior vertebral body.[15] This fracture is frequently associated with spinal cord injury, especially when posterior dislocation is present. A **clay-shoveler's fracture** can also occur with hyperflexion; it is an avulsion fracture of a spinous process, most often at C7. Serious hyperextension fracture-dislocations also occur and may appear radiographically similar to the hyperflexion injuries. Subluxation may be anterior or posterior, and fracture fragments may be seen at the anterosuperior or anteroinferior aspect of the vertebral body. These hyperflexion and hyperextension forces can also result in ligamentous tears and disruptions without radiographic evidence of fracture. The radiographic appearance may range from loss of normal lordosis to locked (overriding) facets with anterior subluxation.

Fractures of the upper and middle thoracic spine are infrequent in comparison with the incidence of cervical and thoracolumbar injury. Two thirds of thoracolumbar fractures occur at T12, L1, and L2.[16] However, there is a higher incidence of spinal cord injury with thoracic spine fractures. Most fractures of the thoracolumbar spine are caused by compression-flexion forces, resulting in a wedge fracture of the vertebral body.[17] Extreme force may, in addition, result in fracture of the posterior elements, which is termed a **flexion-distraction injury**.

Pure axial compression results in a comminuted burst fracture of the vertebral body. If a fragment is displaced posteriorly into the spinal canal, spinal cord or nerve injury results in approximately two thirds of the cases.[8] Fifty percent of burst fractures occur at L1.[18] Fracture-dislocations result from a combination of flexion, axial compression, rotation, and shear forces.[19] These injuries commonly consist of anterior displacement above the level of injury, coupled with anterior wedging and an anterosuperior shear fragment of the vertebral body below,[20] and they most commonly occur in the upper thoracic spine (T4 to T5 or T5 to T6)[21] or at the thoracolumbar junction.[22] There is a high incidence of spinal cord injury in association with thoracolumbar fracture-dislocations.

Distraction injuries of the thoracolumbar region are most commonly the result of a head-on auto collision while a lap seat belt is worn. The **chance fracture**[23] is a distraction injury involving transverse fracture through the posterior elements; this fracture may extend into the posterosuperior or posteroinferior portion of the vertebral body. If the transverse fracture of the posterior elements is associated with a transverse fracture of the vertebral body, it is termed a **fulcrum fracture**.[24] Distraction injury can result in disruption of the posterior spinous ligaments, articular facets, and intervertebral discs, without fracture. Intra-abdominal trauma is frequently associated with this type of injury, especially in children.[25]

Fracture of the posterior elements of the lumbar spine may be acute or chronic in nature. Fracture of the transverse processes is common and results from traction by the quadratus lumborum muscles or a direct blow.[8] The fracture line is usually vertical or oblique. Acute fractures of the pars interarticularis occasionally occur and may be caused by hyperextension.[26] However, most defects seen in the pars interarticularis are the manifestations of **spondylolysis**. This defect is differentiated from an acute fracture by the presence of sclerotic margins. Spondylolysis was previously thought to be congenital, but now there is almost unanimous agreement that the pars defects are chronic stress fractures. Bilateral pars defects may separate and allow subluxation (usually anterior) of the vertebral body; this disorder is termed **spondylolisthesis**. Such subluxation is more commonly associated with severe degenerative disease of the facet joints.[27] Spondylolisthesis occurs most often at L4 to L5 and L5 to S1. The pars defect may be demonstrated on lateral or oblique radiographs.

Sacral fractures are often associated with trauma to the pelvis, and so discussion of these injuries is included in the Pelvis and Hip Joint chapter.

A number of arthritic conditions manifest in the axial skeleton. Their radiographic appearance and patterns of involvement often help in differentiation of the particular disease. AP and lateral spine radiographs are usually sufficient; oblique, axial, and flexion-extension radiographs are reserved for specific cases. Ankylosing spondylitis is usually a bilateral symmetrical disease beginning in the sacroiliac joints and thoracolumbar spine.[28] It is characterized by inflammatory changes in the sacroiliac joints and calcification of the anterior longitudinal ligaments of the spine. The posterior interspinous and capsular ligaments may also become calcified. As the disease progresses, the involvement ascends to include the entire thoracolumbar and cervical spine, although the thoracolumbar spine may be spared in women.[29] In ankylosing spondylitis, the anterior longitudinal ligament calcifications (syndesmophytes) are thin. This feature allows differentiation between the thick and bulky anterior calcifications of diffuse idiopathic skeletal hyperostosis (DISH), which is a benign disease resulting in anterior and lateral bony bridging between vertebral bodies.

Radiographic changes in the spine and sacroiliac joints are similar in psoriatic arthritis and Reiter's syndrome. These changes include unilateral or bilateral inflammatory sacroiliitis and spondylitis with thick, vertical unilateral syndesmophytes. These two conditions differ in pattern, in that Reiter's syndrome often results in asymmetrical sacroiliitis and less frequent vertebral involvement.[30, 31]

Rheumatoid arthritis is a highly inflammatory disease that frequently involves the upper cervical spine (occipito-atlanto-axial complex).[32] It may be found in the sacroiliac joints but is uncommon in the remainder of the spine. Anterior atlanto-axial subluxation is the most common radiographic finding of rheumatoid arthritic involvement in the cervical spine. It is usually caused by laxity or disruption of the transverse ligament.[33] Cranial settling, with the odontoid process projecting into the foramen magnum, may also occur. The apophyseal joints of the lower cervical vertebra may be involved, and osteopenia increases the risk of vertebral fracture. Subluxation and instability of the cervical spine in association with rheumatoid arthritis may necessitate evaluation with flexion-extension lateral radiographs because the abnormality may not be evident in the neutral lateral position.

Primary osteoarthritis most often results in degenerative changes in the midcervical, midthoracic, and L3-to-L4 areas.[34] Radiograph features include intervertebral disc space narrowing, spur formation at the vertebral body margins, apophyseal joint space narrowing, and bony sclerosis in the area of degeneration.[35]

Crystal deposition disorders may manifest in the spine. Gout, although rarely found in the spine, may involve the cervical spine and sacroiliac joints.[36] Calcium pyrophosphate dihydrate deposition disease (CPPD), or pseudogout, most commonly affects the cervical spine, with intervertebral disc calcification and degeneration.[37]

Radiography is commonly used to evaluate abnormal spinal curvature, including scoliosis and kyphosis. Scoliosis, or lateral curvature of the spine, has many potential causes. Adolescent idiopathic (unknown cause) scoliosis is the most prevalent and is present in 80% of patients seeking treatment for the condition.[38] Right thoracic curves predominate.[39] Other causes of scoliosis include congenital malformation, neuromuscular disorders, tumors, and trauma. The AP/posteroanterior (PA) scoliosis radiograph is helpful in curve measurement for initial evaluation, treatment planning, and follow-up examination. The PA projection is recommended for reducing the radiation dose to the breast and thyroid.[40] Lateral-bending AP/PA scoliosis radiographs are used to demonstrate the degree of curve flexibility.[38] The lateral scoliosis position is used to evaluate degree of kyphosis, to demonstrate presence of a spondylolisthesis, and for postoperative examination.

The spine is affected by a significant number of other conditions and diseases. These include malignant and benign tumors, infections, congenital anomalies, and metabolic or endocrine disorders. Although many of these conditions have radiographic manifestations, they cannot, for the sake of brevity, be discussed here.

Routine Spine Radiography

Routine AP Cervical Spine Projection

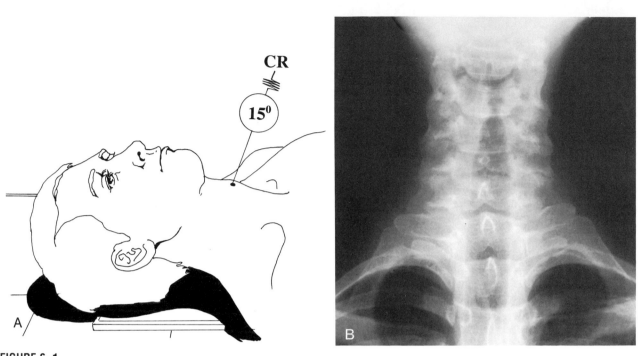

□ **FIGURE 6–1.**

POSITION DESCRIPTION

Part Position: The patient is supine or upright, facing the tube. The neck is extended sufficiently to form an imaginary line, between the lower border of the upper teeth and the mastoid tip, that is perpendicular to the plane of the cassette. The midsagittal plane of the head and neck should be vertical (no rotation).

Central Ray: Angled 15°–20° cephalad, entering the midline at the superior border of the thyroid cartilage (Adam's apple).

IMAGE EVALUATION

An AP projection of the lower five cervical and several upper thoracic vertebrae should be demonstrated without rotation, as evidenced by central location of the spinous processes. The intervertebral and interpedicular joint spaces are usually open. The atlas and axis are obscured by the mandible and occiput.

Routine AP Open-Mouth Cervical Spine Position

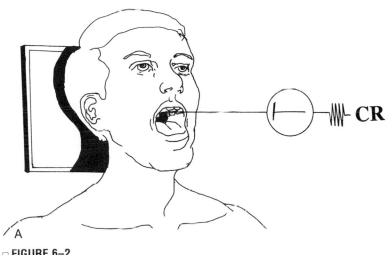

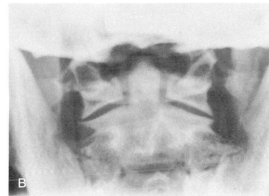

□ **FIGURE 6–2.**

POSITION DESCRIPTION

Part Position: The patient is supine or upright, facing the tube. The mouth is open, and the chin is elevated to form an imaginary line, between the lower border of the upper incisors and the mastoid tip, that is perpendicular to the cassette. The midsagittal plane of the head and neck should be vertical (no rotation).

Central Ray: Perpendicular to the cassette, passing through the center of the open mouth.

IMAGE EVALUATION

An AP projection of the atlas and axis, seen within the open mouth, should be demonstrated. The odontoid process and atlanto-axial joint should be well visualized. The lower border of the upper incisors and the cranial base should be superimposed. The head should not be rotated, as evidenced by the atlas and axis located equidistant from the mandibular rami.

Routine AP Oblique Cervical Spine Position

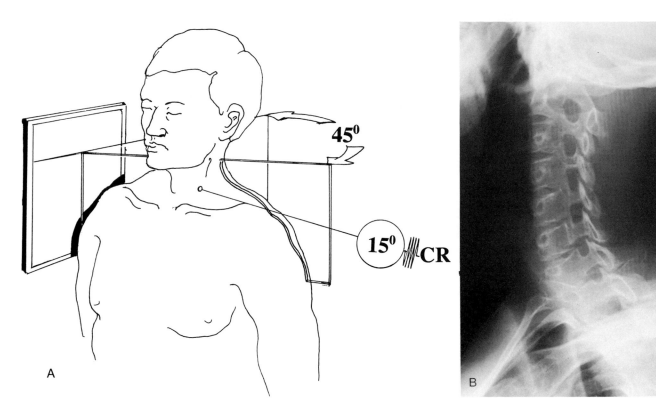

□ **FIGURE 6–3.**

POSITION DESCRIPTION

Part Position: The patient is supine or upright, facing the tube. The body and head are rotated 45°. The chin is extended sufficiently to prevent superimposition of the mandibular rami on the vertebrae.

Note: Alternatively, the head may be further rotated to the lateral position.

Central Ray: Angled 15° cephalad, entering the middle of the neck at the level of the superior border of the thyroid cartilage (Adam's apple).

Note: Alternatively, the central ray may be directed perpendicular to the cassette.

IMAGE EVALUATION

The cervical intervertebral foramina and pedicles farthest from the cassette should be well demonstrated. The entire cervical spine should be visualized, and the intervertebral joint spaces should be open.

Routine PA Oblique Cervical Spine Position

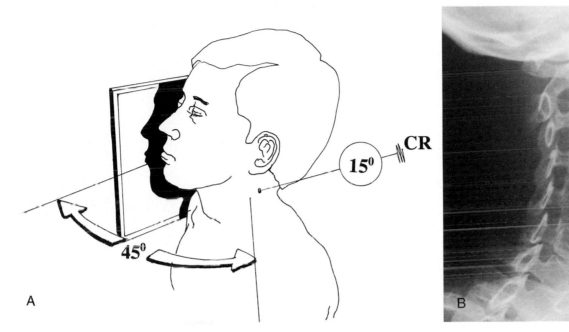

□ **FIGURE 6–4.**

POSITION DESCRIPTION

Part Position: The patient is prone or upright, facing the bucky/cassette holder. The body and head are rotated 45°. The chin is extended sufficiently to prevent superimposition of the mandibular rami on the vertebrae.

Note: Alternatively, the head may be further rotated to the lateral position.

Central Ray: Angled 15° caudad, entering the middle of the neck at the level of the superior border of the thyroid cartilage (Adam's apple).

Note: Alternatively, the central ray may be directed perpendicular to the cassette.

IMAGE EVALUATION

The cervical intervertebral foramina and pedicles closest to the cassette should be well demonstrated. The entire cervical spine should be visualized, and the intervertebral joint spaces should be open.

Routine Lateral Cervical Spine Position

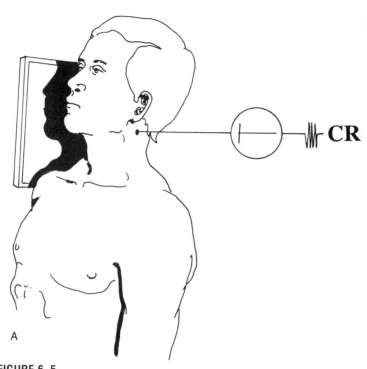

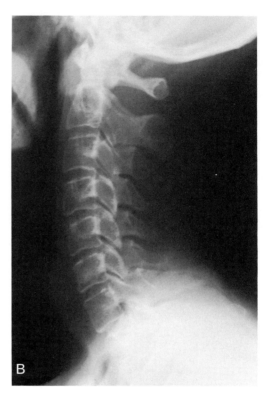

□ **FIGURE 6–5.**

POSITION DESCRIPTION

Part Position: The patient is sitting or standing, with the midcoronal plane of the head and body perpendicular to the cassette and the adjacent shoulder against the bucky/cassette. The neck is extended sufficiently to prevent superimposition of the mandibular rami on the upper cervical vertebrae. The shoulders should be depressed as much as possible.

Note: When severe trauma is suspected, this position should be assumed cross-table with the patient supine. The neck should be moved *only* by the attending physician.

Central Ray: Perpendicular to the cassette (horizontal), entering the side of the neck at the level of the thyroid cartilage.

Note: A 72-inch source-to-image receptor distance (SID) is required.

IMAGE EVALUATION

The vertebral bodies and posterior elements of the entire cervical spine should be demonstrated in lateral position without rotation or tilt, as evidenced by superimposition of the mandibular rami. The intervertebral and apophyseal joints should be well visualized. If C7 is not demonstrated after use of maximal arm traction, a swimmer's lateral position should be imaged.

Routine AP Thoracic Spine Projection

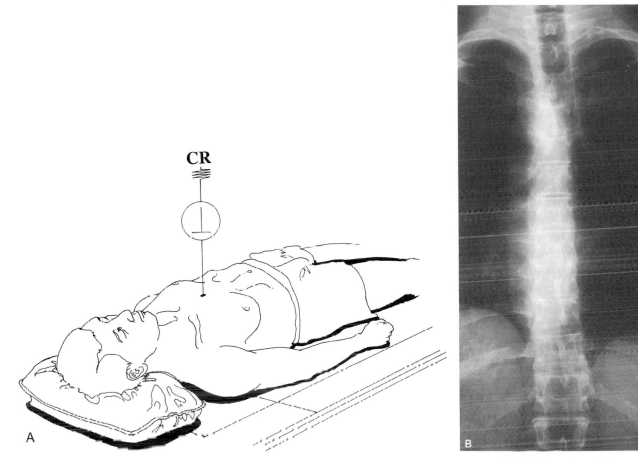

□ **FIGURE 6–6.**

POSITION DESCRIPTION

Part Position: The patient is supine, without body rotation. The patient's head should be oriented toward the anode end of the tube to take advantage of the "heel effect."

Central Ray: Perpendicular to the cassette, entering the midline approximately 3 inches inferior to the sternal notch or slightly inferior to the sternal angle.

IMAGE EVALUATION

The entire thoracic spine should be demonstrated in AP projection without rotation, as evidenced by the spinous processes visible in the center of the vertebral bodies.

Routine Lateral Thoracic Spine

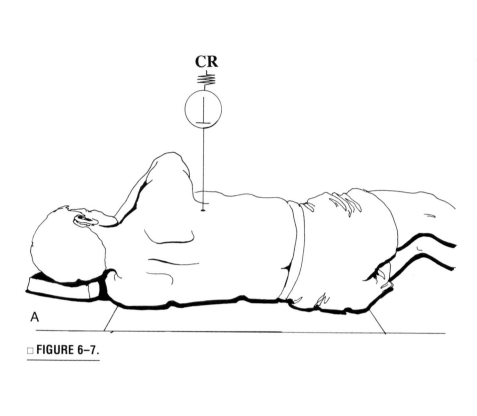

□ **FIGURE 6–7.**

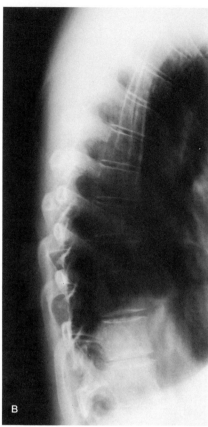

POSITION DESCRIPTION

Part Position: The patient is in the left lateral recumbent position, without forward or backward rotation. The head and waist should be elevated so that the entire spine is in the same plane. The arms should be extended in front of the body.

Note: A long exposure (3 seconds or longer) should be made during shallow breathing, to obscure pulmonary vasculature. The patient's head should be oriented toward the cathode end of the tube to take advantage of the "anode heel affect."

Central Ray: Perpendicular to the cassette, entering the midaxillary line at T7 (7 to 8 inches inferior to the C7 spinous process).

Note: If the entire thoracic spine is not in the same plane, the central ray should be angled perpendicular (cephalad) to the long axis of the spine.

IMAGE EVALUATION

The thoracic spine should be demonstrated in lateral position without rotation, as evidenced by superimposition of the posterior ribs. The intervertebral foramina and intervertebral disc spaces should be open. The upper two or three thoracic vertebrae are usually obscured by the shoulders. Use of the anode heel affect helps, but a swimmer's lateral position is often necessary to visualize these upper vertebrae.

Routine AP Lumbar Spine Projection

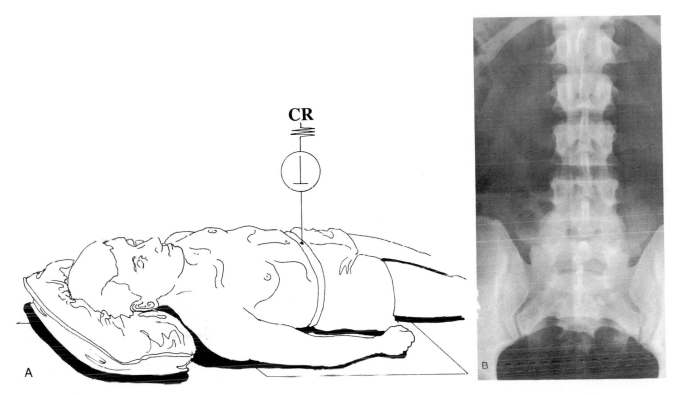

□ **FIGURE 6–8.**

POSITION DESCRIPTION

Part Position: The patient is supine with the hips and knees flexed so that the lower back is in contact with the table.

Central Ray: Perpendicular to the cassette, entering the midline at the level of the crest, to include the sacrum when a 14 × 17 inch film is used.

Note: If a smaller film (11 × 14 or 10 × 12 inches) is used, the central ray should be directed 1½ inches above the crest.

IMAGE EVALUATION

An AP projection of the entire lumbar spine should be demonstrated without rotation, as evidenced by the spinous processes visible in the center of the vertebral bodies.

Routine AP Oblique Lumbar Spine Position

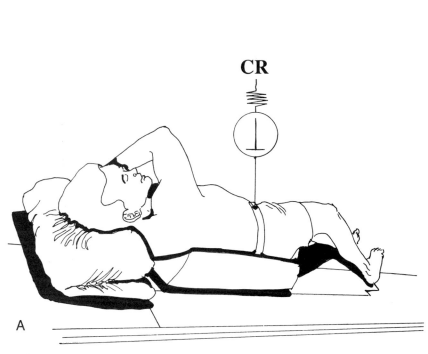

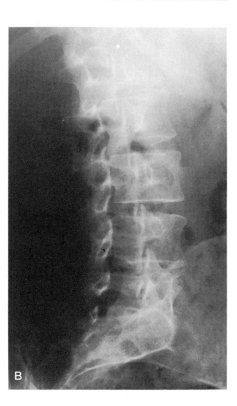

□ FIGURE 6–9.

POSITION DESCRIPTION

Part Position: The patient is in a 45° supine oblique position, with the arm of the side up across the chest. The hip and knee of the side up is flexed to help maintain the position or a 45° angle sponge is used.

Central Ray: Perpendicular to the cassette, entering at a point 2 inches medial to the elevated anterior superior iliac spine and 1½ inches superior to the crest.

IMAGE EVALUATION

The lumbar spine should be demonstrated in an oblique position. The apophyseal joints nearest the film should be well visualized. Correct obliquity has been obtained if the apophyseal joints are seen in the center of the vertebral bodies.

Routine Lateral Lumbar Spine Position

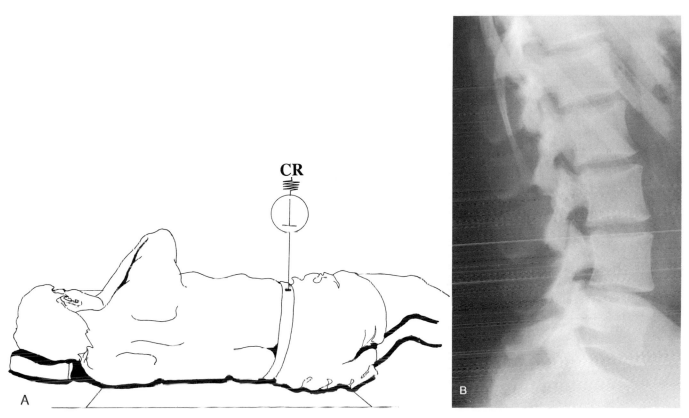

□ FIGURE 6–10.

POSITION DESCRIPTION

Part Position: The patient is in the lateral recumbent position, without forward or backward rotation. The waist should be elevated to place the entire thoracolumbar spine in the same plane, if necessary. A support may be placed between the superimposed knees to maintain proper body position.

Central Ray: Perpendicular to the cassette, entering the midaxillary line at the level of the crest, to include the sacrum when a 14 × 17 inch film is used.

Note: If a smaller film (11 × 14 or 10 × 12 inches) is used, the central ray should be directed 1½ inches above the crest.

IMAGE EVALUATION

The entire lumbar spine should be demonstrated in lateral position, without rotation. The intervertebral foramina of L1 to L4 should be well visualized. The lumbar intervertebral disc spaces should be open.

Routine Lateral Lumbosacral Joint (L5 To S1) Position

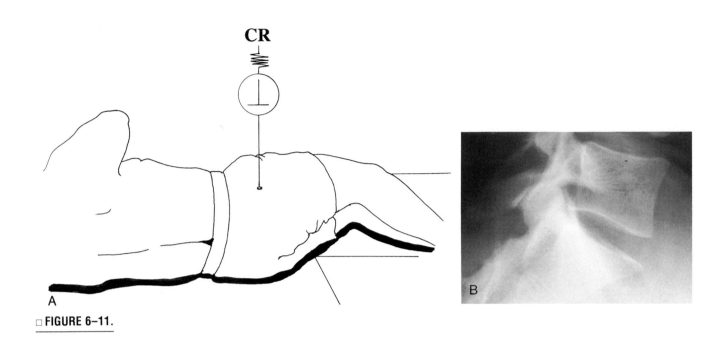

CR

A

B

□ **FIGURE 6–11.**

POSITION DESCRIPTION

Part Position: The patient is in the lateral recumbent position, without forward or backward rotation. The waist should be elevated to place the entire thoracolumbar spine in the same plane, if necessary. A support may be placed between the super-imposed knees, to maintain proper body position.

Central Ray: Perpendicular to the cassette, entering at a point 1½ inches inferior to the crest and 1½ inches anterior to the tip of the L5 spinous process.

Note: If the waist is not elevated, it may be necessary to angle slightly caudad (which is common) or cephalad, depending on the tilt of the pelvis.

IMAGE EVALUATION

The area of the lumbosacral junction should be demonstrated in lateral position, without rotation. The L5-to-S1 intervertebral joint space should be open.

Routine AP Sacrum Projection

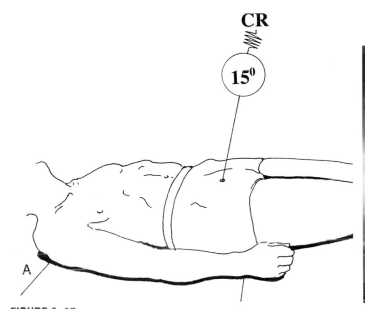

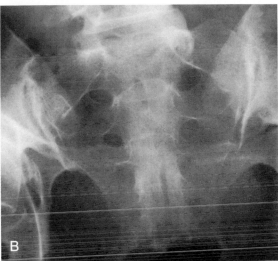

□ FIGURE 6–12.

POSITION DESCRIPTION

Part Position: The patient is supine, without rotation and with the knees slightly flexed and resting on a sponge.

Central Ray: Angled 15° cephalad, entering the midline halfway between the pubic symphysis and the anterior superior iliac spines.

IMAGE EVALUATION

A true AP projection of the entire sacrum should be demonstrated without rotation, as evidenced by symmetry of the sacroiliac joints.

Routine Lateral Sacrum Position

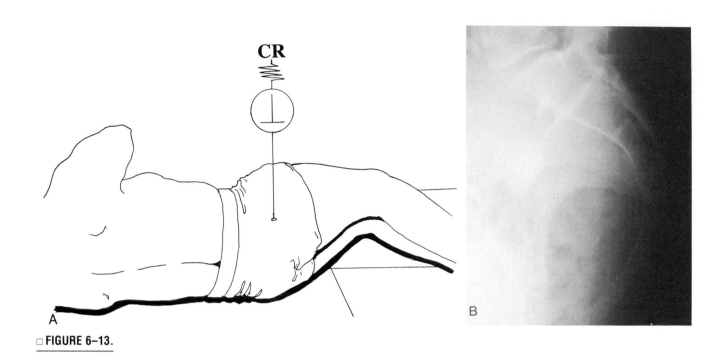

□ **FIGURE 6–13.**

POSITION DESCRIPTION

Part Position: The patient is in the lateral recumbent position, without forward or backward rotation of the pelvis. A support may be placed between the superimposed knees to maintain proper body position.

Central Ray: Perpendicular to the cassette, entering 2 inches anterior to the posterior sacral surface at the level of the anterior superior iliac spine.

IMAGE EVALUATION

The entire sacrum should be demonstrated in lateral position without rotation, as evidenced by superimposition of the ilial and ischial portions of the pelvis.

Routine AP Coccyx Projection

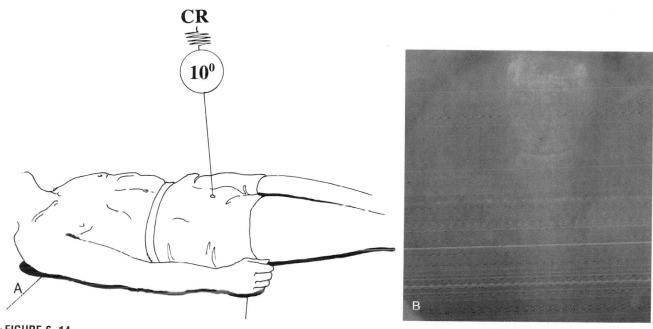

CR

10⁰

A

B

□ **FIGURE 6–14.**

POSITION DESCRIPTION

Part Position: The patient is supine, without rotation and with the slightly flexed knees resting on a sponge.

Central Ray: Angled 10° caudad, entering the midline 2 inches superior to the pubic symphysis.

IMAGE EVALUATION

An AP projection of the entire coccyx should be demonstrated superior to the pubic symphysis. The coccygeal segments should not be overlapped.

Routine Lateral Coccyx Position

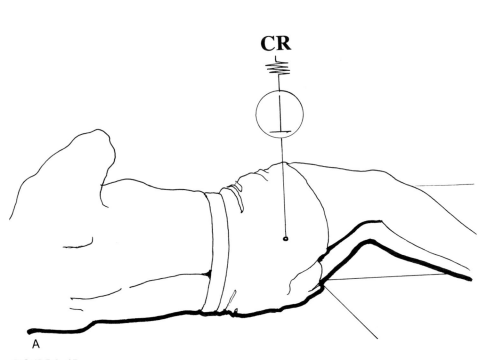

A

□ **FIGURE 6-15.**

B

POSITION DESCRIPTION

Part Position: The patient is in the lateral recumbent position, without forward or backward rotation of the pelvis. A support may be placed between the superimposed knees to maintain proper body position.

Central Ray: Perpendicular to the cassette, entering at a point 1½ inches superior to the greater trochanter and on a coronal plane passing through the posterior surface of the sacrum.

IMAGE EVALUATION

The entire coccyx should be demonstrated in lateral position without rotation, as evidenced by superimposition of the ilial and ischial portions of the pelvis.

Specialized Cervical Spine Radiography

AP Axial Oblique (Pillars) Cervical Spine Position

RATIONALE FOR USE

This position enables evaluation of the *cervical articular pillars (lateral masses) and posterior arches.* It is used most commonly to assess whiplash-type injuries with negative or incomplete findings on routine cervical spine radiographs. Because this projection requires neck extension and head rotation, it is *not* recommended for initial use in cases of acute cervical spine trauma.

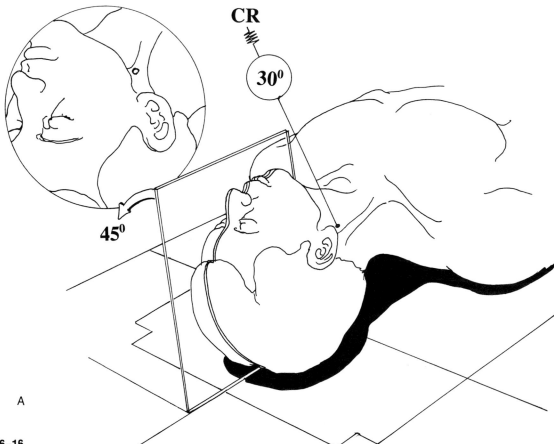

CR

30⁰

45⁰

A

□ **FIGURE 6–16.**

POSITION DESCRIPTION

Part Position: The patient is in the same position as for a routine AP cervical spine radiograph. The neck is then extended and the head rotated to one side as much as the patient's condition allows (45° is sufficient). A second radiograph is taken with the head rotated to the opposite side.

Note: Greater head rotation (up to 70°) is necessary in order that the lower cervical pillars are oblique.

Central Ray: Angled 30° caudad, entering at the top of the thyroid cartilage.

AP Axial Oblique (Pillars) Cervical Spine Position *(continued)*

IMAGE EVALUATION

The cervical articular pillars (lateral masses) on the side away from head rotation should be demonstrated. Portions of the posterior arches should also be visualized. The pillars will exhibit varying degrees of rotation (obliquity): the greatest, superiorly, and the least, inferiorly. If the head and neck are sufficiently rotated and extended, the mandible should not obscure the upper pillars on the side of interest.

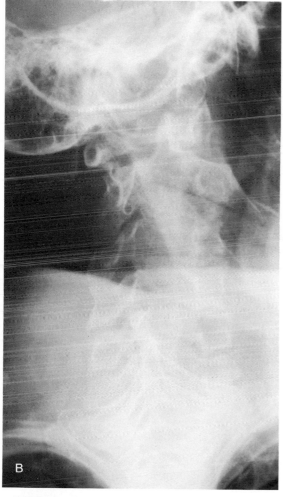

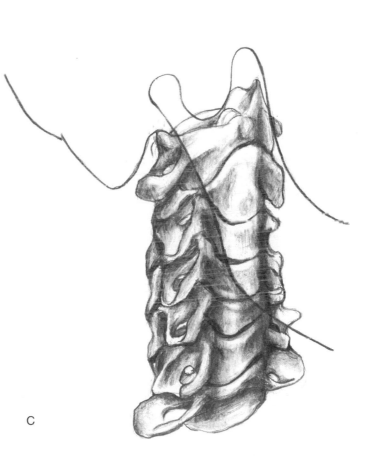

□ **FIGURE 6–16.** *(continued)*

Exaggerated Supine Oblique Cervical Spine Position*

RATIONALE FOR USE

This position may be used to *evaluate the cervical articular processes, pedicles, and intervertebral foramina in cases of acute injury*. Like the trauma oblique position, this position enables the patient to remain supine, and the head does not need to be turned. The increased tube angulation results in greater separation of anterior and posterior cervical structures.

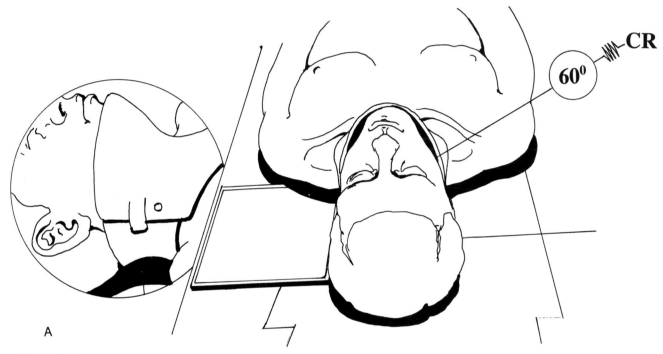

A

☐ **FIGURE 6–17.**

POSITION DESCRIPTION

Part Position: The patient is supine. The cassette is slid under the patient's head and neck (while the head is supported) or under the backboard. The cassette is crosswise and off-centered so that the medial edge of the cassette is even with the midsagittal plane of the neck. The cephalic edge of the cassette should be slightly above the top of the patient's ear.

Central Ray: Angled 60° lateromedially, entering the side of the neck at the level of the thyroid cartilage and passing through C4.

Exaggerated Supine Oblique Cervical Spine Position* *(continued)*

IMAGE EVALUATION

All cervical anatomy will appear elongated, but the articular processes, pedicles, and intervertebral foramina on the tube side should be well demonstrated.

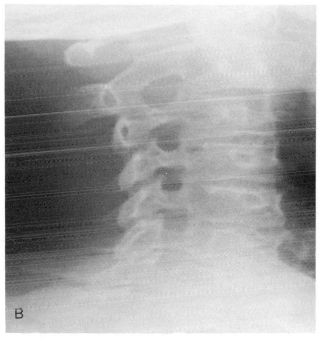

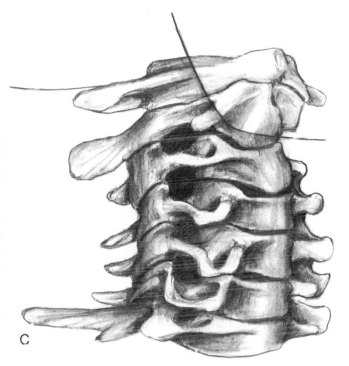

⊔ **FIGURE 6–17.** *(continued)*

*Abel MS. The exaggerated supine oblique view of the cervical spine. *Skeletal Radiol* 1982; 8:213–219.

Extension Lateral Cervical Spine Position

RATIONALE FOR USE

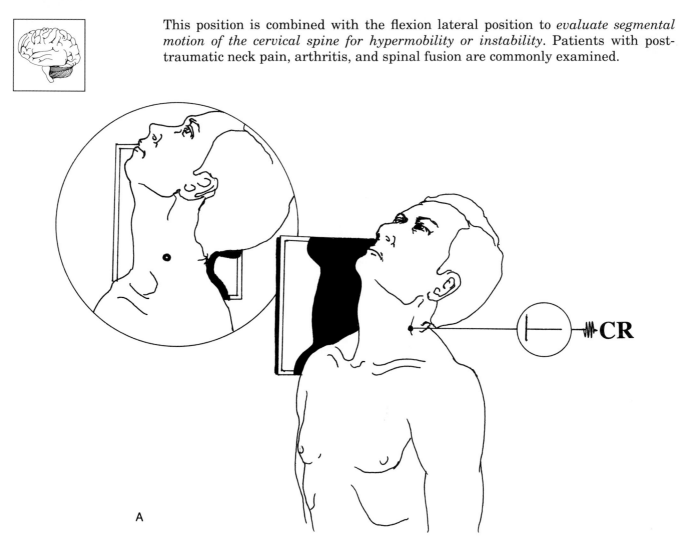

This position is combined with the flexion lateral position to *evaluate segmental motion of the cervical spine for hypermobility or instability.* Patients with post-traumatic neck pain, arthritis, and spinal fusion are commonly examined.

A

□ **FIGURE 6–18.**

POSITION DESCRIPTION

Part Position: The patient is in the same position as for a routine upright lateral cervical spine radiograph. The patient then leans the head back as far as possible. The back should remain straight.

Central Ray: Perpendicular to the cassette (horizontal), entering the side of the neck at the level of the thyroid cartilage.

Note: A 72-inch SID is required.

Extension Lateral Cervical Spine Position *(continued)*

IMAGE EVALUATION

The cervical spine should be demonstrated in lateral projection with maximal extension. The C7 spinous process may be obscured by the shadow of the shoulders.

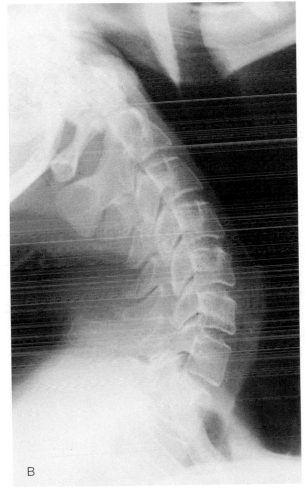

B

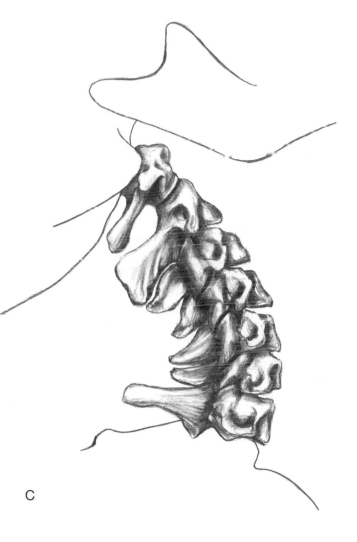

C

□ **FIGURE 6–18.** *(continued)*

Flexion Lateral Cervical Spine Position

RATIONALE FOR USE

This position is combined with the extension lateral position to *evaluate segmental motion of the cervical spine for hypermobility or instability*. Patients with post-traumatic neck pain, arthritis, and spinal fusion are commonly examined.

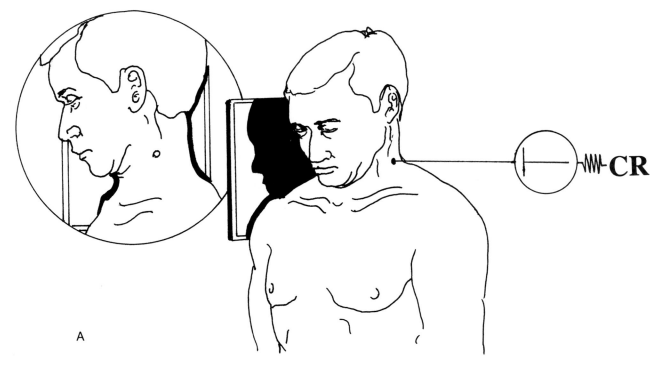

A

□ **FIGURE 6–19.**

POSITION DESCRIPTION

Part Position: The patient is in the same position as for a routine upright lateral cervical spine radiograph. The patient then bows the head, bringing the chin as close to the chest as possible. The back should remain straight so the thoracic spine is not flexed.

Note: If the C7 vertebral body is obscured by the shoulders, the shoulders should be rolled back without being raised.

Central Ray: Perpendicular to the cassette (horizontal), entering the side of the neck at the level of the thyroid cartilage.

Note: A 72-inch SID is required.

Flexion Lateral Cervical Spine Position *(continued)*

IMAGE EVALUATION

The cervical spine should be demonstrated in lateral projection with maximal flexion. The C7 vertebral body may be obscured by the shadow of the shoulders.

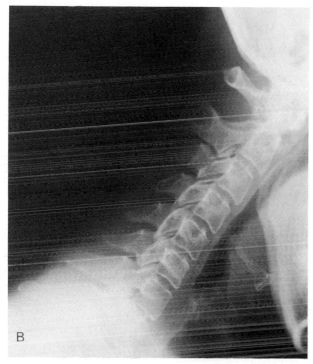

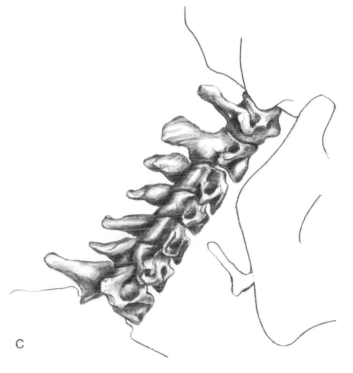

□ **FIGURE 6–19.** *(continued)*

Fuchs* Odontoid Process Position

RATIONALE FOR USE

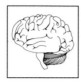

This position may be used to *demonstrate the entire odontoid process when it is not well visualized on the routine AP open-mouth radiograph.* The Fuchs odontoid process position also enables evaluation of the anterior and posterior arches of the atlas (C1). Because this position requires neck extension, it is *not* recommended for initial use in cases of acute cervical spine trauma or in patients with severe arthritis.

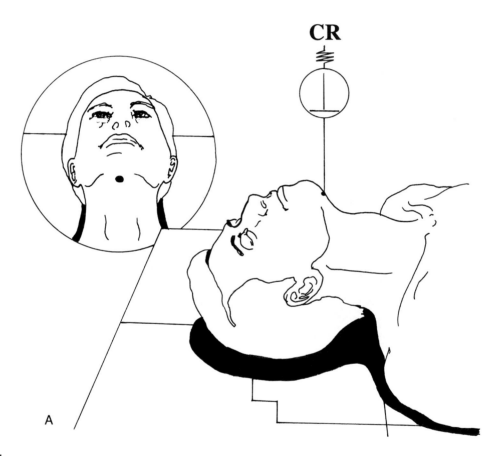

A

□ **FIGURE 6–20.**

POSITION DESCRIPTION

Part Position: The patient is supine with the head tipped back so that the mento-meatal line is perpendicular to the cassette.

Central Ray: Perpendicular to the cassette, entering at the mental point of the mandible.

Note: This position may be achieved on patients in cervical collars by angling 30° cephalad to the thyroid cartilage without extending the head.

Fuchs* Odontoid Process Position *(continued)*

IMAGE EVALUATION

The odontoid process should be seen within the foramen magnum. The anterior and posterior arches of C1 should also be demonstrated. Insufficient head and neck extension will result in the mandible's obscuring the tip of the odontoid process.

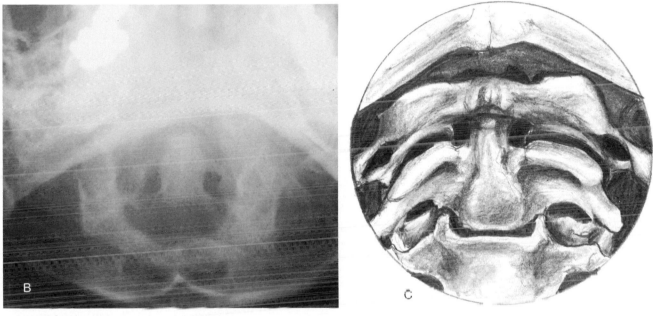

⊔ **FIGURE 6-20.** *(continued)*

---

*Fuchs AW. Cervical vertebra (Part one). *Radiog Clin Photog* 1940; 16(1):2–11.

Lateral Cervicothoracic (Swimmer's) Position*

RATIONALE FOR USE

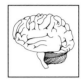

The swimmer's position (also called "flying angel") is used to obtain a *lateral radiograph of the lower cervical and upper thoracic vertebral in cases in which the shoulders obscure this region on the routine lateral radiograph.* The position was originally developed to image the lung apices in the lateral position.

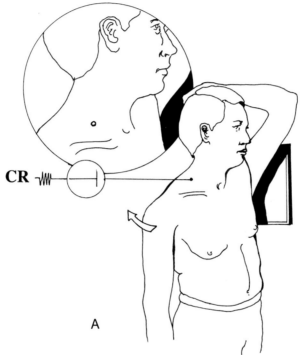

CR

A

□ **FIGURE 6–21.**

POSITION DESCRIPTION

Part Position: The patient is in the lateral position against the upright bucky/cassette holder or recumbent on the table. The arm nearest the film is raised above the head, and the opposite shoulder depressed. The shoulders are rolled slightly in opposite directions to prevent superimposition of the humeral heads on the vertebral column. The shoulder closest to the film is usually rolled forward, and the opposite shoulder is rolled back. The head and neck and the hips must be maintained in lateral position during the shoulder roll. The cassette is centered to the dependent axilla.

Note: This position may be performed as a cross-table lateral position on trauma patients. However, a patient's arm should not be raised over the head without permission from the attending physician. Also, the shoulder roll is not possible, and caudad tube angulation should be used.

Central Ray: Perpendicular to the cassette, entering the side of the neck just above the clavicle, passing through the lower cervical region and exiting the dependent axilla.

Note: The beam is angled 5°–10° caudad when the tube-side shoulder cannot be depressed (5° is recommended).

Lateral Cervicothoracic (Swimmer's) Position* *(continued)*

IMAGE EVALUATION

The lower cervical and upper thoracic vertebra should be demonstrated in a lateral projection. The humeral heads should be slightly anterior and posterior to the vertebral bodies.

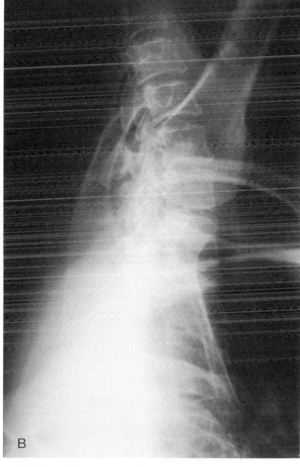

B

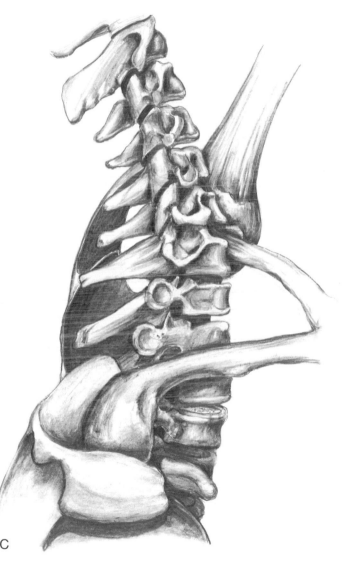

C

□ **FIGURE 6–21.** *(continued)*

*Twining EW. Lateral view of the lung apices (interclavicular projection of the thoracic inlet). *Br J Radiol* 1937; 10(110):123–131.

Trauma Oblique Cervical Spine Position

RATIONALE FOR USE

This position is used to *obtain an oblique cervical spine radiograph in cases of acute injury*. The patient remains supine, and the head does not need to be turned.

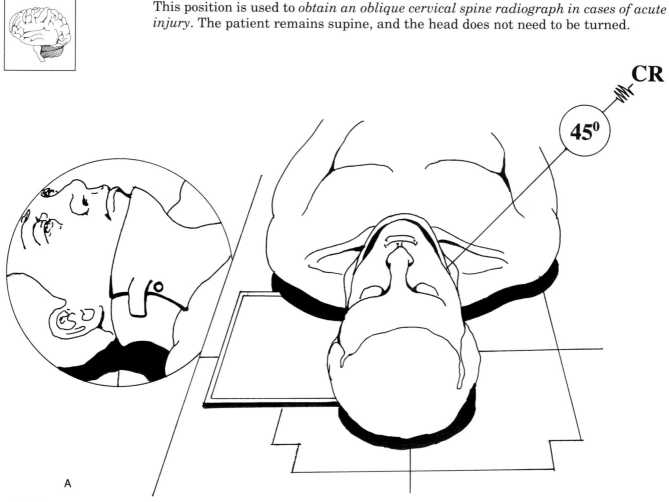

A

□ **FIGURE 6–22.**

POSITION DESCRIPTION

Part Position: The patient is supine. The cassette is slid under the patient's head and neck (while the head is supported) or under the backboard. The cassette is off-centered so that the lateral edge of the cassette is even with the lateral border of the shoulder. The cephalic edge of the cassette should be slightly above the top of the patient's ear.

Central Ray: Angled 45° lateromedially, entering the side of the neck at the level of the thyroid cartilage and passing through C4.

Note: In addition, the central ray may be angled 15° cephalad, if desired.

Trauma Oblique Cervical Spine Position *(continued)*

IMAGE EVALUATION

The pedicles and intervertebral foramina on the tube side should be well demonstrated. The vertebral bodies and articular pillars will be projected obliquely.

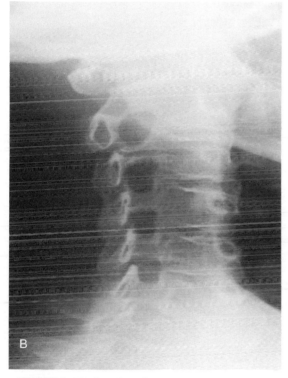

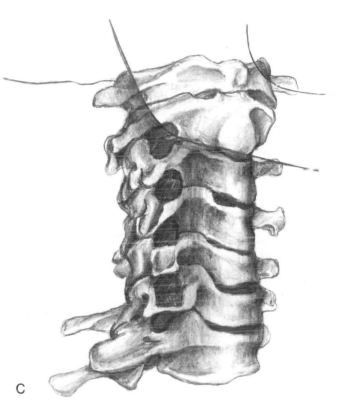

B

C

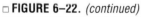

□ **FIGURE 6–22.** *(continued)*

Specialized Lumbar Spine Radiography

AP Axial (Ferguson*) Lumbosacral Projection†

RATIONALE FOR USE

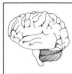

This projection may be used to demonstrate the *L4 and L5 pars interticularis for evaluation of spondylolysis, as well as the relationship of structures at the lumbosacral junction*. The sacrum and sacroiliac joints are also well visualized.

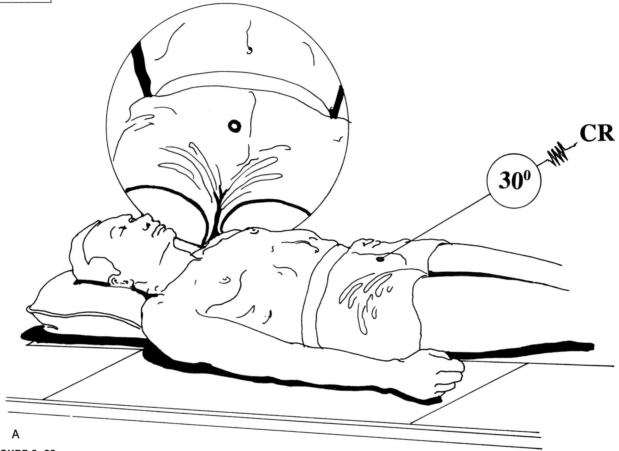

A

□ **FIGURE 6–23.**

POSITION DESCRIPTION

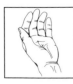

Part Position: The patient is supine with the legs fully extended to allow the normal mechanics of the region to be visualized.

Central Ray: Angled 30° cephalad, entering the midsagittal plane at the level of the anterior-superior iliac spine.

Note: Ferguson* originally recommended an angle of 45°.

AP Axial (Ferguson*) Lumbosacral Projection† (continued)

IMAGE EVALUATION

The pars interarticularis and pedicles of the L4 and L5 vertebrae should be well demonstrated in AP projection, with minimal overlap by the vertebral bodies. The lumbosacral intervertebral joint space should be open. The relationship of the L5 transverse processes with the sacrum should be seen. The sacrum and sacroiliac joints should be well demonstrated.

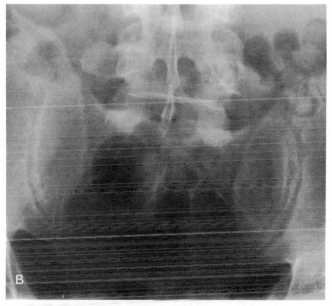

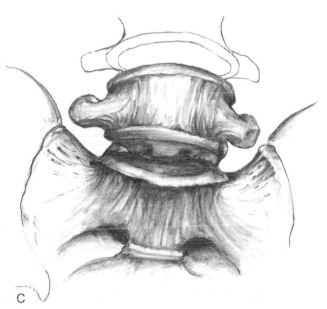

◻ **FIGURE 6–23.** (continued)

---

*Ferguson AB. The clinical and roentgenographic interpretation of lumbosacral anomalies. *Radiology* 1934; 22:548–558.
†Libson E, Bloom RA. Anteroposterior angulated view. *Radiology* 1983; 149:315–316.

AP Axial Oblique Lumbar Spine Position*

RATIONALE FOR USE

This position may be used for *more accurate demonstration of the L4 and L5 pars interarticularis for evaluation of spondylolysis.*

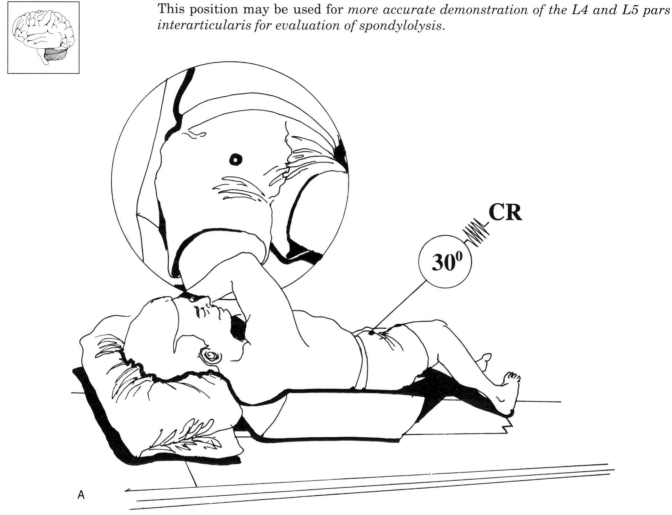

A

□ **FIGURE 6–24.**

POSITION DESCRIPTION

Part Position: The patient is in a 45° supine oblique position.

Central Ray: Angled 30° cephalad, entering 2 inches medial to the anterior-superior iliac spine of the elevated ilium.

AP Axial Oblique Lumbar Spine Position* *(continued)*

IMAGE EVALUATION

The L4 and L5 pars interarticularis (which looks like the neck of a Scotty dog) on the elevated side should be well demonstrated.

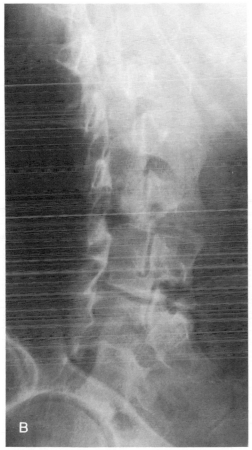

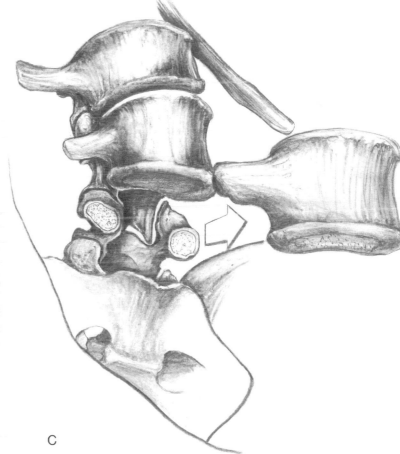

□ **FIGURE 6–24.** *(continued)*

---

*Dubowitz B, Friedman L, Papert B. The oblique cranial tilt view for spondylolysis. *J Bone Joint Surg* 1987; 69B(3):421.

Extension Lateral Lumbar Spine Position

RATIONALE FOR USE

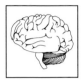

This position is combined with the flexion lateral position to *evaluate motion of the lumbar spine for segmental instability*. Patients with post-traumatic lower back pain, arthritis, and spinal fusion are commonly examined with this position. There are differing opinions regarding whether the radiographs should be taken with the patient upright or recumbent.

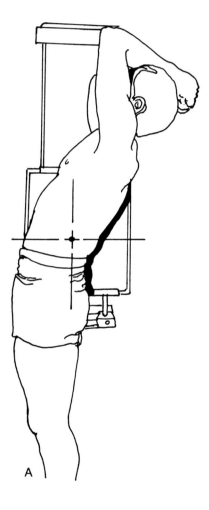

A

☐ **FIGURE 6–25.**

POSITION DESCRIPTION

Part Position: The patient is placed in the lateral position, either upright (standing or sitting) or recumbent, depending on the physician's preference. The patient is then instructed to arch the lower back as much as possible.

Note: It is a good idea to have patients practice the position, so that they can be assisted to achieve maximal extension.

Central Ray: Perpendicular to the cassette, entering the midaxillary line at the level of the iliac crest.

Extension Lateral Lumbar Spine Position *(continued)*

IMAGE EVALUATION

A lateral projection of the lumbar spine in maximal extension should be demonstrated.

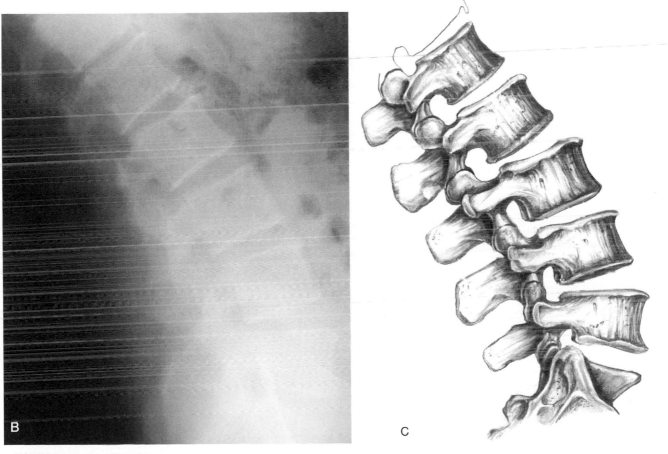

B

C

□ **FIGURE 6–25.** *(continued)*

Flexion Lateral Lumbar Spine Position

RATIONALE FOR USE

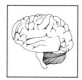

This position is combined with the extension lateral position to *evaluate motion of the lumbar spine for segmental instability*. Patients with post-traumatic lower back pain, arthritis, and spinal fusion are commonly examined. There are differing opinions regarding whether the radiographs should be taken with the patient upright or recumbent.

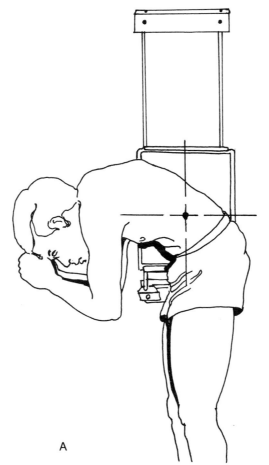

A

□ **FIGURE 6–26.**

POSITION DESCRIPTION

Part Position: The patient is placed in the lateral position, either upright (standing or sitting) or recumbent, depending on the physician's preference. The patient is then instructed to bend the lower back forward as much as possible.

Note: It is a good idea to have patients practice the position, so they can be assisted to achieve maximal flexion.

Central Ray: Perpendicular to the cassette, entering the midaxillary line at the level of the iliac crest.

Flexion Lateral Lumbar Spine Position *(continued)*

IMAGE EVALUATION

A lateral projection of the lumbar spine in maximal flexion should be demonstrated.

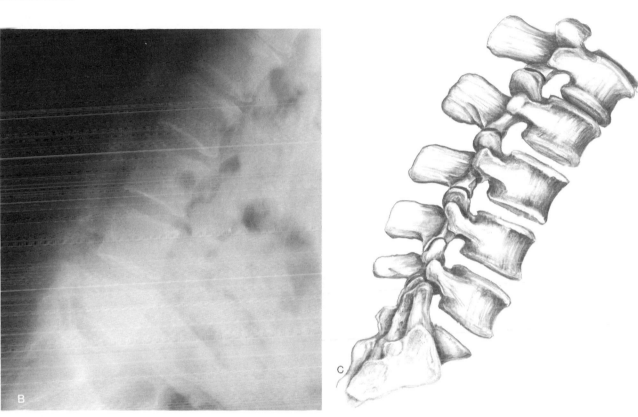

□ **FIGURE 6–26**. *(continued)*

Lateral-Bending AP Lumbar Spine Positions

RATIONALE FOR USE

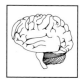

These positions may be used to *evaluate motion of the lumbar spine for segmental instability*. Patients with post-traumatic lower back pain, arthritis, and spinal fusion are commonly examined. There are differing opinions regarding whether the radiographs should be performed with the patient upright or recumbent.

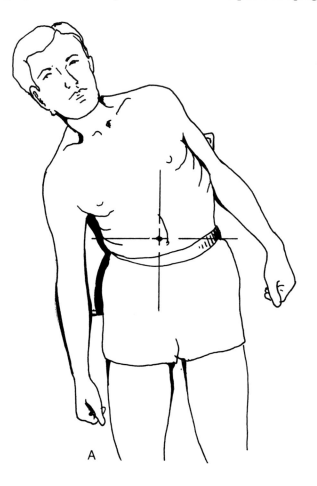

□ **FIGURE 6–27.**

A

POSITION DESCRIPTION

Part Position: The patient is in the same position as for an AP lumbar spine radiograph, either upright (standing or sitting) or recumbent, depending on the physician's preference. The patient is then instructed to bend the lower back to one side as much as possible. A second radiograph is taken with the patient bending to the other side.

Note: It is a good idea to have patients practice the positions, so they can be assisted to achieve maximal lateral bending.

Central Ray: Perpendicular to the cassette, entering the midline at the level of the iliac crest.

Lateral-Bending AP Lumbar Spine Positions *(continued)*

IMAGE EVALUATION

AP projections of the lumbar spine in maximal right and left bending should be demonstrated.

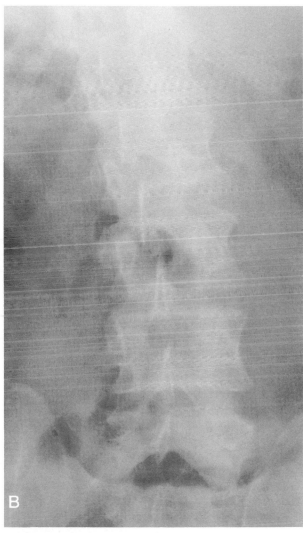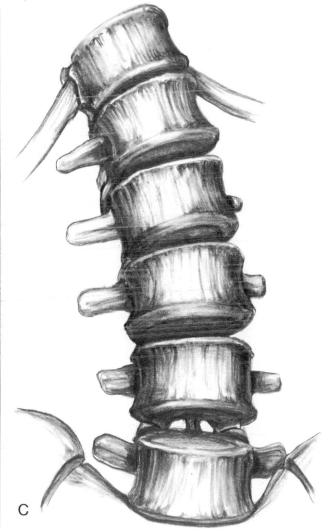

□ **FIGURE 6–27.** *(continued)*

Vertebral Arch Lumbar Spine Position*

RATIONALE FOR USE

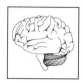

This position may be used to *better demonstrate the laminae and articular processes of the lumbar spine in the supine position.* Acutely injured patients may be evaluated with this position, because they need not be moved from the supine position. The position may also be used to assess patients with chronic lower back pain.

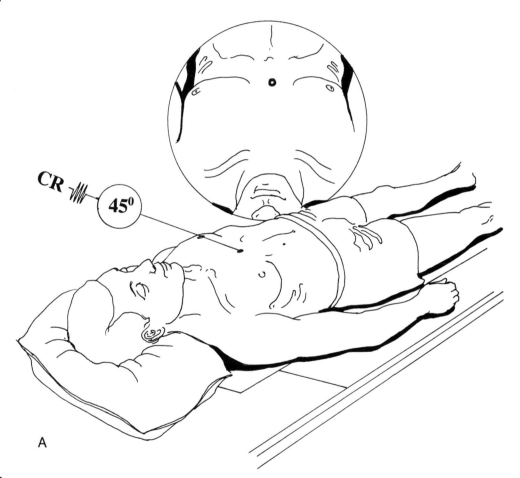

CR — 45°

A

□ **FIGURE 6–28.**

POSITION DESCRIPTION

Part Position: The patient is supine.

Central Ray: Angled 45° caudad, entering the midline 2 inches above the xiphoid process.

Vertebral Arch Lumbar Spine Position* *(continued)*

IMAGE EVALUATION

The vertebral arches (articular processes, laminae, spinous processes) of the lumbar spine should be well demonstrated. The vertebral bodies and intervertebral disc spaces will not be visible.

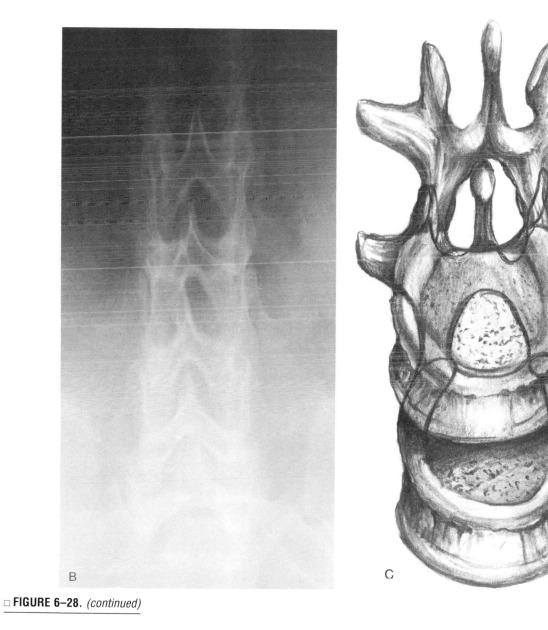

B

C

□ **FIGURE 6–28.** *(continued)*

*Abel MS, Smith GR. Visualization of the posterior elements of the lumbar vertebrae in the anteroposterior projection. *Radiology* 1977; 122:824–825.

Radiography of Abnormal Spinal Curvature

AP Scoliosis Projection

RATIONALE FOR USE

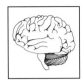

This AP projection is used to *assess the thoracolumbar spine for abnormal curvature or rotation*. Although use of the AP scoliosis projection is common, the PA projection is recommended because of decreased radiation exposure to breast and thyroid.

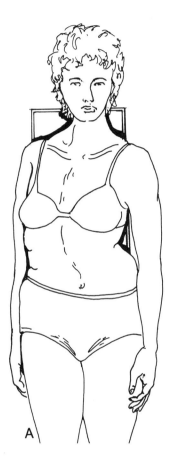

□ **FIGURE 6–29.**

POSITION DESCRIPTION

Part Position: The patient is sitting or standing upright with the back against the upright cassette holder. The midsagittal plane of the body is centered to the cassette, and the arms are allowed to hang relaxed at the sides. The cassette and collimated field is adjusted to include the C7 vertebra at the top, the anterior superior iliac spine at the bottom, and the apex of the abnormal vertebral curve or curves at the sides.

Note: In addition to gonadal shielding, breast and thyroid shielding should be used.

Central Ray: Perpendicular to the cassette (horizontal), entering the midline halfway between the levels of the thyroid cartilage and the anterior superior iliac spine.

Note: A 72-inch SID is recommended.

AP Scoliosis Projection *(continued)*

IMAGE EVALUATION

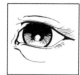

An AP projection of the thoracic and lumbar spines should be demonstrated. The superior portion of the sacroiliac joints and iliac crests should be included.

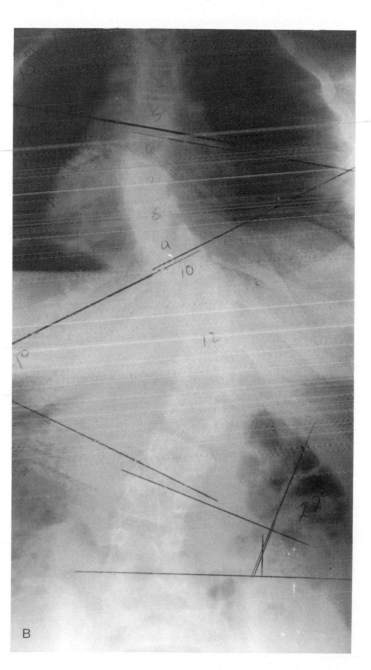

□ **FIGURE 6–29.** *(continued)*

Lateral-Bending AP/PA Scoliosis Projections

RATIONALE FOR USE

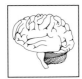

The lateral-bending AP or PA projections are used to *assess the flexibility of the scoliotic curvature, in order to determine degree of surgical straightening possible.* Although use of the AP projection is common, the PA projection is recommended because of decreased radiation exposure to breast and thyroid.

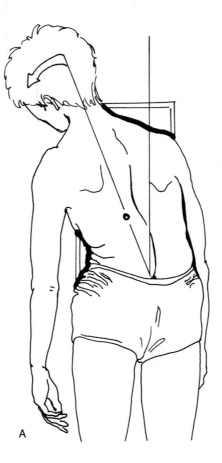

□ **FIGURE 6–30.**

A

POSITION DESCRIPTION

Part Position: The patient is standing, either facing (PA) or with the back against (AP) the upright cassette holder. The midsagittal plane of the body is centered to the cassette, and the arms are allowed to hang relaxed at the sides. The cassette is adjusted to include the C7 vertebra at the top and the anterior superior iliac spine at the bottom. The patient's position is adjusted to offset the lumbar spine to the side of the cassette opposite the direction of side bending. The patient then bends as far as possible to the side. A second radiograph is taken during bending to the other side.

Central Ray: Perpendicular to the cassette (horizontal), to the midline of the cassette.

Lateral-Bending AP/PA Scoliosis Projections *(continued)*

IMAGE EVALUATION

The thoracic and lumbar spine should be demonstrated in AP or PA projection with maximal right and left lateral bending.

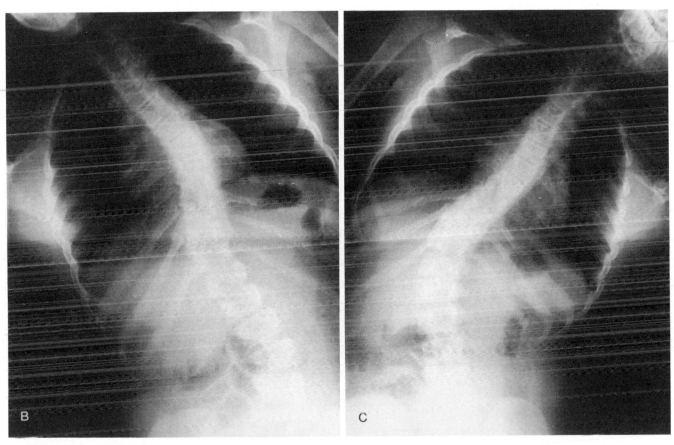

□ **FIGURE 6–30.** *(continued)*

Lateral Kyphosis-Lordosis Position

RATIONALE FOR USE

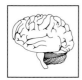

This lateral position may be used during radiographic scoliosis screening to *assess the thoracolumbar spine for an abnormal degree of kyphosis or lordosis*, as well as to evaluate the *presence of a spondylolisthesis.*

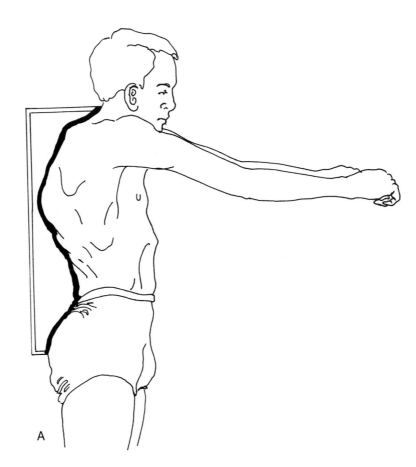

A

□ **FIGURE 6–31.**

POSITION DESCRIPTION

Part Position: The patient is in a sitting or standing upright lateral position, with the primary curve side (if known) against the bucky/cassette holder. The arms should be extended over the head or out in front (holding a support). The cassette is adjusted to include the C7 vertebra at the top and the anterior superior iliac spine at the bottom. The spine is centered to the midline of the cassette.

Note: In addition to gonadal shielding, breast shielding should be used.

Central Ray: Perpendicular to the cassette (horizontal), entering the midline halfway between the levels of the thyroid cartilage and the anterior superior iliac spine.

Note: A 72-inch SID is recommended.

Lateral Kyphosis-Lordosis Position *(continued)*

IMAGE EVALUATION

The thoracic and lumbar spines should be demonstrated in the lateral position. The superior portion of the iliac crest should be included.

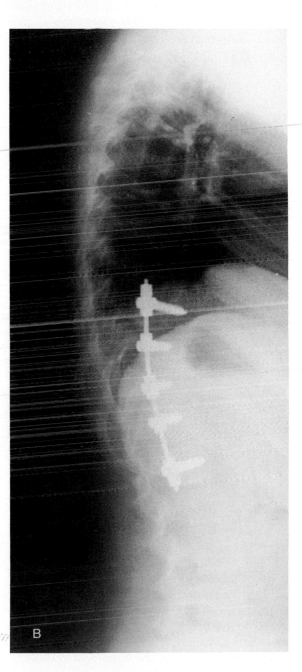

□ **FIGURE 6–31.** *(continued)*

PA Scoliosis Projection

RATIONALE FOR USE

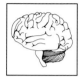

This PA projection is used to *assess the thoracolumbar spine for abnormal curvature or rotation.* Although use of the AP scoliosis projection is common, the PA projection is recommended because of decreased radiation exposure to breast and thyroid. The patient's position for the PA projection enables more precise collimation, because the spinous processes can often be palpated to assess the location of the abnormal curve or curves.

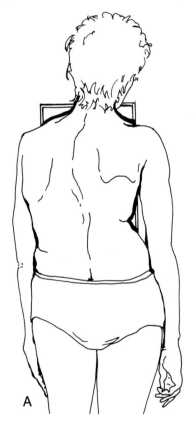

□ **FIGURE 6–32.**

POSITION DESCRIPTION

Part Position: The patient is sitting or standing upright, facing the upright cassette holder. The midsagittal plane of the body is centered to the cassette, and the arms are allowed to hang relaxed at the sides. The cassette and collimated field are adjusted to include the C7 vertebra at the top, the anterior superior iliac spine at the bottom, and the apex of the abnormal vertebral curve or curves at the sides.

Central Ray: Perpendicular to the cassette (horizontal), entering the midline halfway between the levels of the thyroid cartilage and the anterior-superior iliac spine.

Note: A 72-inch SID is recommended.

PA Scoliosis Projection *(continued)*

IMAGE EVALUATION

A PA projection of the thoracic and lumbar spines should be demonstrated. The superior portion of the sacroiliac joints and iliac crests should be included.

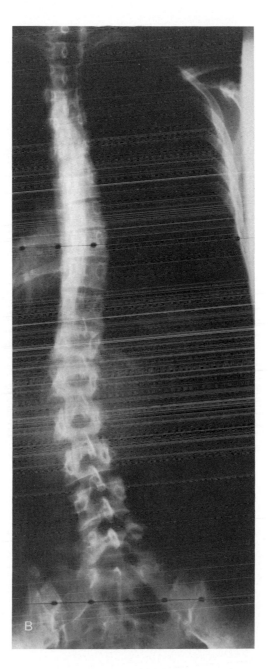

□ **FIGURE 6–32.** *(continued)*

Sacroiliac Joint Radiography

AP Axial Sacroiliac Joints Projection

RATIONALE FOR USE

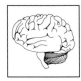

This projection *clearly demonstrates the sacroiliac joints.* The projection also demonstrates the sacrum, the state of fusion of the sacral wings, the relationship of the L5 spinous processes with the sacrum, and the L5 vertebral arch.

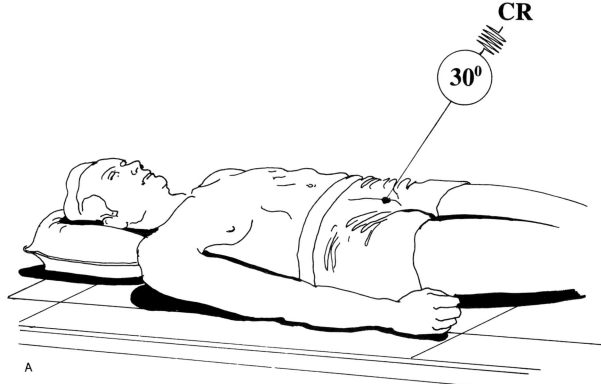

A

□ **FIGURE 6–33.**

POSITION DESCRIPTION

Part Position: The patient is supine with the legs fully extended to allow the normal mechanics of the region to be visualized.

Central Ray: Angled 30°–35° cephalad, entering 1 inch cephalad to the pubic symphysis.

Note: Ferguson* recommended an angle of 45° cephalad.

AP Axial Sacroiliac Joints Projection *(continued)*

IMAGE EVALUATION

The sacroiliac joints should be well demonstrated in an AP projection. The lumbo-sacral intervertebral joint space will probably be open. The relationship of the L5 transverse processes with the sacrum should be seen. The pars interarticularis and pedicles of the L5 vertebra should be well demonstrated, with minimal overlap by the vertebral body

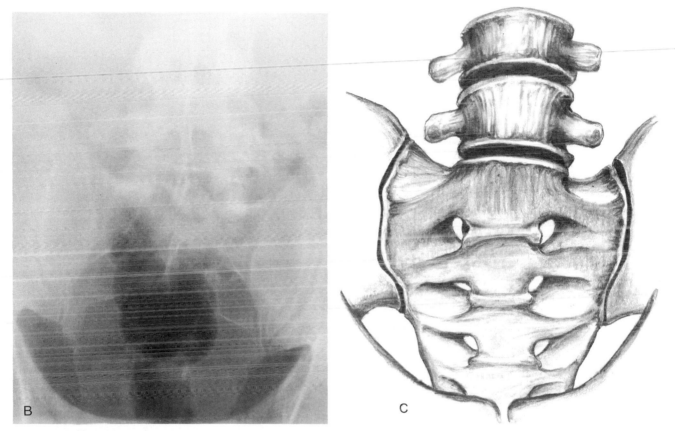

□ **FIGURE 6–33.** *(continued)*

*Ferguson AB. The clinical and roentgenographic interpretation of lumbosacral anomalies. *Radiology* 1934; 22:548–558.

AP Oblique Sacroiliac Joint Position

RATIONALE FOR USE

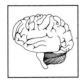

This position demonstrates a *profile of the sacroiliac joint on the elevated side.* The oblique body position places the sacroiliac joint space approximately parallel to the central ray.

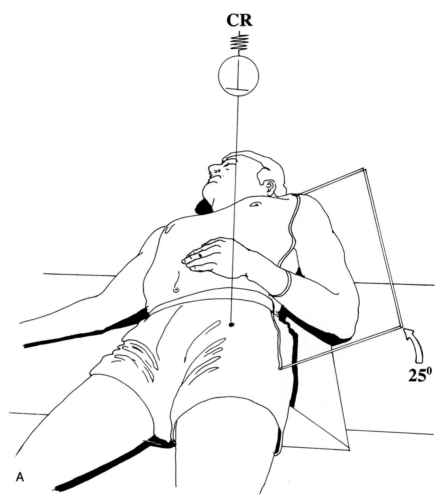

CR

25°

A

□ **FIGURE 6–34.**

POSITION DESCRIPTION

Part Position: The patient is in a 25°–30° supine oblique position, with the side of interest elevated.

Central Ray: Perpendicular to the cassette, entering 1 inch medial to the elevated anterior superior iliac spine.

AP Oblique Sacroiliac Joint Position *(continued)*

IMAGE EVALUATION

The sacroiliac joint space should be demonstrated with minimal overlap. The remainder of the sacrum and ilium will be obliquely oriented.

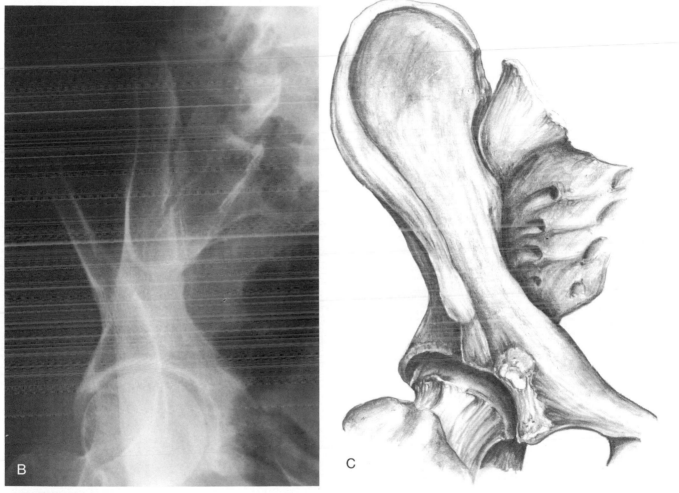

B

C

☐ **FIGURE 6–34.** *(continued)*

AP Sacroiliac Joints Projection

RATIONALE FOR USE

This projection is used to *demonstrate the sacroiliac joints*. This position may be used in conjunction with the AP axial projection.

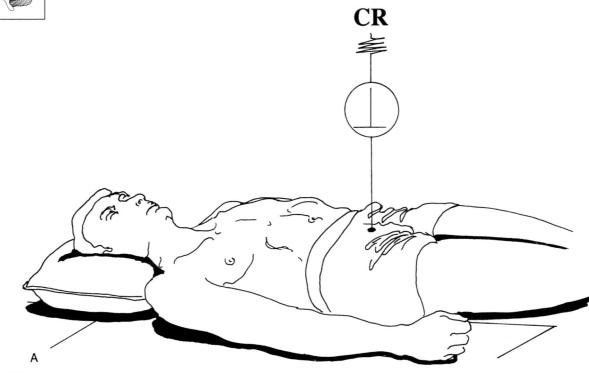

□ **FIGURE 6–35.**

POSITION DESCRIPTION

Part Position: The patient is supine with the legs fully extended, to allow the normal mechanics of the region to be visualized.

Central Ray: Perpendicular to the cassette, entering the midline at the level of the anterior superior iliac spine.

AP Sacroiliac Joints Projection *(continued)*

IMAGE EVALUATION

The sacroiliac joints should be demonstrated in anatomical position.

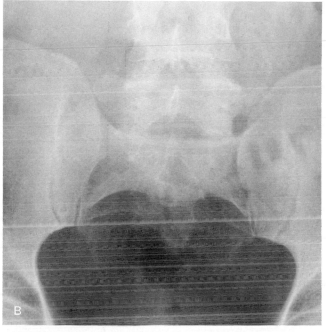

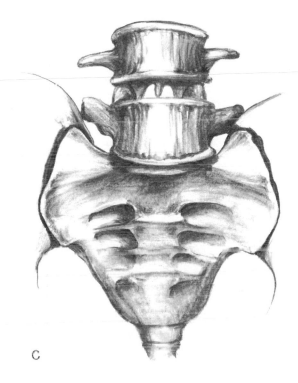

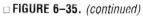
□ **FIGURE 6–35.** *(continued)*

References

1. Daffner RH. "Fingerprints" of vertebral trauma—a unifying concept based on mechanism. *Skeletal Radiol* 1986; 15:518.
2. Greenspan A. *Orthopedic Radiology: A Practical Approach,* 2nd ed. New York: Gower Medical; 1992.
3. Calenoff L, Chessare JW, Rogers LF, et al. Multiple level spinal injuries: importance of early recognition. *AJR* 1978; 130:665.
4. Hadley MN, Zabramski JM, Browner CM, et al. Pediatric spinal trauma. Review of 122 cases of spinal cord and vertebral column injuries. *J Neurosurg* 1988; 8:18–24.
5. Ducker T, Perot P. *National Spinal Cord Injury Registry.* Charleston, SC: U.S. Department of Defense; 1974–1975.
6. Castellano V, Bocconi FL. Injuries of the cervical spine with spinal cord involvement (myelic fractures): statistical considerations. *Bull Hosp Joint Dis* 1970; 31:188.
7. Del Bigio MR, Johnson GE. Clinical presentation of spinal cord concussion. *Spine* 1989; 14:37.
8. Rogers LF. *Radiology of Skeletal Trauma,* 2nd ed. New York: Churchill Livingstone; 1992.
9. Bohlman HH. Pathology and current treatment concepts of cervical spine injuries. *Instructional Course Lectures,* vol 21, The American Academy of Orthopedic Surgeons. St. Louis: CV Mosby; 1972:108–115.
10. Jefferson G. Fracture of the atlas vertebra: report of four cases and a review of those previously reported. *Br J Surg* 1920; 7:407–422.
11. Firooznia H, Rafii M, Golimbu C, Gulfo VJ. Radiographic diagnosis of fracture-dislocations of the spine. *In* Errico TJ, Bauer RD, Waugh T (eds). *Spinal Trauma.* Philadelphia: JB Lippincott; 1991:11–54.
12. Seimon LP. Fracture of the odontoid in young children. *J Bone Joint Surg* 1977; 59A:943–948.
13. Elliot JM, Rogers LF, Wissinger JP, et al. The hangman's fracture. Fractures of the neural arch of the axis. *Radiology* 1972; 104:303–307.
14. Seljeskog EL, Chou SN. Spectrum of the hangman's fracture. *J Neurosurg* 1976; 45:3–8.
15. Scheider RC, Kahn EA. Chronic neurological sequelae of acute trauma to the spine and spinal cord. *J Bone Joint Surg* 1956; 38A:985.
16. Young MH. Long-term consequences of stable fractures of the thoracic and lumbar vertebral bodies. *J Bone Joint Surg* 1973; 55B:295.
17. Holdsworth FW. Fractures, dislocations, and fracture-dislocations of the spine. *J Bone Joint Surg* 1963; 45B:6–20.
18. Atlas SW, Regenbogen V, Rogers LF, Kim KS. The radiographic characterization of burst fractures of the spine. *AJR* 1986; 147:575.
19. Denis F. The three-column spine and its significance in the classification of acute thoracolumbar spinal injuries. *Spine* 1983; 8:817–831.
20. Keene JS. Radiographic evaluation of thoracolumbar fractures. *Clin Orthop* 1984; 189:58.
21. Hanley EN, Eskay ML. Thoracic spine fractures. *Orthopedics* 1989; 12:689.
22. Nicoll EA. Fractures of the dorso-lumbar spine. *J Bone Joint Surg* 1949; 31B:376.
23. Chance GQ. Note on a type of flexion fracture of the spine. *Br J Radiol* 1948; 21:452.
24. Howland WJ, Curry JL, Buffington CB. Fulcrum fractures of the lumbar spine. *JAMA* 1965; 193:240.
25. Kolowich P, Phillips W. Seat belt lumbar fractures in children. *Orthop Trans* 1986; 10:566.
26. Farrandez L, Usabiaga J, Curto JM, et al. Atypical multivertebral fracture due to hyperextension in an adolescent girl. *Spine* 1989; 14:645.
27. Epstein BS, Epstein JA, Jones MD. Lumbar spondylolisthesis with isthmic defects. *Radiol Clin North Am* 1977; 15:261–274.
28. Braunstein EM, Martel W, Moidel R. Ankylosing spondylitis in men and women: a clinical and radiographic comparison. *Radiology* 1982; 144:91–94.
29. Resnick D, Dwosh IL, Goergen TG, et al. Clinical and radiographic abnormalities in ankylosing spondylitis: a comparison of men and women. *Radiology* 1976; 119:293–297.
30. Killebrew K, Gold RH, Sholkoff SD. Psoriatic spondylitis. *Radiology* 1973; 108:9–16.
31. Sholkoff SD, Glickman MG, Steinbach HL. Roentgenology of Reiter's syndrome. *Radiology* 1970; 97:497–503.
32. Martel W. The occipito-atlanto-axial joints in rheumatoid arthritis and ankylosing spondylitis. *AJR* 1961; 86:223–240.
33. Lipson SJ. Rheumatoid arthritis of the cervical spine. *Clin Orthop* 1984; 182:143–149.
34. Moskowitz RW. Osteoarthritis. *In* Katz WA (ed). *Diagnosis and Management of Rheumatic Diseases,* 2nd ed. Philadelphia: JB Lippincott; 1988:569–581.
35. Resnick D. Degenerative diseases of the vertebral column. *Radiology* 1985; 156:3–14.
36. Jajic I. Gout in the spine and sacroiliac joints: radiological manifestations. *Skeletal Radiol* 1982; 8:209–212.
37. Resnick D, Niwayama G, Goergen TG, et al. Clinical, radiographic, and pathologic abnormalities in calcium pyrophosphate dihydrate deposition disease (CPPD): pseudogout. *Radiology* 1977; 122:1–15.
38. McAlister WH, Shackelford GD. Classification of spinal curvatures. *Radiol Clin North Am* 1975; 13:93–112.
39. Goldstein LA, Waugh TR. Classification and terminology of scoliosis. *Clin Orthop* 1973; 93:10–22.
40. Gary JE, Hoffman AD, Peterson HA. Reduction of radiation exposure during radiography for scoliosis. *J Bone Joint Surg* 1983; 65A:5–12.

SEVEN

The Pelvis and
Hip Joint

THE PELVIS AND HIP JOINT: AN OVERVIEW

ROUTINE PELVIS AND HIP JOINT RADIOGRAPHY

Pelvis
Routine AP Pelvis Projection
Hip Joint
Routine AP Hip Projection
Routine Frog-Leg Lateral Hip Position

SPECIALIZED PELVIS RADIOGRAPHY

AP Frog-Leg (Modified Cleaves) Pelvis Projection
Inlet Pelvis Position
Outlet (Tangential) Pelvis Position
Judet Oblique Acetabulum Positions

SPECIALIZED HIP JOINT RADIOGRAPHY

Axiolateral (Trauma/Surgical Lateral) Hip Position
Modified Lauenstein Lateral Hip Position

The Pelvis and Hip Joint: An Overview

The pelvis serves several functions. It transmits upper body weight to the lower extremities, protects the pelvic viscera, and provides attachment sites for trunk and lower extremity muscles. In the seated position, upper body weight is primarily borne by the pelvis (ischial tuberosities). The ilium, ischium, and pubis contribute to the structure of the acetabulum, a somewhat round depression located on the lateral aspect of each hemipelvis. The bone-rimmed acetabulum accepts the femoral head to form the enarthrodial (ball and socket) joint of the hip. The polyaxial hip joint allows a great deal of lower extremity motion, including flexion-extension, abduction-adduction, and medial-lateral rotation.

When the pelvis and hip joints are injured or diseased, quality of life may be affected because of their involvement in locomotion and weight-bearing functions. Incongruity or instability of the pelvic ring and its articulations may result in chronic pain or a decrease in motion, if treatment is inappropriate. Accurate diagnosis is essential to ensure proper treatment and optimal results. Radiography plays an important role in evaluation of pelvic or hip conditions and in the course of their treatment.

Fractures of the pelvis account for approximately 2% to 3% of all fractures.[1] These fractures have been classified by degree of stability and amount or direction of impact forces. Direction of force is usually classified as anteroposterior, lateral, or vertical (shear). Identifying relative stability of pelvic fractures is important because it is generally recognized that there is a greater incidence of hemorrhage and soft-tissue injury in association with the more severe, unstable fractures.

Fractures of an individual bone or single breaks in the pelvic ring are usually stable[2] and are identified in the majority (up to two thirds) of pelvic fractures.[3] They frequently occur as a result of floor-level falls, low-impact motor vehicle accidents, and apophyseal avulsion in adolescent athletes.[4] Pelvic injury with two or more breaks in the pelvic ring are generally considered unstable and are frequently associated with motor vehicle accidents, automobile-pedestrian accidents, industrial accidents, and falls from heights.[5-8]

There is a great variety of stable fractures of the pelvis. The patterns seen are related to age, activity, amount of force, and direction of force. Avulsion injury is most frequently seen in adolescent athletes and commonly occurs at the anterior superior iliac spine, the anterior inferior iliac spine, and the ischial tuberosity.[9] Numerous fractures involve an individual bone of the pelvis. The majority are fractures of one pubic ramus.[10] These are followed, in frequency, by **Duverney's fracture** (lateral margin of iliac wing) and isolated transverse sacral fracture.[3] A single break in the pelvic ring may occur without instability. The fracture most often occurs near the pubic symphysis and, less frequently, near the sacroiliac joints.[11] When widening of the anterior pelvic arch occurs, it is termed an **"open book"** injury.

Two or more breaks in the pelvic ring usually result in instability. Great force is necessary and may result in complex, multiple fractures. There is often disruption of both the anterior and posterior pelvic arches, termed **Malgaigne's fractures,** and commonly are on the same side.[12] When they occur on opposite sides, they are termed **bucket-handle fractures.** The double break in the pelvic ring may also result from **straddle fractures**, which consist of bilateral fracture of both pubic rami.

Acetabular fractures usually occur as a result of forces driving the femoral head into the pelvis. The common mechanisms include blows to the knee with the hip in flexion and blows to the greater trochanter or lateral pelvis. Fracture of the posterior acetabular wall, often with posterior hip dislocation, is prevalent with blows to the flexed knee.[9] Blows to the greater trochanter or lateral pelvis cause impact on the acetabulum and femoral head. The resulting fracture depends on the direction of force and the position of the leg at impact. The fracture may be isolated to the anterior, superior, or posterior portions. More complex fractures may involve both anterior and posterior columns and may have transverse, "T", or vertical orientations. These complex fractures are more likely to result in central (medial) displacement of the femoral head.[13]

Radiography to assess pelvic trauma should at a minimum include an anteroposterior (AP) pelvic radiograph. Evaluation of anteroposterior displacement or mediolateral rotation requires addition of the axial inlet and outlet (tangential) pelvis radiographs.[7, 9] If acetabular involvement is suspected, Judet[14] oblique radiographs of the affected side or entire pelvis are recommended.

Fractures of the proximal femur are usually termed **hip fractures**. These fractures occur predominantly in the elderly, and osteoporotic women are more frequently affected.[15, 16] Hip fractures may be either intracapsular or extracapsular. Intracapsular fractures may involve the femoral head or, more commonly, the neck. The majority of intracapsular femoral neck fractures in adults are subcapital, usually consisting of a short spiral fracture at the junction of the femoral head and neck.[17] In children, transcervical (midneck) fractures are more commonly seen.[18]

Extracapsular hip fractures may be intertrochanteric or subtrochanteric. As the name implies, the **intertrochanteric** fracture traverses the trochanteric portion of the proximal femur. The main fracture line usually extends obliquely from the greater to the lesser trochanter. Nearly half of these fractures are unstable, consisting of three or more fragments.[19] **Subtrochanteric** fractures involve the area just distal to the lesser trochanter. They often extend into the trochanteric area or into the shaft. Those caused by trauma are usually oblique, whereas pathological fractures in this area tend to be transverse.[20] Trochanteric avulsion fractures are also classified as extracapsular. The greater trochanter is most commonly avulsed in the elderly, as the result of a fall on the trochanter. The lesser trochanter is more commonly avulsed in adolescents, during sports such as football, basketball, or running.[21]

Radiography of hip trauma is dependent on the extent of injury. Initial films often include an AP projection of the pelvis or affected hip and a lateral radiograph of the affected hip. If the hip can be flexed, the frog-leg lateral position is obtained. If the leg must remain in extension, the axiolateral (trauma/surgical lateral) position is obtained. Suspected acetabular involvement may be evaluated with Judet oblique radiographs.

A variety of nontraumatic conditions affect the pelvis and hip joint in children, adolescents, and adults. These conditions may affect the congruity and/or mobility of the joints, thereby affecting the quality of the patient's life. Radiographic examination may aid in the diagnosis or staging of the condition.

Conditions of the pelvis and hip in young patients may manifest at different ages. Congenital dislocation of the hip is most often detected during neonatal examination. The hip dislocation may be irreducible, reducible with force, or manually dislocatable and reducible by means of provocation tests (Ortolani,[22] Barlow[23]). The importance of radiography in the diagnosis of congenital hip dislocation has not been clearly established, but several methods have been advocated. The pelvis may be radiographed with the hips in full extension, in 30° of flexion,[24] or in 45° of abduction, full extension, and internal rotation (von Rosen's view[25]).

Legg-Calve-Perthes disease (Perthes' disease) manifests as osteonecrosis of the capital femoral epiphysis, with frequent involvement of the adjacent capital femoral physis. The age of most frequent incidence is 4 to 9 years; boys are four times more likely than girls to be affected.[26] Radiographic examination may include AP projection of the pelvis or affected hip and a frog-leg or Lauenstein lateral position of the affected hip.

Slipped capital femoral epiphysis manifests as displacement of the immature femoral head at the capital femoral physis. The extent of the slip may range from physeal widening to marked displacement. The condition predominantly affects adolescents, and no single causative factor has been identified. Endocrine dysfunction and heredity have been identified as possible causes.[27] The onset of pain has not been conclusively linked to a traumatic event. Radiography may include an AP projection and modified Cleaves position of the pelvis. The lateral radiograph is important because the direction of displacement is often posterior and may not be visible on the AP radiograph.[28]

A variety of arthritides affect the pelvis (sacroiliac joints and pubic symphysis) and hip joints. Rheumatoid arthritis manifests in the hip as diffuse joint space narrowing and axial migration of the femoral head.[29] Ankylosing spondylitis may affect the sacroiliac joints, pubic symphysis, and hip joints. The sacroiliitis of ankylosing spondylitis is usually bilateral and symmetrical. Both the sacroiliac joints and pubic symphysis may exhibit erosion, sclerosis, and bony ankylosis.[30] In the hip, the manifestations of ankylosing spondylitis appear similar to those of rheumatoid arthritis with the addition of femoral head osteophytes.[31] In psoriatic arthritis and Reiter's syndrome, hip and pelvis involvement is similar to that of ankylosing spondylitis, but the sacroiliac joint damage is more likely to be unilateral or asymmetrical. Crystal-induced arthritis, such as gout or pseudogout, may involve the hip or pelvis. Gout is infrequently seen, but pseudogout is found in the symphysis pubis almost as frequently as in the knee.[32]

Osteoarthritis of the hip may be primary or associated with an underlying cause such as Perthes' disease, slipped capital femoral epiphysis, or pseudogout.[33] The radiographic appearance includes joint space narrowing, subchondral sclerosis, subchondral cyst formation, and osteophyte development.[34] Resnick[35] found these changes in the weight-bearing, superior aspect of the joint in approximately 80% of patients with primary osteoarthritis.

Radiography for arthritic involvement may consist of an AP projection and a modified Cleaves position of the pelvis to determine pattern and extent of involvement. Additional radiographs of affected areas, including AP and lateral hip or AP and AP axial sacroiliac joint radiographs, may also be taken.

A great number and variety of other congenital, developmental, or acquired conditions may affect the pelvis and hips. They necessitate no special radiographic techniques for demonstration, and space does not allow their inclusion in this overview.

Routine Pelvis and Hip Joint Radiography

Routine AP Pelvis Projection

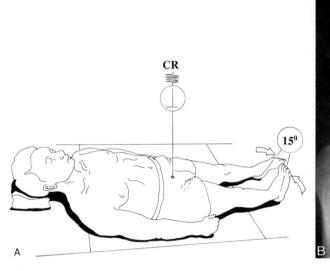

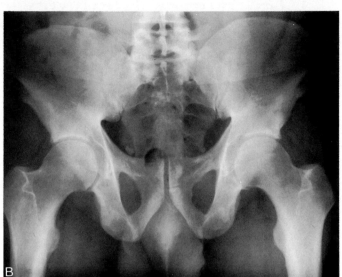

☐ **FIGURE 7–1.**

POSITION DESCRIPTION

Part Position: The patient is supine with the legs extended and internally rotated 15°.

Note: The legs should not be internally rotated if fracture of the proximal femur is suspected.

Central Ray: Perpendicular to the cassette (vertical), entering the midline 2 inches superior to the pubic symphysis.

IMAGE EVALUATION

The pelvic girdle and proximal femurs should be demonstrated in AP projection. The pelvis should not be rotated, as evidenced by symmetry of the obturator foramina and iliac wings. The femoral necks should be fully demonstrated without foreshortening (because of inversion). The greater trochanters should be well demonstrated on the lateral aspect of the proximal femurs. A small portion of the lesser trochanters may be visible on the medial aspect of the proximal femurs.

Routine AP Hip Projection

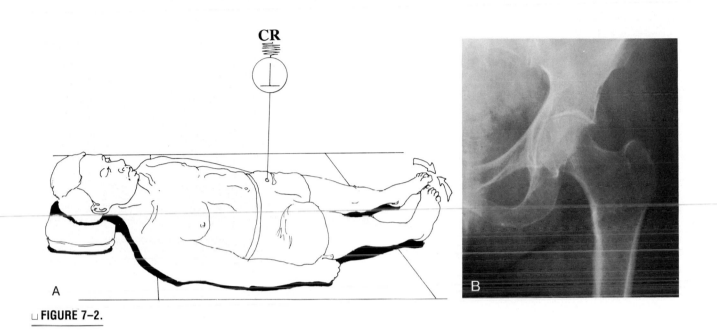

A

B

□ **FIGURE 7–2.**

POSITION DESCRIPTION

Part Position: The patient is supine with the affected leg extended and internally rotated 15°.

Note: The leg should not be internally rotated if fracture of the proximal femur is suspected.

Central Ray: Perpendicular to the cassette (vertical), entering the groin area 2 inches medial and 2 inches inferior to the anterior superior iliac spine.

IMAGE EVALUATION

The pelvis, hip joint, and proximal femur of the affected side should be demonstrated in AP projection. The femoral neck should be fully demonstrated without foreshortening (because of inversion). The greater trochanter should be well demonstrated on the lateral aspect of the proximal femur. A small portion of the lesser trochanter may be visible on the medial aspect of the proximal femur.

Routine Frog-Leg Lateral Hip Projection

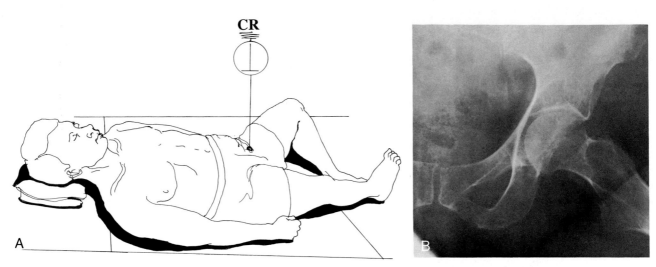

□ **FIGURE 7–3.**

POSITION DESCRIPTION

Part Position: The patient is supine with the affected hip and knee flexed as much as can be achieved comfortably. The affected femur is abducted, to place its long axis approximately 50° to the plane of the table. The lateral side of the foot usually rests on the table.

Central Ray: Perpendicular to the cassette (vertical), entering the groin area 2 inches medial and 2 inches inferior to the anterior superior iliac spine.

IMAGE EVALUATION

The acetabular area should be seen in AP projection, whereas the proximal femur (head, neck, trochanters) should be demonstrated in the lateral position. The lesser trochanter should be visible on the medial aspect of the proximal femur, and the femoral neck should be well demonstrated.

Specialized Pelvis Radiography

AP Frog-Leg (Modified Cleaves*) Pelvis Projection

RATIONALE FOR USE

The frog-leg pelvis projection may be used in conjunction with the routine AP pelvis projection to *evaluate the pelvis and upper femora.*

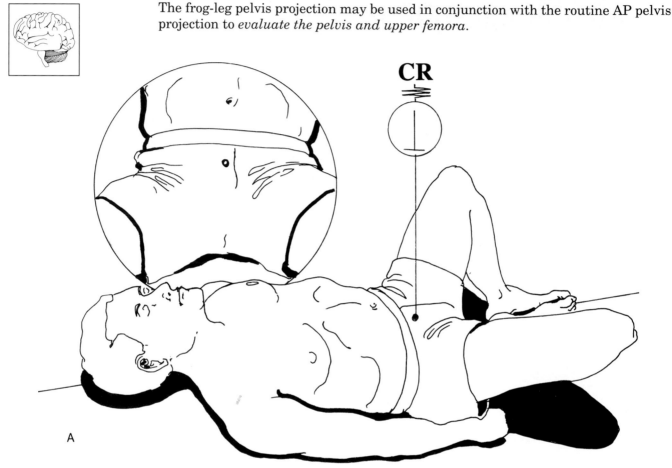

CR

A

□ **FIGURE 7–4.**

POSITION DESCRIPTION

Part Position: The patient is supine with the hips and knees flexed and the soles of the feet together. The feet are brought as close as possible to the buttocks, and the thighs are equally abducted to place the long axis of the femurs approximately 50° to the plane of the table (40° from vertical).

Central Ray: Perpendicular to the cassette, entering the midline 2 inches below the level of the anterior superior iliac spine.

AP Frog-Leg (Modified Cleaves*) Pelvis Projection *(continued)*

IMAGE EVALUATION

The pelvis is seen in AP projection. The upper femora are demonstrated in lateral position.

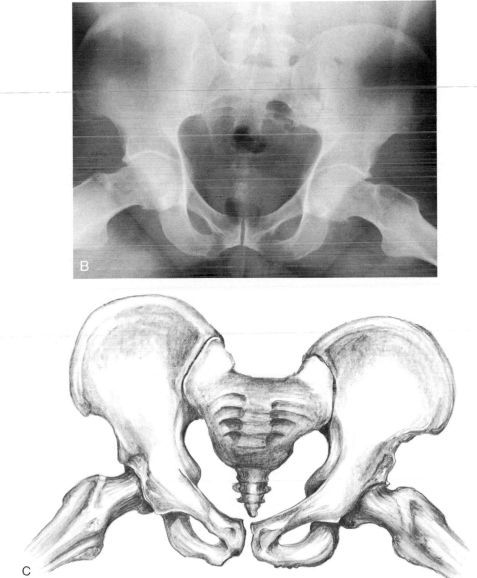

☐ **FIGURE 7–4.** *(continued)*

---

*Cleaves EN. Observations on lateral views of hips. *AJR* 1941; 39(6):964–966.

Inlet* Pelvis Position

RATIONALE FOR USE

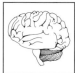

This position may be used in cases of pelvic trauma to *assess posterior displacement of the hemipelvis and inward or outward rotation of the anterior portion of the pelvis.*

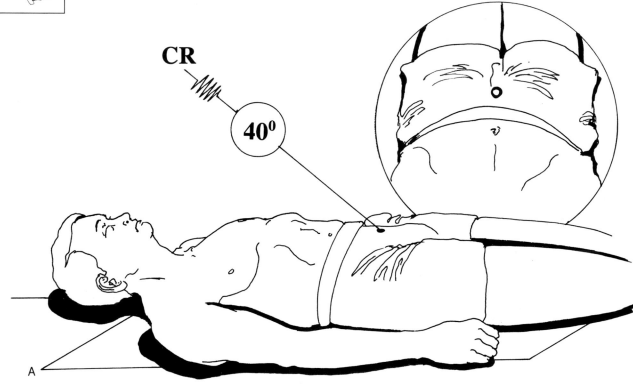

CR

40⁰

A

□ **FIGURE 7–5.**

POSITION DESCRIPTION

Part Position: The patient is supine, with the legs extended.

Central Ray: Angled 40° caudad, entering the midline at the level of the anterior superior iliac spine.

Note: An angle of 35° was recommended by Bridgman† in his original introduction of this position, as a modification of the original positions of Lilienfeld‡ and Staunig.§

Inlet* Pelvis Position *(continued)*

IMAGE EVALUATION

An axial projection of the pelvic ring should be demonstrated. When the anterior and posterior portions are properly exposed, the iliac wings are often obscured by excessive radiographic density.

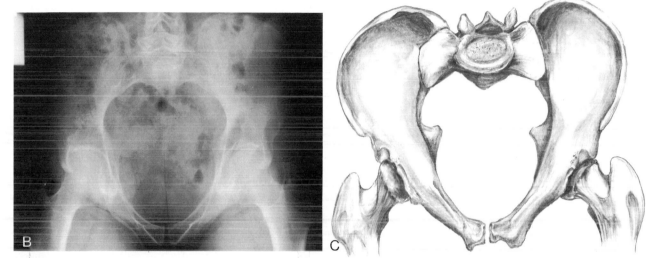

□ **FIGURE 7–5.** *(continued)*

---

*Pennal GF. Pelvic disruption: assessment and classification. *Clin Orthop* 1980; 151:12–21.
†Bridgman CF. Radiography of the hip bone. *Med Radiog Photog* 1952; 28(2):41–46.
‡Lilienfeld L. Die axiale Aufnahme der Regio pubica. *Fortschr Roentgenstr* 1918–1919; 24:285–290.
§Staunig K. Die axiale Aufnahme der Regio pubica. *Fortschr Roentgenstr* 1919–1921; 27:514–517.

Outlet (Tangential)* Pelvis Position

RATIONALE FOR USE

This position may be used in cases of pelvic trauma to assess *superior displacement of the posterior half of the pelvis and superior or inferior displacement of anterior pelvic structures.*

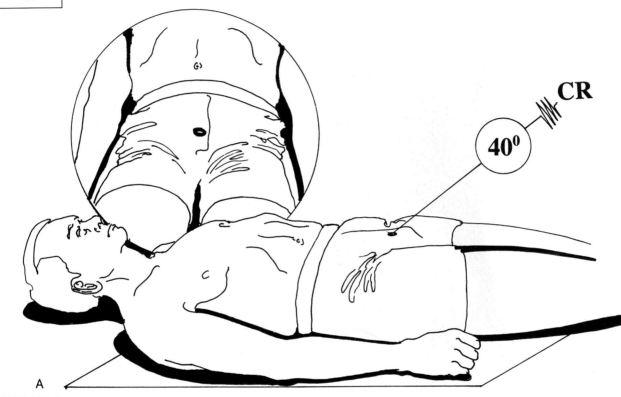

□ **FIGURE 7–6.**

POSITION DESCRIPTION

Part Position: The patient is supine with the legs extended.

Central Ray: Angled 40° cephalad, entering at the inferior aspect of the pubic symphysis.

Note: Taylor† recommended an angle of 30°–45° for females and 20°–35° for males.

Outlet (Tangential)* Pelvis Position *(continued)*

IMAGE EVALUATION

Orientation of the central ray perpendicular to the plane of the anterior pelvic bones reduces foreshortening and results in a true AP projection of the anterior pelvic structures. Much of the iliac wings are obscured by superimposition of the acetabular portions.

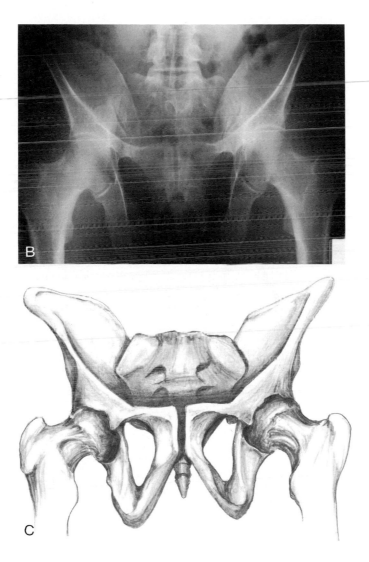

☐ **FIGURE 7–6.** *(continued)*

---

*Pennal GF. Pelvic disruption: assessment and classification. *Clin Orthop* 1980; 151:12–21.
†Taylor R. Modified anteroposterior projection of the anterior bones of the pelvis. *Radiog Clin Photog* 1941; 17:67–69.

Judet* Oblique Acetabulum Positions

Iliac Oblique Position

RATIONALE FOR USE

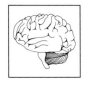

This position is used to *demonstrate fractures of the posterior (ilioischial) column and anterior rim of the acetabulum.* The iliac wing is also well visualized.

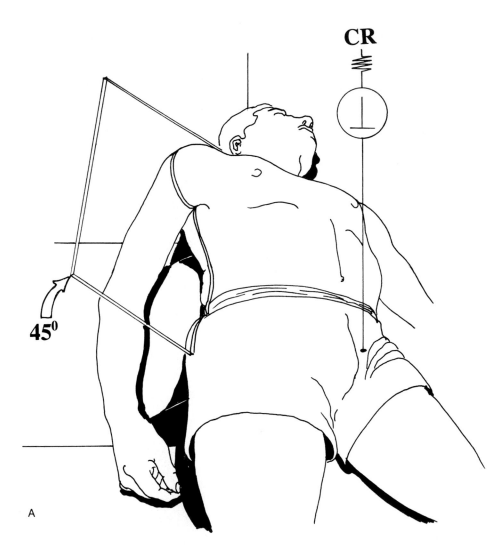

CR

45⁰

A

□ **FIGURE 7–7.**

POSITION DESCRIPTION

Part Position: The patient is placed in a 45° posterior oblique body position, with the side of interest down (closest to the table).

Central Ray: Perpendicular to the cassette, entering at the pubic symphysis.

Judet* Oblique Acetabulum Positions *(continued)*

Obturator Oblique Position

RATIONALE FOR USE

This position is used to *demonstrate fractures of the anterior (iliopubic) column and posterior rim of the acetabulum.* The obturator ring is also well visualized

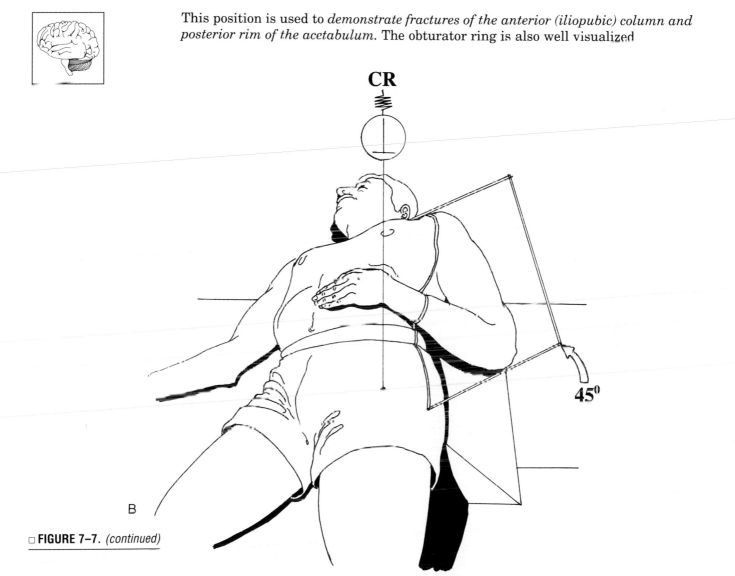

□ **FIGURE 7–7.** *(continued)*

POSITION DESCRIPTION

Part Position: The patient is placed in a 45° posterior oblique body position, with the side of interest up (farthest from table).

Central Ray: Perpendicular to the cassette, entering 2 inches inferior to the anterior superior iliac spine of the side up (affected side).

---

*Judet R, Judet J, Letournel E. Fractures of the acetabulum: classification and surgical approaches for open reduction. *J Bone Joint Surg* 1964; 46A(8):1615–1675.

Judet* Oblique Acetabulum Positions *(continued)*

Cross-Table Iliac Oblique Position

RATIONALE FOR USE

This position is used when patient's condition does not allow placement on the affected side. It *results in an iliac oblique radiograph with the affected side up.*

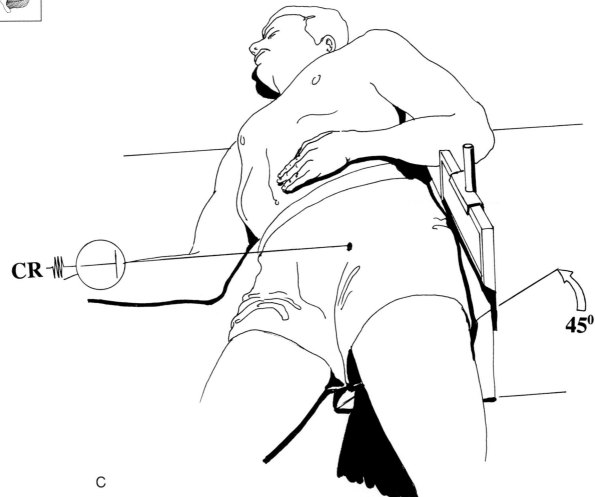

C

☐ **FIGURE 7–7.** *(continued)*

POSITION DESCRIPTION

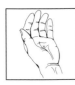

Part Position: The patient is placed in a 45° posterior oblique body position with the affected side up. The vertically oriented grid cassette is placed against the affected hip.

Central Ray: Horizontal and perpendicular to the cassette, entering at the pubic symphysis.

Judet* Oblique Acetabulum Positions *(continued)*

IMAGE EVALUATION

The affected side down (iliac oblique) position should demonstrate the posterior (ilioischial) column and anterior rim of the affected acetabulum. The iliac wing of the affected side should be seen without foreshortening.

The affected side up (obturator oblique) position should demonstrate the anterior (iliopubic) column and posterior rim of the affected acetabulum. The obturator foramen of the affected side should be seen without foreshortening and maximally open.

The cross-table iliac oblique position will have the same appearance as the affected side down iliac oblique position.

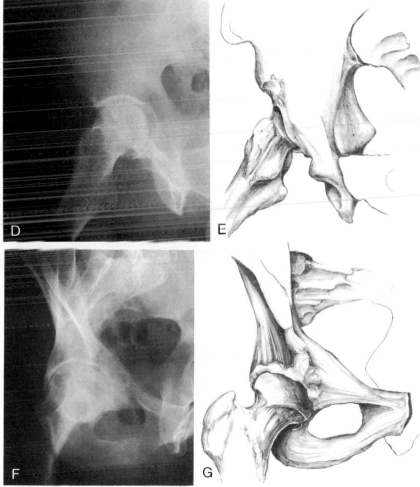

□ **FIGURE 7–7.** *(continued)*

(*D, E,* iliac oblique. *F, G,* obturator oblique.)

*Judet R, Judet J, Letournel E. Fractures of the acetabulum: classification and surgical approaches for open reduction. *J Bone Joint Surg* 1964; 46A(8):1615–1675.

Judet Oblique Acetabulum Positions *(continued)*

CASE STUDY

The patient presented with an obvious deformity to the right knee, after having been struck by an automobile.

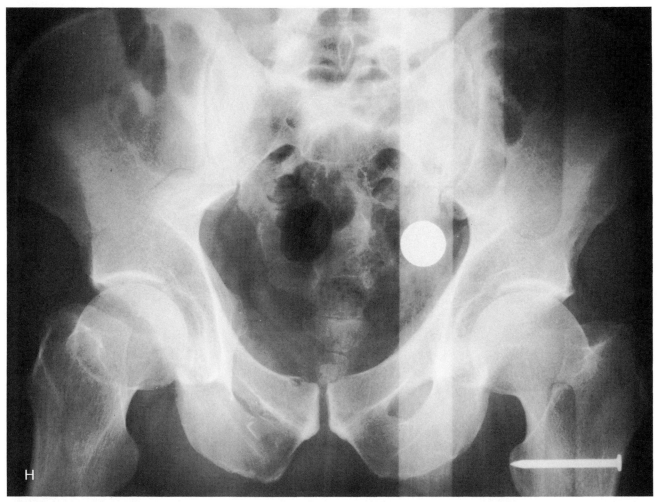

□ **FIGURE 7–7.** *(continued)*

A routine AP pelvis projection was taken in the trauma room and revealed no defects except a small line density on the right iliac wing.

Judet Oblique Acetabulum Positions *(continued)*

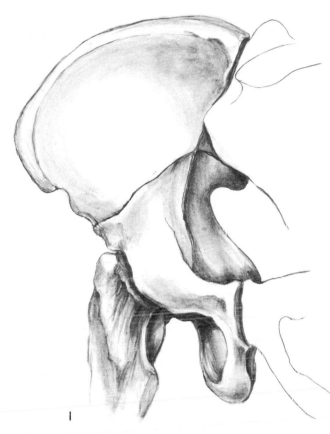

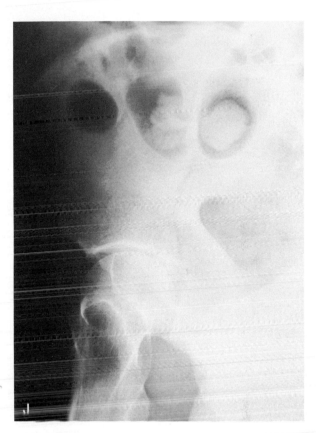

□ **FIGURE 7–7.** *(continued)*

Judet oblique acetabulum radiographs were taken, and the iliac oblique demonstrated a nondisplaced fracture involving the iliac wing and the right acetabulum.

Specialized Hip Joint Radiography

Axiolateral (Trauma/Surgical Lateral) Hip Position*,†

RATIONALE FOR USE

This position is used to obtain a lateral hip radiograph when the affected leg cannot be moved.

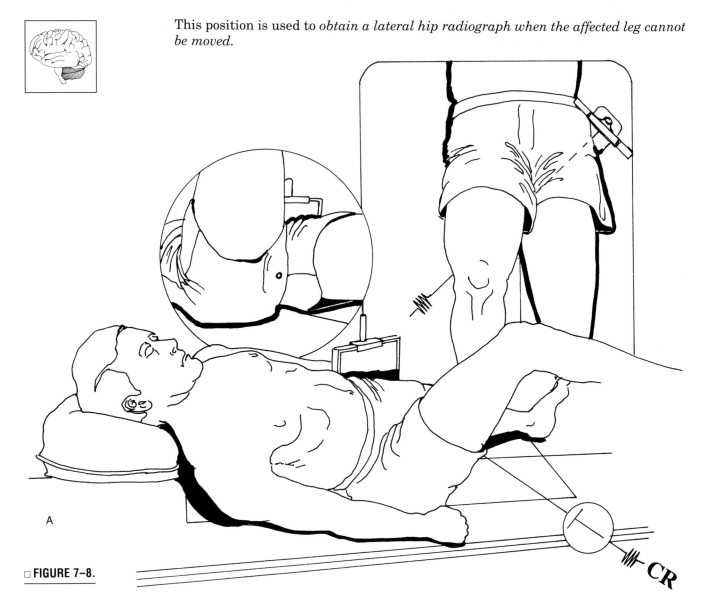

□ **FIGURE 7–8.**

POSITION DESCRIPTION

Part Position: The patient is in the supine position. The unaffected leg is flexed and elevated to prevent superimposition of the unaffected femur on the affected hip. The unaffected leg must be supported in the elevated position. A vertically oriented grid cassette is placed against the affected hip and angled so that it is parallel to the femoral neck. The cephalic edge of the cassette is gently pushed against the flank just above the crest.

Central Ray: Horizontal and perpendicular to the cassette, entering the perineal crease of the thigh midway between the anterior and posterior thigh surfaces.

Axiolateral (Trauma/Surgical Lateral) Hip Position*,† *(continued)*

IMAGE EVALUATION

The hip joint and proximal femur (head, neck, trochanters) should be seen in lateral position. The greater trochanter should be seen superimposed on the distal portion of the femoral neck. A small portion of the lesser trochanter should be seen on the posterior aspect of the femur. The position of the trochanters may vary with leg rotation.

Note: The axiolateral position was originated by Lorenz.* His technique has been modified by a number of authors, but the method currently in use is credited to Danelius and Miller.†

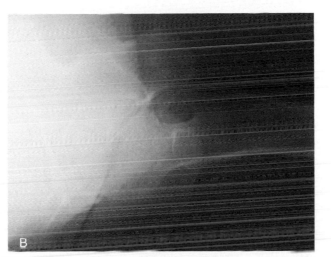

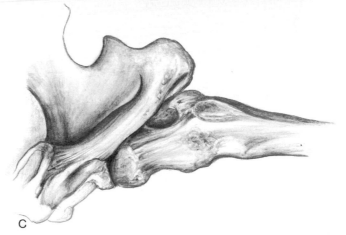

□ **FIGURE 7–8.** *(continued)*

---

*Lorenz. Die röntgenographische Darstellung des subskapularen Raumes und des Schenkelhalses im Querschnitt. *Fortschr Roentgenstr* 1917–1918; 25:342–343.
†Danelius G, Miller LF. Lateral view of the hip. *AJR* 1936; 35(2):282–284.

Modified Lauenstein* Lateral Hip Position

RATIONALE FOR USE

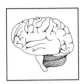

This lateral position is used to *assess the upper femur and hip joint when severe injury is not suspected.*

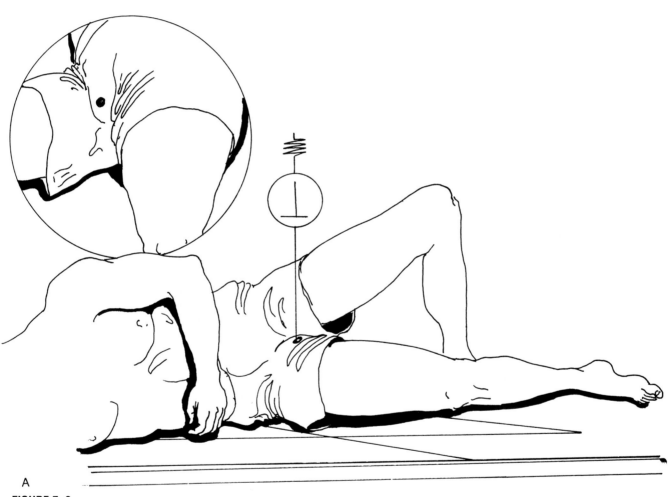

A

□ **FIGURE 7–9.**

POSITION DESCRIPTION

Part Position: The patient is placed in a near lateral position on the affected side. The affected hip and knee are flexed as much as possible (up to 90°). The pelvis is adjusted slightly backwards to prevent superimposition of the hip joints.

Central Ray: Perpendicular to cassette, entering at a point halfway between the anterior-superior iliac spine and the pubic symphysis.

Modified Lauenstein* Lateral Hip Position *(continued)*

IMAGE EVALUATION

The hip joint and proximal femur should be demonstrated in lateral position. The greater trochanter should be seen superimposed on the femoral neck.

Note: An article by Bridgman† indicates that Lauenstein's original flexed and abducted lateral position was to be performed with the patient supine and the central ray angled cephalad at an angle equal to that of the long axis of the femur. This corresponds to the Cleaves‡ position published in 1938. The earliest reference that we could find concerning modifying the position to a steep oblique position was Hickey.§ We could not ascertain the origin of the perpendicular central ray modification.

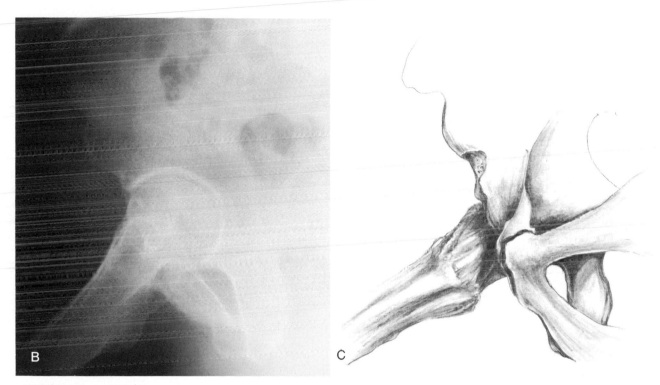

B C

□ **FIGURE 7–9.** *(continued)*

*Lauenstein C. Nachweis der "Kocher'schen Verbiegung" des Schenkelhalses bei der Coxa vara durch Röntgen-Strahlen. *Fortschr Röntgenstr* 1899–1900; 3–4:61–64.
†Bridgman CF. Radiography of the hip joint. Part four: lateral projection—extremity flexed and abducted. *Med Radiogr Photogr* 1951; 27(1):2–11.
‡Cleaves EN. Observations on lateral views of hips. *AJR* 1938; 39:964–966.
§Hickey PM. The value of the lateral view of the hip. *AJR* 1916; 3:308–309.

References

1. Berquist TH. *Imaging of the Acutely Injured Patient.* Baltimore: Urban & Schwartzenburg; 1985.
2. Berquist TH, Coventry MB. The pelvis and hips. *In* Berquist TH (ed). *Imaging of Orthopedic Trauma,* 2nd ed. New York: Raven Press; 1992:207–310.
3. Rogers LF. *Radiology of Skeletal Trauma,* 2nd ed. New York: Churchill Livingstone; 1992.
4. Burgess AR, Tile M. Fractures of the pelvis. *In* Rockwood CA, Green DP, Bucholz RW (eds). *Fractures in Adults.* Philadelphia: JB Lippincott; 1991:1399–1479.
5. Key JA, Conwell HE. *Management of Fractures, Dislocations, and Sprains.* St. Louis: CV Mosby; 1951.
6. Dunn AW, Morris HD. Fractures and dislocations of the pelvis. *J Bone Joint Surg* 1968; 50A:1639–1648.
7. Pennal GF, Tile M, Wadell JP, Garside H. Pelvic disruption: assessment and classification. *Clin Orthop* 1980; 151:12–21.
8. Young JWR, Resnick CS. Fractures of the pelvis: current concepts of classification. *AJR* 1990; 155:1169–1175.
9. Tile M. *Fractures of the Pelvis and Acetabulum.* Baltimore: Williams & Wilkins; 1984.
10. Huittinen VM, Slatis P. Fractures of the pelvis. Trauma mechanism, types of injury, and principles of treatment. *Acta Chir Scand* 1972; 138:563.
11. Tile M. Pelvic fractures: operative vs. non-operative treatment. *Orthop Clin North Am* 1980; 11:423–464.
12. Trunkey DD, Chapman MW, Lim RC, Dunphy JE. Management of pelvic fractures in blunt trauma injury. *J Trauma* 1974; 14:912.
13. Dunn AW, Russo CL. Central acetabular fractures. *J Trauma* 1973; 13:1568.
14. Judet R, Judet J, Letournel E. Fractures of the acetabulum: classification and surgical approaches for surgical reduction. *J Bone Joint Surg* 1964; 46A:1615–1647.
15. Alffram PA. An epidemiologic study of cervical and trochanteric fractures of the femur in an urban population. *Acta Orthop Scand (Suppl)* 1964; 65:1–109.
16. Atkins JM. Relevance of osteoporosis in women with fracture of the femoral neck. *Br Med J (Clin Res)* 1984; 288:597–601.
17. Garden RS. Reduction and fixation of subcapital fractures of the femur. *Orthop Clin North Am* 1974; 5:683–712.
18. Lam SF. Fractures of the neck of the femur in children. *J Bone Joint Surg* 1971; 53A:1165–1179.
19. Dimon JH, Hughston JC. Unstable intertrochanteric fractures of the hip. *J Bone Joint Surg* 1967; 49A:440–450.
20. Watson HK, Campbell RD, Wade PA. Classification, treatment, and complications of the adult subtrochanteric fracture. *J Trauma* 1964; 4:457–480.
21. Karlin LI. Injuries to the hip and pelvis in the skeletally immature athlete. *In* Nicholas JA, Hershman EB (eds). *The Lower Extremity and Spine in Sports Medicine.* St. Louis: CV Mosby; 1986:1292–1329.
22. Ortolani M. The classic congenital hip dysplasia in the light of early and very early diagnosis. *Clin Orthop* 1976; 119:6–10.
23. Barlow TG. Early diagnosis and treatment of congenital dislocation of the hip. *J Bone Joint Surg* 1962; 44B:292–301.
24. Coleman SS. *Congenital Dysplasia and Dislocation of the Hip.* St. Louis: CV Mosby; 1978.
25. Andren L, von Rosen S. The diagnosis of dislocation of the hip in newborns and the primary results of immediate treatment. *Acta Radiol (Stockh)* 1958; 49:89–95.
26. Catterall M. Perthes' disease. *In* Steinberg ME (ed). *The Hip and Its Disorders.* Philadelphia: WB Saunders; 1991:419–439.
27. Pizzutillo P. Slipped capital femoral epiphysis. *In* Balderton RA, Rothman RH, Booth RE, Hozack WJ (eds). *The Hip.* Philadelphia: Lea & Febiger; 1992:152–160.
28. Busch MT, Morrissy RT. Slipped capital femoral epiphysis. *Orthop Clin North Am* 1988; 18:636–647.
29. Glick EN, Mason RM, Wenley WG. Rheumatoid arthritis affecting the hip joint. *Ann Rheum Dis* 1963; 22:416–423.
30. McEwen C, DiTata D, Lingg C, et al. Ankylosing spondylitis and spondylitis accompanying ulcerative colitis, regional enteritis, psoriasis, and Reiter's disease: a comparative study. *Arthritis Rheum* 1971; 14:291–318.
31. Dwosh IL, Resnick D, Becker MA. Hip involvement in ankylosing spondylitis. *Arthritis Rheum* 1976; 19:683–692.
32. Resnick D, Niwayama G, Goergen TG, et al. Clinical, radiographic and pathologic abnormalities in calcium pyrophosphate dihydrate deposition disease (CPPD): pseudogout. *Radiology* 1977; 122:1–15.
33. Solomon L. Patterns of osteoarthritis of the hip. *J Bone Joint Surg* 1976; 58B:176–185.
34. Stewart IM. Radiological changes in primary osteoarthritis of the hip. *J Rheumatol* 1983; 10(Suppl 9):70–71.
35. Resnick D. Patterns of migration of the femoral head in osteoarthritis of the hip. Roentgenographic-pathologic correlation and comparison with rheumatoid arthritis. *AJR* 1975; 124:62–74.

EIGHT

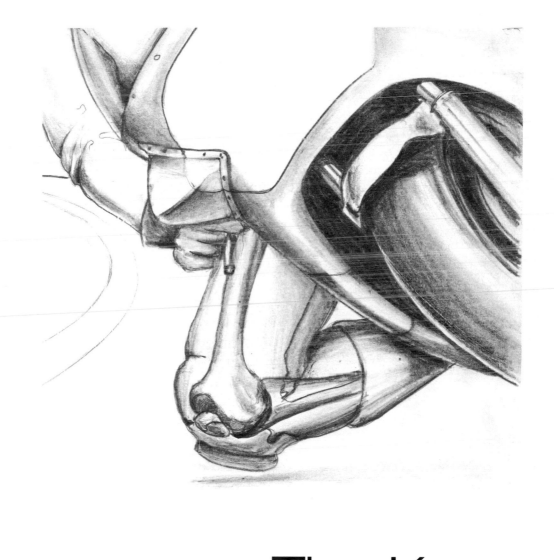

The Knee

THE KNEE: AN OVERVIEW

ROUTINE KNEE RADIOGRAPHY

Routine AP Knee Projection
Routine Lateral Knee Position

SPECIALIZED KNEE RADIOGRAPHY

AP Weight-Bearing Knee Position
AP External (Lateral) Oblique Knee Position
AP Internal (Medial) Oblique Knee Position
Intercondylar Fossa (Tunnel/Notch) Positions
Camp-Coventry
Holmblad
PA Weight-Bearing Flexed Knee Position

PATELLOFEMORAL JOINT RADIOGRAPHY

Axial (Sunrise/Skyline) Patella Projections
Merchants
Hughston
Settegast
Ficat

The Knee: An Overview

The knee is a principal joint of locomotion, serving as the fulcrum for the thigh and lower leg. The bony components of the knee joint are the femoral condyles, tibial plateaus, and the patella. A complex arrangement of ligaments, tendons, and muscles provide stability for the joint, which must withstand significant stress during motion. The knee is susceptible to a variety of injuries because of its location and biomechanical characteristics. These injuries may be caused directly, by impact, or indirectly, by torsional or angular forces. The knee is also involved in a variety of conditions that may cause pain or a reduction in joint motion.

Radiography plays an important role in the diagnosis of injury or disease affecting the knee. Many of these conditions produce features that are evident on radiographs. Fractures, joint effusions, calcifications, and joint-space changes can be demonstrated. This information may aid in decisions related to treatment.

Fractures of the knee occur in all component bones. The type and location of the fracture is often related to a patient's age or condition or to the mechanism of injury. Young patients may present with physeal or apophyseal involvement. Significant injury can occur in the elderly as a result of seemingly minor trauma.

Knee fractures involving the distal femur are commonly designated **supracondylar** and may be extra- or intra-articular. The extra-articular type is often transversely oriented, with varying degrees of comminution. Those involving the articular surface may have "T" or "Y" configurations involving the intercondylar notch or may be vertically oriented through one condyle. Supracondylar fractures are more common in older, osteoporotic adults because less force is required to initiate the injury;[1] a fall may be all that is required. Fracture in the supracondylar area is rare in children and adolescents, but if it is present, separation of the distal femoral epiphysis is often involved.[2]

Fractures of the proximal tibia may involve the plateaus, condyles, subcondylar region, anterior tubercle, intercondylar eminence, or tibial spines. The tibial plateaus are frequently involved in adults; the lateral plateau is most commonly affected.[3] Medial, posterior, and bicondylar fractures also occur. Tibial plateau fractures may be classified as local compression, split, split-compression, total depression, rim (avulsion or compression), and bicondylar.[4, 5] Subcondylar fractures usually require significant force and are often associated with bicondylar fractures of the tibial plateau.[6] Fracture of the subcondylar area in children usually involves the proximal tibial epiphysis.[2]

Avulsion fracture of the tibial tubercle most commonly occurs in adolescents participating in jumping sports.[7] All or part of the tubercle may be avulsed, and the fracture line may extend into the proximal tibial epiphysis.[8] A more chronic form of this injury is the **Osgood-Schlatter** lesion. The displaced fragments are fully corticated, and usually no single traumatic event is identified.[9, 10] Isolated avulsion of the tibial tubercle is uncommon in adults and is most often associated with subcondylar fractures of the proximal tibia.[6] Avulsion fractures of the anterior tibial spine or intercondylar eminence are more common in children and adolescents.[11] This fracture occurs at the origin of the anterior cruciate ligament (ACL). In adults, the ACL is more likely to tear than the intercondylar eminence is to avulse.[12] Other avulsion fractures in the knee may be associated with the posterior cruciate ligament, medial or lateral collateral ligaments, medial meniscus, lateral capsular ligament (Segond fracture), or iliotibial band. Recognition of the insignificant-appearing **Segond fracture** on the margin of the lateral tibial condyle is important because a very high percentage of these fractures are associated with ACL tears.[13]

Osteochondral fractures often involve the patella or femoral condyles. Lateral patellar dislocation may result in an osteochondral fracture on the medial patellar facet and/or the lateral femoral condyle.[14] The articular surface of the femoral condyles may also be damaged by a rotary stress or impaction of the patella against the condylar surface.[15] Adults are more likely to have pure chondral fractures without involvement of subchondral bone, whereas children and adolescents more often present with true osteochondral fractures.[16]

Fractures of the patella are fairly common, involving approximately 1% of all skeletal injuries.[17] Most are caused by direct blows to the patella, either from falls or automobile accidents. These fractures may occur at any age but are rare in children. If present, a pediatric patellar fracture is more likely to be an avulsion or osteochondral injury related to patellar dislocation.[14] Most patellar fractures are transversely oriented and located in the central or lower third.[18] The next most common fractures are stellate and comminuted fractures.[6]

Most fractures of the knee can be diagnosed on routine anteroposterior (AP) and lateral radiographs. Oblique positions enable further assessment when the presence or extent of a fracture is questioned. Intercondylar (tunnel/notch) positions are helpful for demonstration of osteochondral fractures, loose bodies, or osteochondritis dissecans. Axial patellar projections may be used to assess vertical or osteochondral fractures, subluxation, anatomical abnormalities, and articular degeneration.

Ligamentous and meniscal injuries are frequently seen in adults but are much less common in skeletally immature children. The ACL is most frequently injured, followed by the medial collateral ligament (MCL).[19] These ligaments are commonly torn during twisting combined with knee flexion and valgus force or by direct valgus force such as the football "clipping" injury.[20] Meniscal tears most often involve the posterior portion of the medial meniscus. Although these soft-tissue structures are radiolucent, AP, lateral, intercondylar fossa (tunnel/notch), and axial patellar radiographs are useful for evaluation of soft-tissue swelling, joint effusion, and osteochondral defects.

The knee may be involved, at least to some degree, in nearly all arthritides. It is the most frequent site of osteoarthritis, and the characteristic joint-space changes are often seen in the medial tibiofemoral compartment.[21] Patellofemoral osteoarthritis is equally common, manifested as subchondral patellar sclerosis and erosion of the anterior femoral cortex proximal to the condyles.[22] Rheumatoid arthritis in the knee may result in chronic intracapsular effusion, accumulating in the suprapatellar or popliteal bursa.[23] Joint-space narrowing tends to be uniform and may involve all three compartments (medial and lateral tibiofemoral, patellofemoral).[24] The knee is commonly involved in juvenile rheumatoid arthritis. In addition to adult rheumatoid changes, overgrowth of epiphyses and squaring of the patellar apex may be seen.[25]

The seronegative spondyloarthropathies also affect the knee. Approximately 30% of patients with long-standing ankylosing spondylitis eventually present with knee involvement that appears similar to that of rheumatoid arthritis.[26] Twenty-five to forty percent of patients with Reiter's syndrome manifest joint effusion in the knee. Periarticular tendinous calcification is frequently seen.[27] Soft-tissue swelling of the knee is commonly seen in the enteropathic (ulcerative colitis, Crohn's disease, Whipple's disease) arthropathies.[28] Psoriatic arthritis may also affect the knee; the manifestations appear similar to those of rheumatoid arthritis.

The crystal deposition arthropathies, such as gout and calcium pyrophosphate dihydrate (CPPD) deposition disease, may also involve the knee. Gout is relatively common in the knee and often manifests as soft-tissue swelling without articular involvement. Bone changes are frequently limited to marginal erosions with a relatively intact articular space.[29] CPPD, or pseudogout, most commonly affects the knee, with chondrocalcinosis present in the intra-articular fibrocartilage (meniscus), hyaline cartilage, articular capsule, and periarticular soft tissues. The medial tibiofemoral compartment is most frequently involved, followed by the patellofemoral compartment.[30]

The knee is commonly involved with intra-articular hemorrhage in hemophilia. This results in swelling (early), synovial fibrosis, hyaline cartilage destruction, and secondary osteoarthritis. Widening of the intercondylar fossa, caused by hemorrhage at the cruciate ligament insertions, is a significant indicator of this condition.[31]

Radiographic evaluation of arthritis in the knee includes, at a minimum, AP and lateral radiographs to assess bone changes and determine the presence of soft tissue swelling. Intercondylar fossa (tunnel/notch) positions enable evaluation of the posterior articular surface of the femoral condyles[32] and the presence of loose bodies or osteochondral defects. Axial patella projections are used to assess patellofemoral joint involvement. Weight-bearing AP or posteroanterior (PA) projections may be used to more accurately demonstrate the degree of joint-space narrowing present.[33, 34]

A great variety of other acquired conditions may affect the knee. However, for the sake of brevity, they cannot be covered in this overview.

Routine Knee Radiography

Routine AP Knee Projection

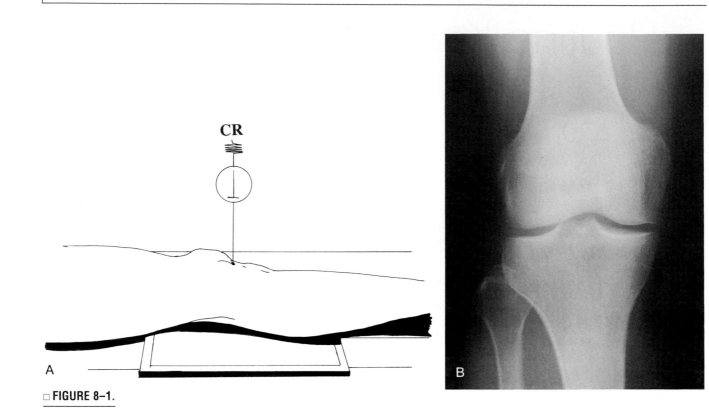

CR

A

B

☐ **FIGURE 8–1.**

POSITION DESCRIPTION

Part Position: The patient is supine with the legs extended. The affected leg is internally rotated slightly so that the coronal plane is through the femoral epicondyles and parallel to the plane of the cassette.

Central Ray: Perpendicular to the cassette, entering ½ inch inferior to the patellar apex.

Note: Martensen* recommended a *5° caudad* angle for slender patients (anterior-superior iliac spine [ASIS] to tabletop distance less than 19 cm) and a *5° cephalad* angle for heavy patients (ASIS-to-tabletop distance greater than 24 cm).

IMAGE EVALUATION

An AP projection of the distal femur and the proximal tibia and fibula should be demonstrated. The tibiofemoral joint space should be open. The patella will be superimposed over the distal femur. The medial third of the fibular head should be partially obscured by the tibia.

*Martensen KM. Alternate AP knee method assures open joint space. *Radiol Technol* 1992; 64(1):19–23.

Routine Lateral Knee Position

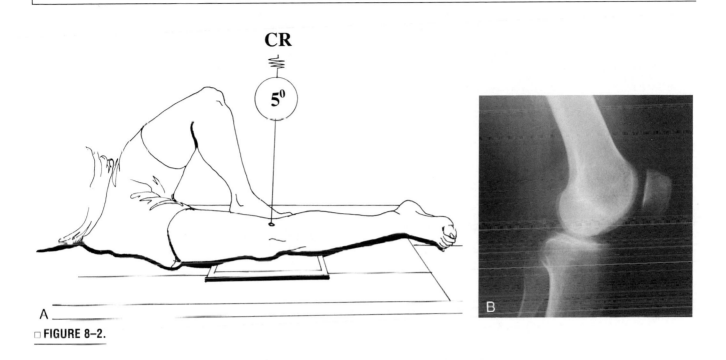

□ **FIGURE 8–2.**

POSITION DESCRIPTION

Part Position: The patient is in the lateral position, on the affected side. The affected knee is flexed approximately 30°, and the leg is rotated so that the coronal plane of the patella is perpendicular to the plane of the cassette. The opposite leg may be placed in front of or behind the affected leg, to prevent superimposition.

Central Ray: Angled 5° cephalad, entering the midpoint of the knee ½ inch distal to the medial epicondyle.

IMAGE EVALUATION

The distal femur, the proximal tibia and fibula, and the patella should be demonstrated in lateral position. The femoral condyles should be superimposed. The patellofemoral joint space should be open. The medial and lateral borders of the tibial plateau should be superimposed.

Specialized Knee Radiography

AP Weight-Bearing Knee Position*

RATIONALE FOR USE

This position may be used to *assess joint-space narrowing in the knee*. The weight-bearing posture may demonstrate the degree of narrowing more accurately than a recumbent position. Both knees are included for comparison.

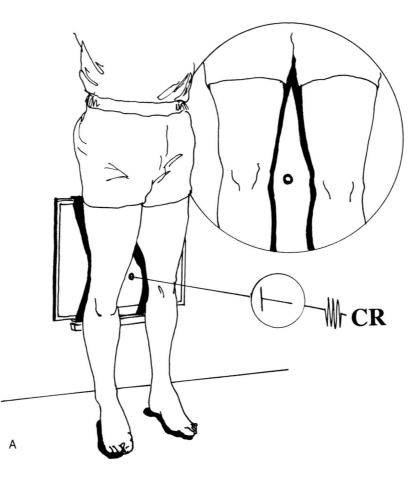

A

□ **FIGURE 8–3.**

POSITION DESCRIPTION

Part Position: The patient stands facing the tube, with the popliteal surface of the knees against the vertically oriented bucky/cassette. The patient should stand with toes pointing forward, knees extended, and equal weight on each foot.

Central Ray: Perpendicular to the cassette (horizontal), passing between the knees at the level of the tibiofemoral joint spaces (½ inch inferior to the patellar apices).

AP Weight-Bearing Knee Position* *(continued)*

IMAGE EVALUATION

An AP projection of both knees should be demonstrated. In the presence of articular cartilage degeneration, the affected tibiofemoral joint space may appear narrowed.

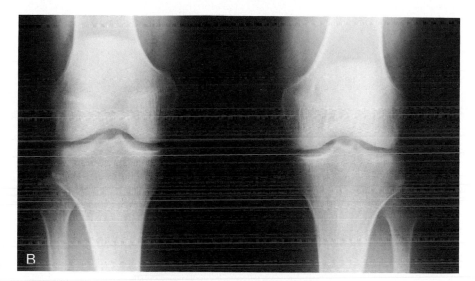

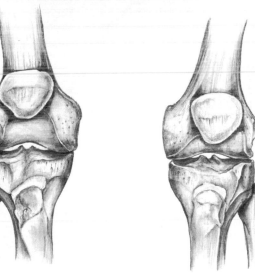

□ **FIGURE 8–3.** *(continued)*

*Ahlbäck S. Osteoarthritis of the knee—a radiographic investigation. *Acta Radiol (Diagn)* 1968; Suppl 277:7–72.

AP External (Lateral) Oblique Knee Position

RATIONALE FOR USE

The position may be used to demonstrate the *anterolateral and posteromedial portions of the knee.*

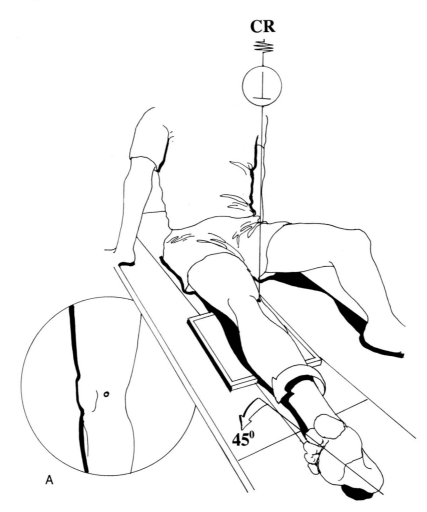

□ **FIGURE 8–4.**

POSITION DESCRIPTION

Part Position: The patient is supine with the leg extended and externally rotated 45°.

Central Ray: Perpendicular to the cassette, entering the knee joint at a level just inferior to the patellar apex.

Note: On heavy patients (ASIS to table distance greater than 24 cm), the central ray may be angled 5° cephalad.

AP External (Lateral) Oblique Knee Position *(continued)*

IMAGE EVALUATION

The medial femoral and tibial condyles should be well demonstrated. The proximal fibula should be superimposed by the tibia. Most of the patella should be superimposed over the lateral condylar area. The medial and lateral tibiofemoral joint space may appear unequal in height.

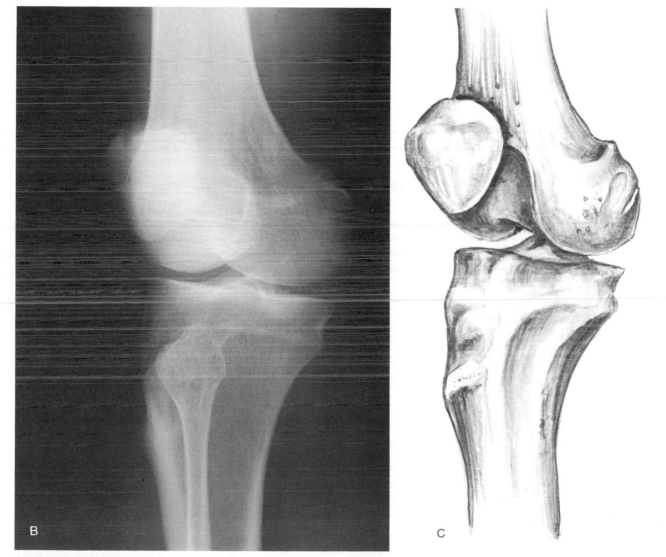

□ **FIGURE 8–4.** *(continued)*

AP Internal (Medial) Oblique Knee Position

RATIONALE FOR USE

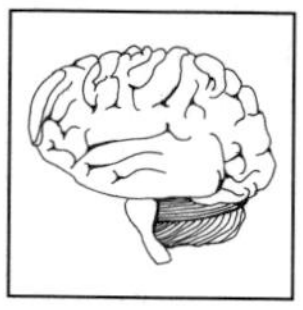

The position may be used to demonstrate the *anteromedial and posterolateral portions of the knee.*

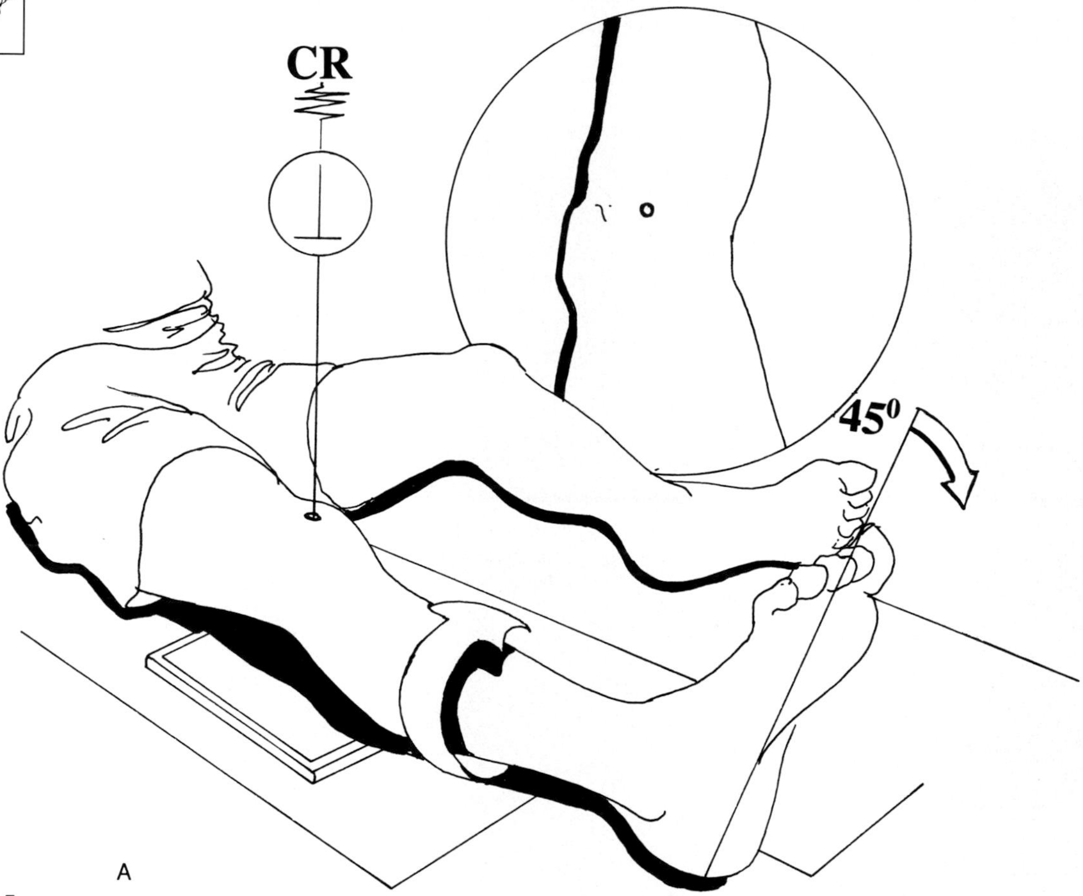

CR

45⁰

□ **FIGURE 8–5.**

A

POSITION DESCRIPTION

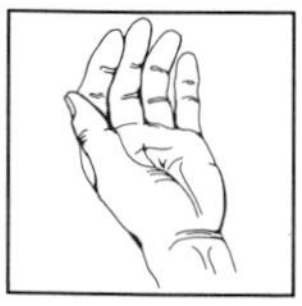

Part Position: The patient is supine with the leg extended and internally rotated 45°.

Central Ray: Perpendicular to the cassette, entering the knee joint at a level just inferior to the patellar apex.

Note: On heavy patients (ASIS to table distance greater than 24 cm), the central ray may be angled 5° cephalad.

AP Internal (Medial) Oblique Knee Position *(continued)*

IMAGE EVALUATION

The lateral femoral and tibial condyles should be well demonstrated. The fibular head and tibiofibular joint should be seen without superimposition. The patella should be partially superimposed over the medial condylar area. The medial and lateral tibiofemoral joint space may appear unequal in height.

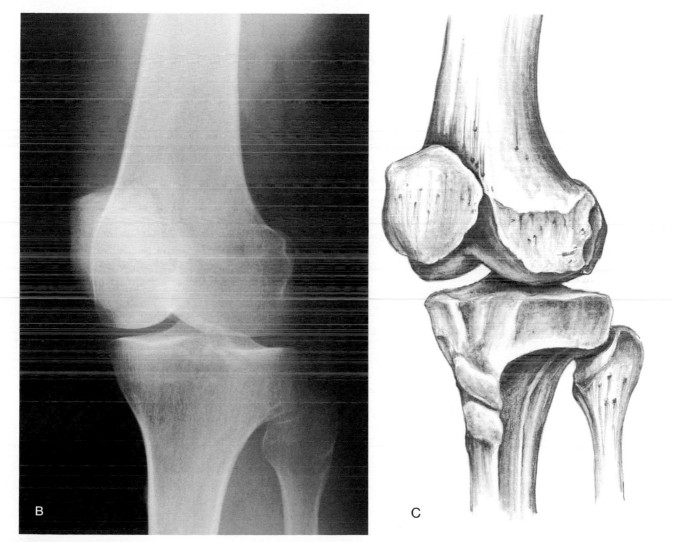

B

C

□ **FIGURE 8–5.** *(continued)*

Intercondylar Fossa (Tunnel/Notch) Positions

Camp-Coventry*

RATIONALE FOR USE

This position may be used to demonstrate the *intercondylar fossa and the posterior articular surface of the femoral condyles.* Osteochondral defects or joint-space narrowing may be evaluated.

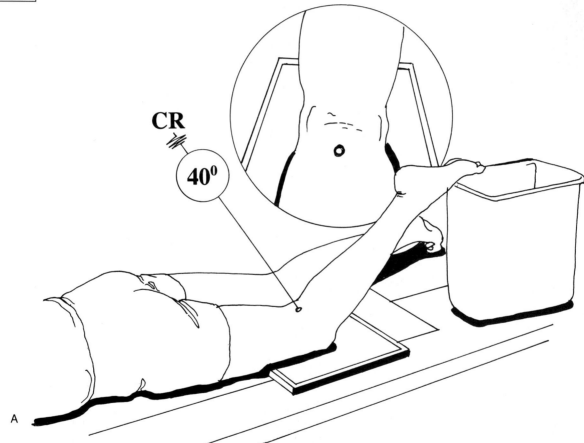

CR

40⁰

A

□ **FIGURE 8–6.**

POSITION DESCRIPTION

Part Position: The patient is prone with the affected knee flexed approximately 40° and the foot supported to maintain the position.

Central Ray: Angled caudad, perpendicular to the long axis of the lower leg, entering the popliteal region and exiting ½ inch inferior to the patellar apex.

Intercondylar Fossa (Tunnel/Notch) Positions *(continued)*

Camp-Coventry*

IMAGE EVALUATION

The intercondylar fossa (tunnel) and femoral condyles should be well demonstrated. The tibial spines (eminences) should be seen, and the tibiofemoral joint space should be open. The medial third of the fibular head should be partially obscured by the tibia.

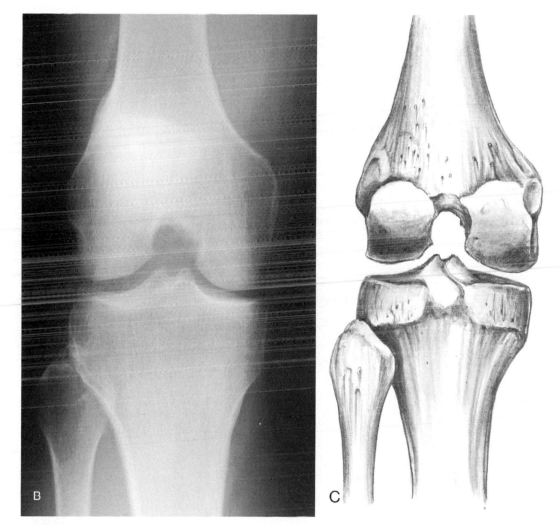

□ **FIGURE 8–6.** *(continued)*

---

*Camp JD, Coventry MB. Use of special views in roentgenography of the knee joint. *U.S. Naval Med Bull* 1944; 42:56–58.

Intercondylar Fossa (Tunnel/Notch) Positions *(continued)*

Holmblad*

RATIONALE FOR USE

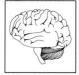

This position may be used to demonstrate the *intercondylar fossa and the posterior articular surface of the femoral condyles.* Osteochondral defects or joint-space narrowing may be evaluated.

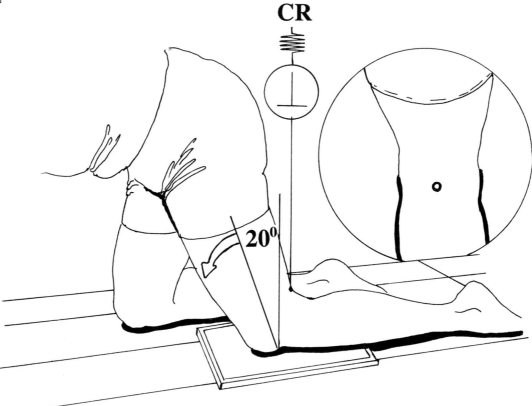

CR

20⁰

A

□ **FIGURE 8–7.**

POSITION DESCRIPTION

Part Position: The patient is in the kneeling position on the table, with the affected knee over the cassette. Knee flexion is adjusted to 70° by having the patient lean forward slightly.

Central Ray: Perpendicular to the cassette, entering the popliteal region and exiting ½ inch inferior to the patellar apex.

Intercondylar Fossa (Tunnel/Notch) Positions *(continued)*

Holmblad*

IMAGE EVALUATION

The intercondylar fossa (tunnel) and femoral condyles should be well demonstrated. The tibial spines (eminences) should be seen, and the tibiofemoral joint space should be open. The medial third of the fibular head should be partially obscured by the tibia.

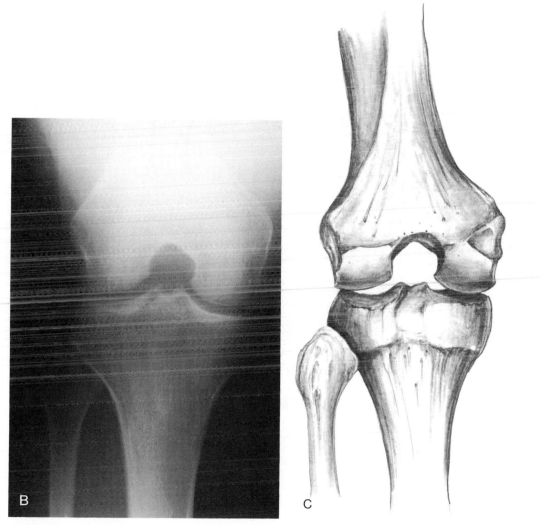

□ **FIGURE 8–7.** *(continued)*

---

*Holmblad EC. Postero-anterior x-ray view of the knee in flexion. *JAMA* 1937; 109:1196–1197.

PA Weight-Bearing Flexed Knee Position*

RATIONALE FOR USE

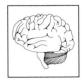

This position may be used to *assess joint-space narrowing in the knee*. The weight-bearing posture may demonstrate the degree of narrowing more accurately than may a recumbent position. The knee flexion enables evaluation of the posterior articular surface of the condyles. Both knees are included for comparison.

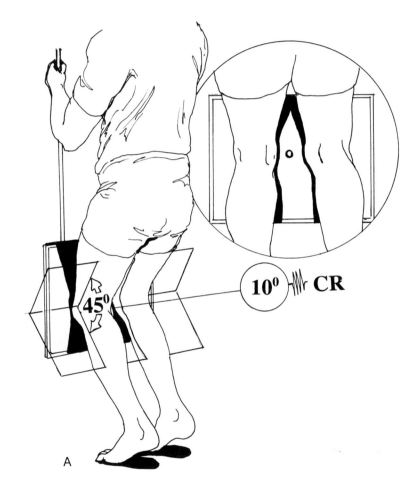

□ **FIGURE 8–8.**

POSITION DESCRIPTION

Part Position: The patient stands facing away from the tube, with the knees flexed 45° and the patellae against the vertically oriented bucky/cassette. The patient should stand with toes pointing forward and equal weight on each foot.

Central Ray: Angled 10° down from horizontal, passing between the knees at the level of the tibiofemoral joint spaces (exiting ½ inch inferior to the patellar apices).

Note: The 10° angle places the central ray parallel to the tibial plateau.

PA Weight-Bearing Flexed Knee Position* *(continued)*

IMAGE EVALUATION

A PA projection of both flexed knees should be demonstrated. A portion of the intercondylar fossa should be visible but not as much as is seen in the intercondylar fossa (tunnel/notch) position. In the presence of articular cartilage degeneration, the affected tibiofemoral joint space may appear narrowed.

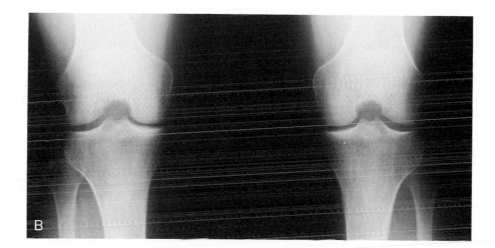

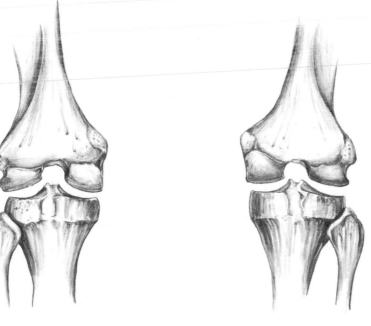

□ **FIGURE 8–8.** *(continued)*

---

*Rosenberg TD, Paulos LE, Parker RD, et al. The forty-five degree posteroanterior flexion weight-bearing radiograph of the knee. *J Bone Joint Surg* 1988; 70A(10):1479–1483.

Patellofemoral Joint Radiography

Axial (Sunrise/Skyline) Patella Projections

Merchant*

RATIONALE FOR USE

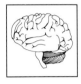

The Merchant axial patella projection may be used to *evaluate abnormalities of the patella and the patellofemoral joint.* The degree of flexion used (45°) allows demonstration of patellar subluxation. Both knees are examined for comparison.

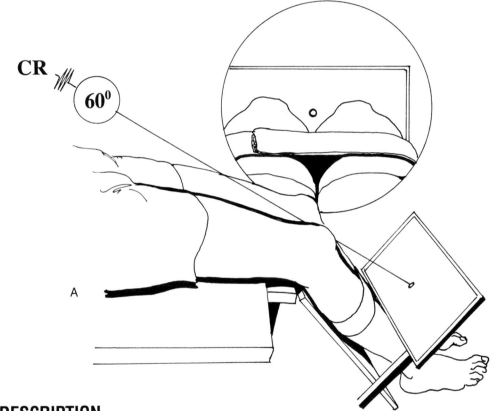

CR

60°

A

☐ **FIGURE 8–9.**

POSITION DESCRIPTION

Part Position: The patient is supine with the lower legs extended over the end of the table and supported by the special positioning device/cassette holder (The Axial Viewer, Orthopedic Products, Mountain View, California). The top of the device should be even with the top of the table and the leg rest adjusted at a 45° angle. The knees may need to be elevated slightly so that the femora are parallel to the tabletop. The legs should be strapped closely together with the attached Velcro strap. The cassette is rested on the swing down holder, with the cassette edge resting against the patient's distal lower legs.

Central Ray: Angled 60° caudad, directed between the knees at a level just proximal to the superior pole of the patella.

Note: A 60-inch source–to–image receptor distance (SID) is recommended, to compensate for the increased object–to–image receptor distance (OID) used with this method.

Axial (Sunrise/Skyline) Patella Projections *(continued)*

Merchant*

IMAGE EVALUATION

An axial projection of both patellae and patellofemoral joints should be demonstrated.

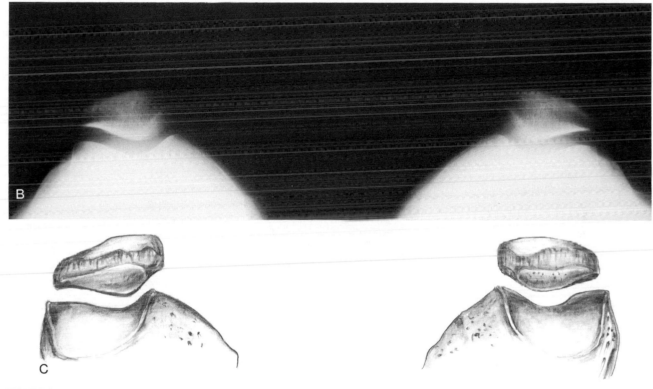

□ **FIGURE 8–9.** *(continued)*

---

*Merchant AC, Mercer RL, Jacobsen RH, Cool CR. Roentgenographic analysis of patellofemoral congruence. *J Bone Joint Surg* 1974; 56A:1391–1396.

Axial (Sunrise/Skyline) Patella Projections *(continued)*

Hughston*

RATIONALE FOR USE

The Hughston axial patella projection may be used to *evaluate abnormalities of the patella and the patellofemoral joint.* The degree of flexion used (55°) allows demonstration of patellar subluxation. Both knees are examined for comparison.

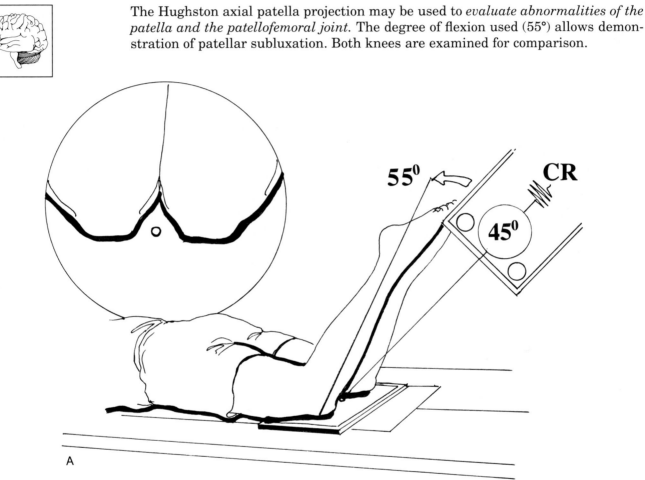

55⁰   45⁰   CR

A

□ **FIGURE 8–10.**

POSITION DESCRIPTION

Part Position: The patient is prone, with the knees flexed 55° and the feet resting on the collimator housing or other suitable support. The cassette is placed on the table under the knees.

Note: A cloth should be placed between the feet and the hot collimator housing.

Central Ray: Angled 45° cephalad, directed between the knees at a level just distal to the patellar apex.

Axial (Sunrise/Skyline) Patella Projections *(continued)*

Hughston*

IMAGE EVALUATION

An axial projection of both patellae and patellofemoral joints should be demonstrated.

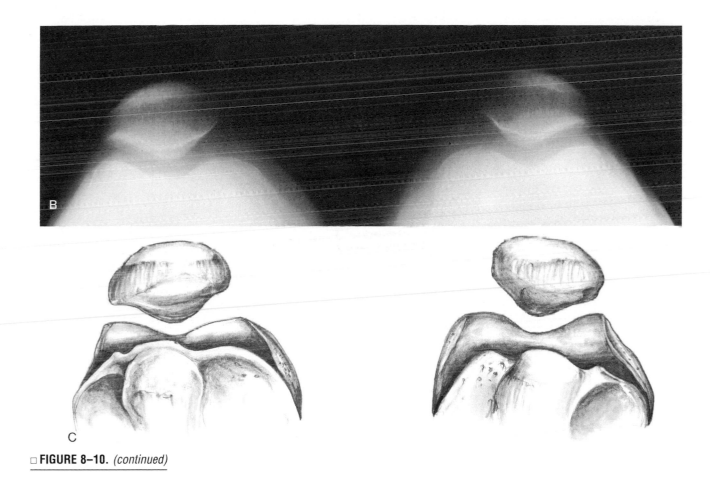

□ **FIGURE 8–10.** *(continued)*

*Hughston JC. Subluxation of the patella. *J Bone Joint Surg* 1968; 50A:1003–1026.

Axial (Sunrise/Skyline) Patella Projections *(continued)*

Settegast*

RATIONALE FOR USE

The Settegast axial patella projection may be used to *evaluate abnormalities of the patella and the patellofemoral joint.*

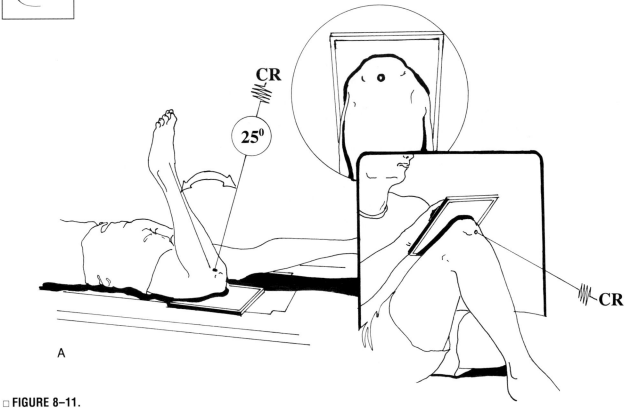

A

☐ **FIGURE 8–11.**

POSITION DESCRIPTION

Part Position: The patient is prone, with the knee acutely flexed (greater than 90°). The flexion may be maintained with a strap around the ankle that is held by the patient. The cassette is placed on the table under the knee.

Note: The position may also be done with the patient supine, knee flexed acutely, and the tube side of the cassette resting against the distal femur. Additional positions (lateral recumbent or sitting at end of table), maintaining the same part-to-cassette orientation, may be used.

Central Ray: Angled cephalad to pass tangentially through the patellofemoral joint (approximately 20°–25° angle between the central ray and the long axis of the tibia), entering just distal to the patellar apex.

Axial (Sunrise/Skyline) Patella Projections *(continued)*

Settegast*

IMAGE EVALUATION

An axial projection of the patella and patellofemoral joint should be demonstrated.

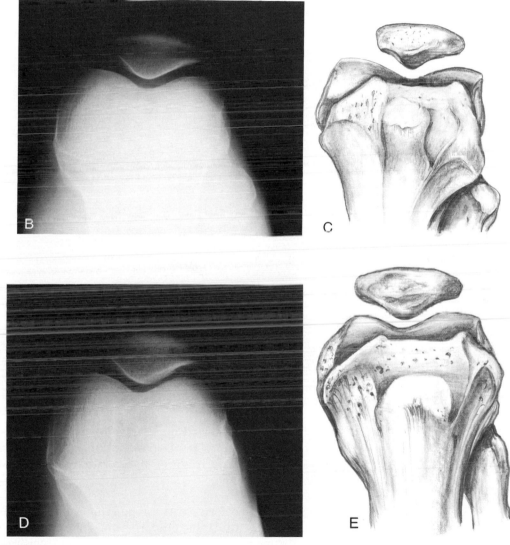

□ **FIGURE 8–11.** *(continued)*

(*B, C,* prone. *D, E,* seated.)

---

*Settegast H. Typische roentgenbilder von normalen menschen. *Lehmanns Med Atlanten* 1921; 5:211.

Axial (Sunrise/Skyline) Patella Projections *(continued)*

Ficat*

RATIONALE FOR USE

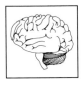

The Ficat axial patella projections may be used to *evaluate abnormalities of the patella and the patellofemoral joint.* The increments of flexion used (30°, 60°, 90°) allow evaluation of the patellofemoral relationship throughout the functional range. Both knees are examined for comparison.

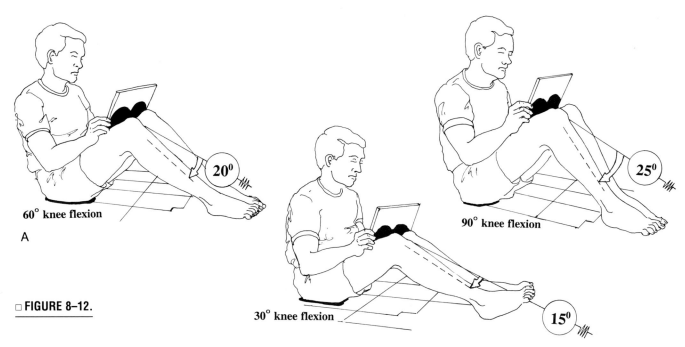

60° knee flexion

20°

A

90° knee flexion

25°

30° knee flexion

15°

□ **FIGURE 8-12.**

POSITION DESCRIPTION

Part Position: The patient is seated on the table with the knees raised in 30° of flexion. The edge of the cassette is placed against the distal femora and angled perpendicular to the central ray. Additional exposures are made with the knees in 60° and 90° of flexion.

Note: Ficat recommended performing these positions with the patient's lower legs extended over the end of the table and resting on an adjustable angle board. However, the inferosuperior projection and tube angles required make this very difficult without equipment modifications.

Central Ray: Directed upward from the feet to the knees and angled to pass tangentially through the patellofemoral joint, passing between the knees at a level just distal to the patellar apex.

Note: The recommended angles between the central ray and the tibia are as follows: 10°–15° for 30° knee flexion; 15°–20° for 60° knee flexion; and 20°–25° for 90° knee flexion.

Axial (Sunrise/Skyline) Patella Projections *(continued)*

IMAGE EVALUATION

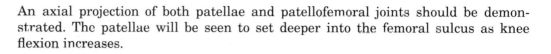

An axial projection of both patellae and patellofemoral joints should be demonstrated. The patellae will be seen to set deeper into the femoral sulcus as knee flexion increases.

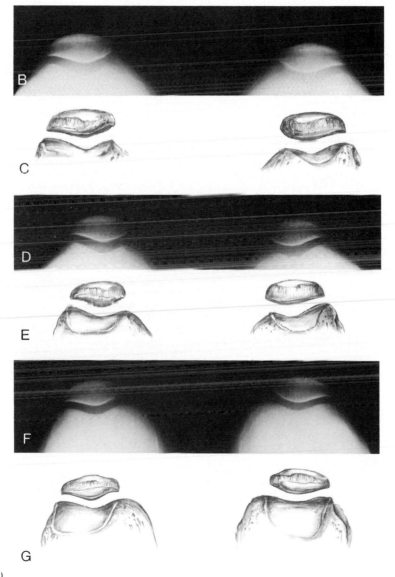

□ **FIGURE 8–12.** *(continued)*

(*B, C,* 30° knee flexion. *D, E,* 60° knee flexion. *F, G,* 90° knee flexion.)

Ficat P, Phillipe J, Bizou H. Le defile femoro-pattellaire. Rev Med Toulouse 1970; 6:241–244.

References

1. Schatzker J, Lambert DC. Supracondylar fractures of the femur. *Clin Orthop* 1979; 109:77–83.
2. Mann DC, Rajmaira S. Distribution of physeal and nonphyseal fractures in 2,650 long-bone fractures in children age 0-16 years. *J Pediatr Orthop* 1990; 10:713–716.
3. Hohl M. Tibial condylar fractures. *J Bone Joint Surg* 1967; 49A:1455–1467.
4. Hohl M. Tibial condylar fractures: long term followup. *Tex Med* 1974; 70:46–56.
5. Moore T. Fracture-dislocation of the knee. *Clin Orthop* 1981; 156:128–140.
6. Hohl M, Johnson, EE, Wiss DA. Fractures of the knee. *In* Rockwood CA, Green DP, Bucholz RW (eds). *Fractures in Adults,* 3rd ed. Philadelphia: JB Lippincott 1991; 2:1725–1797.
7. Mirbey J, Besarcenot J, Chambers RT, et al. Avulsion fractures of the tibial tuberosity in the adolescent athlete. *Am J Sports Med* 1988; 16:336–340.
8. Balmat P, Vichard P, Pem R. The treatment of avulsion fractures of the tibial tuberosity in adolescent athletes. *Sports Med* 1990; 9:311.
9. Osgood RB. Lesions of the tibial tubercle occurring during adolescence. *Boston Med Surg* 1903; 148:114–117.
10. Schlatter C. Verletzungen des Schnabelformigen Fortsatzes der Oberen Tibiaepiphyse. *Beitr Klin Chir* 1903; 38:874–887.
11. Oostvogel HJM, Klasen HJ, Reddingius RE. Fractures of the intercondylar eminence in children. *Arch Orthop Trauma Surg* 1988; 107:242.
12. Feagin JA. The syndrome of the torn anterior cruciate ligament. *Orthop Clin North Am* 1979; 10:81–90.
13. Goldman AB, Pavlov H, Rubenstein D. The Segond fracture of the proximal tibia: a small avulsion that reflects major ligament damage. *AJR* 1988; 151:1163–1167.
14. Rorabeck CH, Bobechko WP. Acute dislocation of the patella with osteochondral fracture. *J Bone Joint Surg* 1976; 58B:237–240.
15. Kennedy JC, Grainger RW, McGraw RW. Osteochondral fractures of the femoral condyle. *J Bone Joint Surg* 1966; 48B:436–440.
16. Johnson-Nurse C, Dandy DJ. Fracture-separation of articular cartilage in the adult knee. *J Bone Joint Surg* 1985; 67B:42.
17. Boström A. Fractures of the patella: a study of 422 patellar fractures. *Acta Orthop Scand* 1972; 143(Suppl):1–80.
18. Nummi J. Fracture of the patella: a clinical study of 707 patellar fractures. *Ann Chir Gynaecol Fenn* 1971; 60(Suppl): 179.
19. Rand JA, Berquist TH. The Knee. *In* Berquist TH (ed). *Imaging of Orthopedic Trauma,* 2nd ed. New York: Raven Press; 1991:333–432.
20. Scott WN. *Ligament and Extensor Mechanism Injuries of the Knee.* St. Louis: Mosby Year Book; 1991.
21. Freeman MAR. The surgical anatomy and pathology of the arthritic knee. *In* Freeman MAR (ed). *Arthritis of the Knee.* New York: Springer-Verlag; 1980:31–56.
22. Norman A. Osteoarthritis. *In* Taveras JM, Ferrucci JJ (eds). *Radiology: Diagnosis-Imaging-Intervention,* vol 5. Philadelphia: JB Lippincott; 1992:1–26.
23. Pastershank SP, Mitchell DM. Knee joint bursal abnormalities in rheumatoid arthritis. *J Can Assoc Radiol* 1977; 28:199–203.
24. Chaplin DM. The pattern of bone and cartilage damage in the rheumatoid knee. *J Bone Joint Surg* 1971; 53B:711–717.
25. Martel W, Holt JF, Cassidy JT. Roentgenologic manifestations of juvenile rheumatoid arthritis. *AJR* 1962; 88:400–423.
26. Resnick D. Patterns of peripheral joint disease in ankylosing spondylitis. *Radiology* 1974; 110:523.
27. Weldon WV, Scalettar R. Roentgen changes in Reiter's syndrome. *AJR* 1961; 86:344.
28. Resnick D. Enteropathic arthropathies. *In* Resnick D, Niwayama G (eds). *Diagnosis of Bone and Joint Disorders,* 2nd ed. Philadelphia: WB Saunders; 1988:1218–1251.
29. Watt I, Middlemiss H. The radiology of gout. *Clin Radiol* 1975; 26:27.
30. Resnick D, Niwayama G, Goergen TG, et al. Clinical, radiographic, and pathologic abnormalities in calcium pyrophosphate dihydrate deposition disease (CPPD): pseudogout. *Radiology* 1977; 122:1.
31. Greenfield GB. *Radiology of Bone Diseases,* 5th ed. Philadelphia: JB Lippincott; 1990.
32. Resnick D, Nint V. The "tunnel" view in assessment of cartilage loss in osteoarthritis of the knee. *Radiology* 1980; 137:547–548.
33. Leach RE, Gregg T, Siber FJ. Weight-bearing radiography in osteoarthritis of the knee. *Radiology* 1970; 97:265–268.
34. Rosenberg TD, Paulos LE, Parker RD, et al. The forty-five-degree posteroanterior flexion weight-bearing radiograph of the knee. *J Bone Joint Surg* 1988; 70A:1479–1483.

NINE

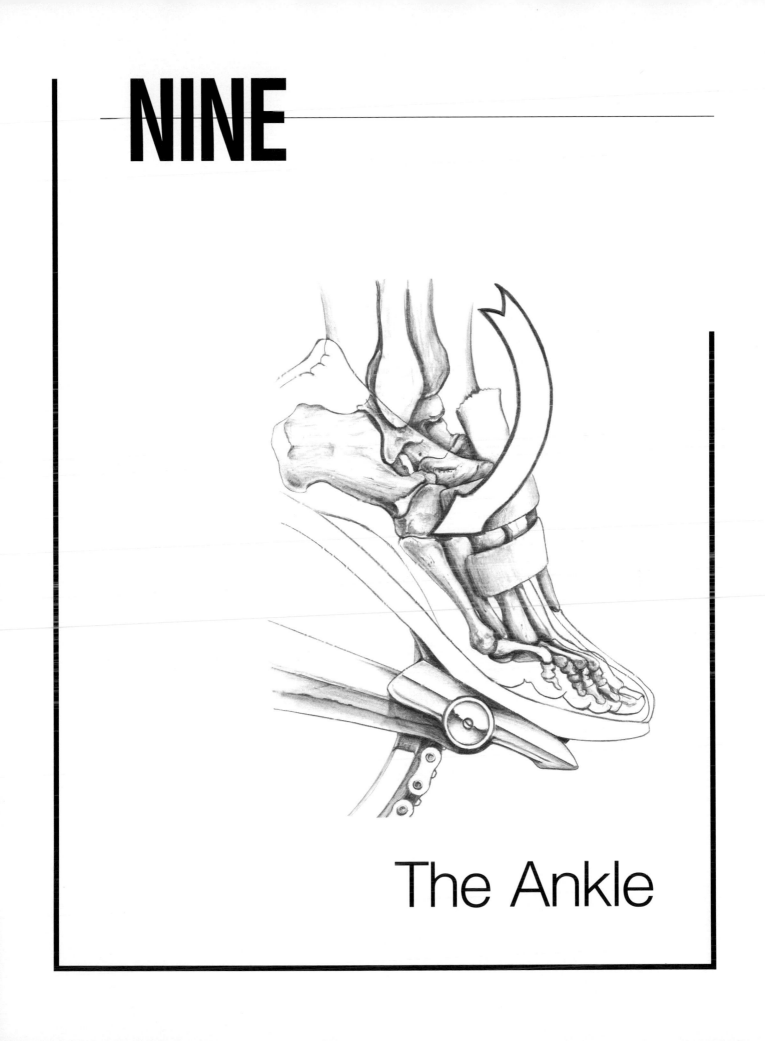

The Ankle

THE ANKLE: AN OVERVIEW

ROUTINE ANKLE RADIOGRAPHY

Routine AP Ankle Projection
Routine Internal (Medial) Oblique Ankle Position
Routine Lateral Ankle Position

SPECIALIZED ANKLE RADIOGRAPHY

External (Lateral) Oblique Ankle Position
Mortise Position
"Poor" Lateral Ankle Position

The Ankle: An Overview

The ankle joint, along with the subtalar joints, allows many movements of the foot. These motions include dorsiflexion, plantarflexion, inversion (supination-adduction), eversion (pronation-abduction), internal rotation, and external rotation. The ankle contributes to locomotion by dorsiflexing and plantarflexing during the gait cycle. Any condition that disrupts the stability or motion of this joint may affect the patients ability to walk effectively. Failure to recognize a destabilizing condition may result in chronic changes in the joint architecture. Radiography has an important role in the assessment of ankle joint congruence.

The ankle is subject to a number of fractures and ligamentous injuries. An ankle sprain consists of injury to the medial or lateral ligamentous structures and is one of the most common joint injuries.[1] The sprain may be a mild stretch (grade 1), a partial tear (grade 2), or a complete tear with instability (grade 3). The lateral ligament complex is most frequently injured as a result of forced inversion of the foot.[2] Tears of the deltoid (medial) ligament complex is associated with eversion injuries and is not often seen without malleolar fractures or tibiofibular diastasis.[3] Routine anteroposterior (AP), mortise, and lateral radiographs are usually taken and may demonstrate soft-tissue swelling, joint effusion, avulsion fracture (grade 4 sprain), or tibiotalar joint asymmetry. Varus and valgus stress radiography may be necessary for demonstrating questionable instability. Other soft tissue injuries, such as tendon ruptures or plantar fascitis, are not effectively assessed with the use of routine radiography.

The patterns of ankle fractures are related to a patient's age, condition of the bone, and mechanism of injury (position of foot and loading force factors). The classification of fracture patterns may be based on the mechanism of injury (Lauge-Hansen[4]) or the level of fibular fracture as an indicator of syndesmosis injury and mortise displacement (Danis[5]/Weber[6, 7] - AO[8]). Most ankle fractures are the result of inversion or eversion injuries, often occurring in combination with adduction, abduction, lateral rotation, or axial forces.[9] Inversion injuries are most common; supination–lateral rotation accounts for over half of ankle fractures.[10]

The patterns of injury progress across the joint and depend on the severity and/ or duration of applied forces. The lateral side (lateral collateral ligaments, lateral malleolus) is injured first with inversion forces and, conversely, the medial side (deltoid ligament, medial malleolus) is affected first in eversion injury. The ligaments under tension may stretch, rupture, or avulse from their bone attachments. In the later stages of injury, the opposite malleolus and/or ligaments are affected. Osteochondral fracture of the talar dome may accompany inversion ankle injury. The lateral surface is usually involved in inversion-dorsiflexion, and the medial surface is affected in inversion-plantarflexion.[11] Mediolateral or anteroposterior shift of the talus, in relation to the tibial plafond, indicates joint instability.

The fibular fracture, if present, tends to have a characteristic radiographic appearance related to the mechanism of injury. A transverse avulsion fracture of the lateral malleolus indicates pure inversion (supination-adduction) injury. A spiral fibular fracture at or just proximal to the tibiotalar joint, best demonstrated on the lateral radiograph, is characteristic of the commonly seen supination–lateral rotation injury. An oblique or comminuted fibular fracture at or just proximal to the tibiotalar joint, best demonstrated on the AP radiograph, is seen as a late-stage occurrence in pure eversion (pronation-abduction) injury. A spiral fibular fracture, often well above the tibiotalar joint, is a late-stage result of pronation–lateral rotation injury.

A variety of fractures occur at the ankle. **Dupytren's fracture,**[12] also called **Pott's fracture,**[13] consists of a fibular fracture proximal to the ankle joint with tibiofibular diastasis and a frequently associated talar shift caused by deltoid ligament tear or medial malleolar fracture. A fracture of the proximal fibula near the head with rupture of the interosseous membrane and distal tibiofibular syndesmosis, often accompanied by deltoid ligament tear or medial malleolus fracture, is termed **Maisonneuve's**[14] **fracture.** Rogers[15] stated that the entire lower leg should be radiographed in order to rule out proximal fibular fracture if an isolated posterior tibial lip fracture is identified or if either clear space (medial or lateral) is widened without evidence of injury to the opposite side of the joint.

A **Tillaux**[16]**-Chaput**[17] **fracture** involves avulsion of either the anterior or posterior tubercle of the lateral tibial articular surface with diastasis of the tibiofibular syndesmosis. This fracture is usually involved in a triad injury that includes the tubercle avulsion fracture with tibiofibular diastasis, deltoid ligament rupture or medial malleolus fracture, and a fibular fracture proximal to the tibiotalar joint.[18] **LaFort**[19]**-Wagstaffe**[20] fractures consist of an avulsion of the anterior fibular tubercle by the anterior tibiofibular ligament.

A **trimalleolar fracture,**[21] or **Cotton's fracture,**[22] consists of a combination of fractures involving the medial malleolus, lateral malleolus, and the posterior lip of the tibia (posterior malleolus[23]). A supramalleolar transverse, oblique, or comminuted fracture of the distal tibia is termed **Malgaigne's fracture.** A fibular fracture accompanies Malgaigne's fracture.[24] **Gosselin's fracture** is a V-shaped fracture of the distal tibia that may extend into the articular plafond.[25] The **pilon fracture**[26] is a comminuted fracture of the tibial plafond caused by impaction of the talus against the plafond.[27] The medial malleolus, lateral malleolus, anterior tibial lip, and the distal tibia proximal to the articular surface are involved. A hallmark of the pilon fracture is an anteriorly displaced fracture of the anterior tibial lip, often maintained in association with the talus.[15]

Dislocations of the ankle joint are usually associated with fractures. A number of the previously mentioned fractures may progress to fracture-dislocation in their later stages. **Bosworth's fracture**[28] consists of a spiral fracture of the distal fibula with posterior dislocation and entrapment of the proximal fragment posterior to the tibia. This injury results from severe external rotation of the foot. The posterior fibular dislocation can also occur without fracture.[29] Pure dislocations of the tibiotalar joint do occur; medial displacement of the talus is most commonly seen.[30]

Ankle injuries in children result from the same forces that cause injury in adults. However, the injury patterns differ because of the presence of the distal tibial and fibular physes. A great number of ankle fractures in children involve these physes. Osseous fractures associated with the physeal injury may be complete or incomplete (greenstick, torus). These physeal fractures are considered equivalent to ligamentous injuries in adults because the physis is two to five times weaker than the ligaments.[31] A minimally displaced Salter-Harris type I fracture of the distal fibula may result from an inversion injury and is equivalent to the adult ankle sprain. Rogers[15] suggested that when this injury is suspected, an external oblique position should be added to the radiographic examination to better demonstrate this minimally displaced fibular fracture.

The commonly occurring supination–lateral rotation injury may result in a Salter-Harris type I or II fracture involving the posterolateral aspect of the distal tibial physis and a greenstick fracture of the distal fibula proximal to the physis.[32] Eversion or pronation injuries may result in Salter-Harris type I or II fracture involving the anterolateral aspect of the distal tibial physis and sometimes includes a fibular fracture.[33] All other Salter-Harris type fractures can be found in the ankle. In addition, juvenile versions of Tillaux's, Bosworth's, and the triplane fractures may occur.

Radiographic evaluation of ankle fractures should include AP, internal (medial) oblique, and lateral radiographs. Although the 45° internal oblique is commonly included, the mortise oblique (15°–20°)[34] is recommended for initial evaluation. The mortise position results in a true AP projection of the ankle mortise and better demonstrates the relationships of joint structures. Additional radiographs should be included when the initial examination is inconclusive. As previously mentioned, the entire lower leg should be radiographed when ankle joint incongruity is seen without a bone injury pattern that is consistent with the instability. The "poor" lateral position[35] may demonstrate fractures of the posterior tibial lip and the anterior surface of the medial malleolus. The external oblique position may demonstrate fracture of the anterior tibial tubercle and Salter-Harris type I or II fractures of the distal fibular physis. Stress radiography (AP or lateral) may assist in evaluation of suspected ligamentous injuries of the ankle.

The ankle may be involved, at least to some degree, in nearly all arthritides. Routine AP, oblique, and lateral radiographs are usually sufficient to evaluate arthritis in the ankle joint. Rheumatoid arthritis is seen in the ankle, but less frequently than in the knee, hand, wrist, and foot.[36] Radiographic manifestation is often limited to soft-tissue swelling and masses caused by synovial hypertrophy[37] but may progress to loss of joint space and bone erosions. The rheumatoid variants or seronegative spondyloarthropathies manifest in the ankle; however, ankylosing spondylitis is rarely seen.[38] Radiographic abnormalities of the ankle joint are seen in 30°–50° of patients with Reiter's syndrome.[39] Soft-tissue swelling is most often present, but the bone changes associated with Reiter's syndrome (fluffy periostitis, joint space narrowing, marginal erosions) may occur. Psoriatic arthritis also occurs in the ankle and has a radiographic appearance similar to that of Reiter's syndrome.

Primary osteoarthritis is seldom seen in the ankle. It is more commonly secondary, related to athletics, trauma, other arthritides, and postsurgical or congenital fusion of the subtalar joints.[40] The crystal deposition arthritides (gout, crystal pyrophosphate dihydrate deposition disease [CPPD]) do not frequently affect the ankle. The ankle is second in frequency of involvement in the enteropathic (colitic) arthropathies,[41] manifested radiographically as monoarticular soft-tissue swelling and periarticular osteoporosis.[42]

A great variety of other acquired conditions may affect the ankle. However, for the sake of brevity, they cannot be covered in this overview.

Routine Ankle Radiography

Routine AP Ankle Projection

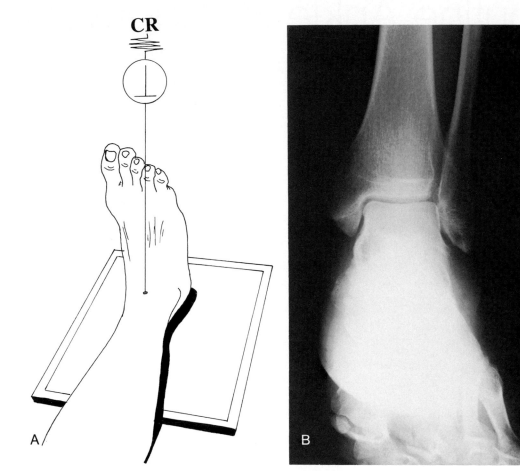

□ **FIGURE 9–1.**

POSITION DESCRIPTION

Part Position: The patient is supine or sitting, with the leg extended. The foot is dorsiflexed so that the plantar surface is perpendicular to the cassette. The ankle is rotated so that the long axis of the foot is vertical.

Central Ray: Perpendicular to the cassette (vertical), entering midway between the medial and lateral malleoli.

IMAGE EVALUATION

An AP projection of the ankle joint should be demonstrated without rotation, as evidenced by an open medial clear space (medial talomalleolar articulation), closed distal tibiofibular articulation, and slight superimposition of the lateral malleolus on the talus.

Routine Internal (Medial) Oblique Ankle Position

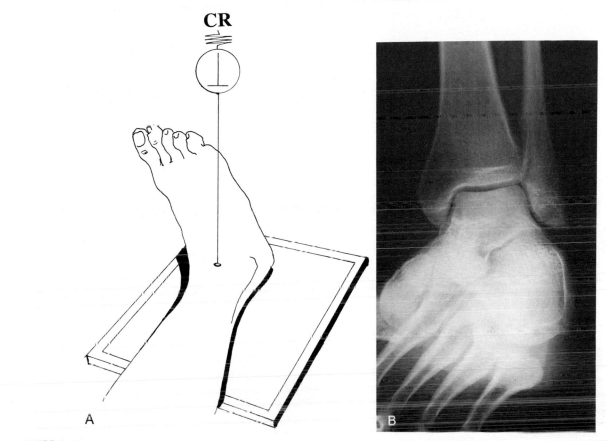

CR

A

B

□ FIGURE 9–2.

POSITION DESCRIPTION

Part Position: The patient is supine or sitting, with the leg extended. The foot is dorsiflexed so that the plantar surface is perpendicular to the cassette. The leg is rotated inward so that the ankle is in a 45° internal (medial) oblique position .

Central Ray: Perpendicular to the cassette, entering midway between the malleoli.

Note: Although the 45° internal (medial) oblique is commonly included in ankle routines, the mortise position is recommended because it demonstrates a "true" AP of the ankle mortise joint.

IMAGE EVALUATION

The lateral malleolus and tibiofibular articulation should be well demonstrated.

Routine Lateral Ankle Position

CR

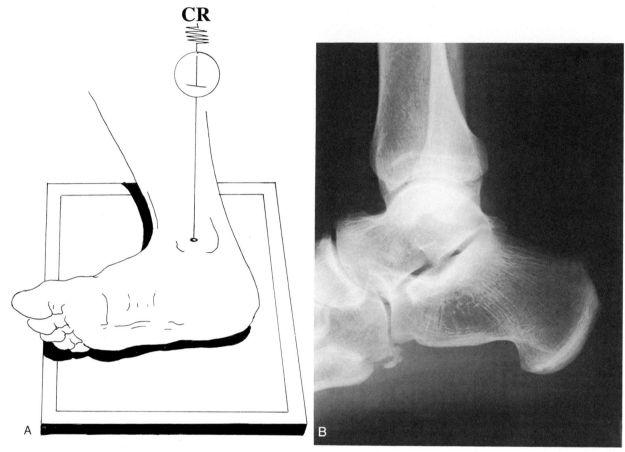

□ **FIGURE 9–3.**

POSITION DESCRIPTION

Part Position: The patient is recumbent on the affected side with the leg in lateral position (knee adjusted so that the transverse axis of the patella is vertical). The plantar surface of the foot should be perpendicular to the plane of the cassette. The foot should be dorsiflexed, if possible.

Central Ray: Perpendicular to the cassette (vertical), passing through the malleoli.

IMAGE EVALUATION

The distal tibia and fibula, the tibiotalar joint, and the tarsals should be demonstrated in lateral position. The fibula should be superimposed over the posterior aspect of the tibia. The sinus tarsi should be seen between the posterior and middle talocalcaneal joints.

Specialized Ankle Radiography

External (Lateral) Oblique Ankle Position

RATIONALE FOR USE

This external oblique position *may be used in cases where presence or extent of ankle injury is unclear* on the routine radiographs.

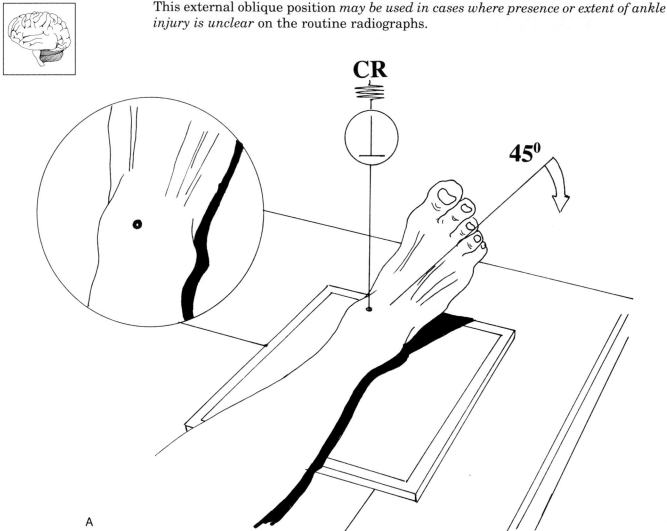

A

□ **FIGURE 9–4.**

POSITION DESCRIPTION

Part Position: The patient is supine or sitting, with the leg extended. The foot is dorsiflexed so that the plantar surface is perpendicular to the cassette. The leg is rotated outward so that the ankle is in a 45° external (lateral) oblique position.

Central Ray: Perpendicular to the cassette, entering midway between the malleoli.

External (Lateral) Oblique Ankle Position *(continued)*

IMAGE EVALUATION

The malleoli should be superimposed on the talus. The fibula should be superimposed on the anterior aspect of the tibia. The talus and calcaneus should be seen, but articulations will be obscured.

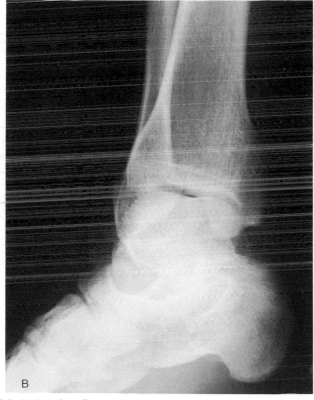

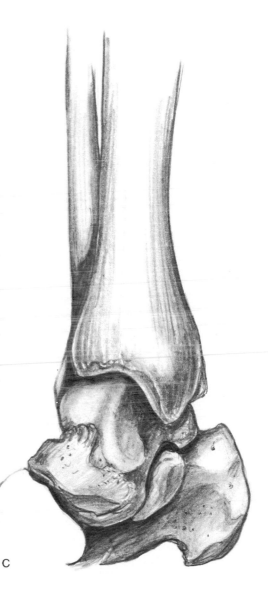

□ **FIGURE 9–4.** *(continued)*

Mortise Position*,†

RATIONALE FOR USE

This position may be used to obtain a *true AP projection of the ankle mortise joint (tibiotalar articulation)*.

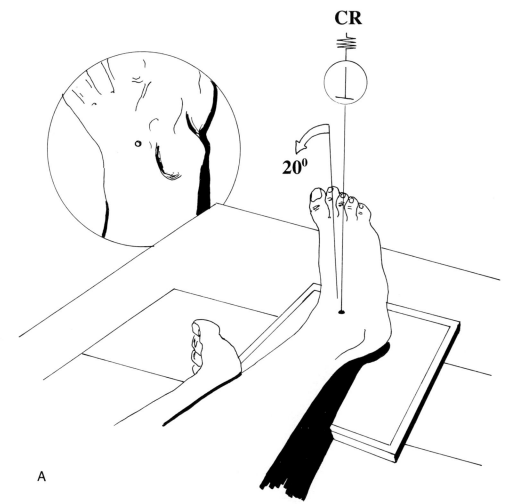

□ **FIGURE 9–5.**

POSITION DESCRIPTION

Part Position: The patient is supine or sitting, with the leg extended. The foot is dorsiflexed so that the plantar surface is perpendicular to the cassette. The leg is rotated inward so that the malleoli are parallel to the plane of the cassette. This usually requires a 15° to 20° internal (medial) oblique position.

Central Ray: Perpendicular to the cassette, entering midway between the malleoli.

Mortise Position*,† *(continued)*

IMAGE EVALUATION

The talotibial joint should be well demonstrated in true AP projection. The medial and lateral talomalleolar articulations should be open. The malleoli should be well visualized.

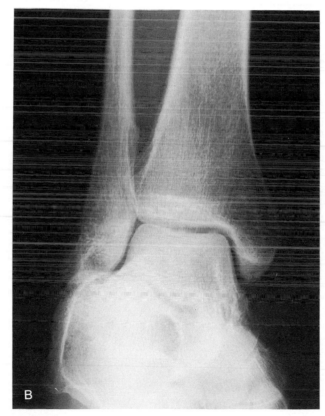

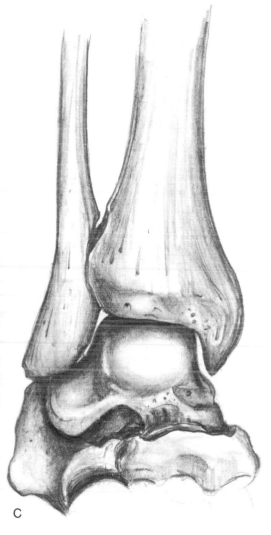

□ **FIGURE 9–5.** *(continued)*

---

*Mukherjee SK, Pringle RM, Baxter AD. Fracture of the lateral process of the talus. *J Bone Joint Surg* 1974; 56B:263–273.
†Goergen TG, Danzig LA, Resnick D, Owen CA. Roentgenographic evaluation of the tibiotalar joint. *J Bone Joint Surg* 1977; 59A(7):874–877.

"Poor" Lateral Ankle Position*

RATIONALE FOR USE

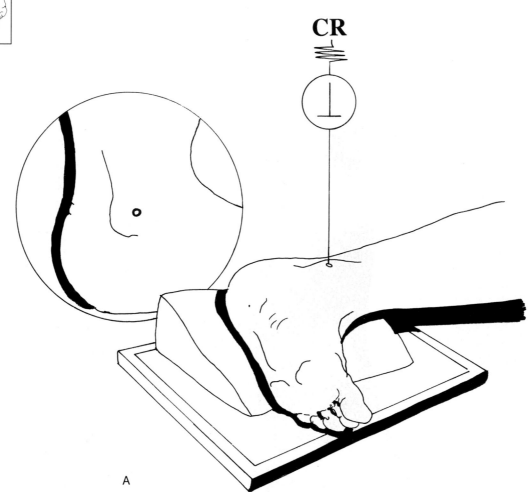

This position may be used to demonstrate *fractures of the posterior tibial lip.*

□ **FIGURE 9–6.**

POSITION DESCRIPTION

Part Position: The patient is positioned as for a routine lateral foot. The long axis of the foot is then tilted approximately 15°, with the toes pointing down and the heel elevated on a sponge.

Central Ray: Perpendicular to the cassette (vertical), passing through the malleoli.

"Poor" Lateral Ankle Position* *(continued)*

IMAGE EVALUATION

The posterior lip of the tibia is superimposed on the fibula, but fractures may nevertheless be demonstrated.

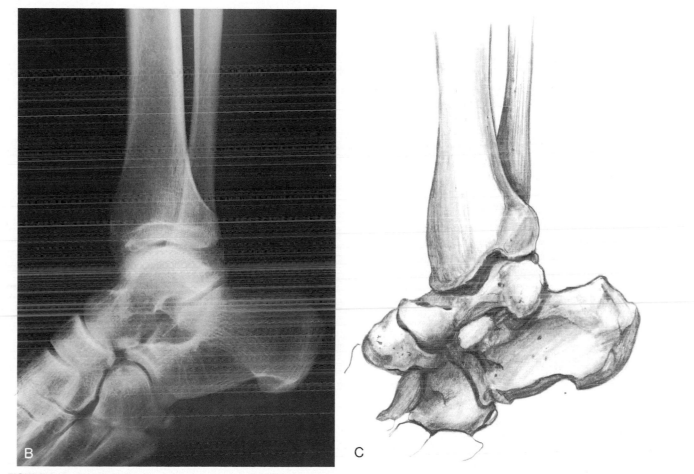

□ **FIGURE 9–6**. *(continued)*

---

*Mandell J. Isolated fractures of the posterior tibial lip at the ankle as demonstrated by an additional projection, the "poor" lateral view. *Radiology* 1971; 101:319–322.

References

1. Cass JR, Morrey BF. Ankle instability: current concepts, diagnosis, and treatment. *Mayo Clin Proc* 1984; 59:165–170.
2. Garrick JG. The frequency of injury, mechanism of injury, and epidemiology of ankle sprains. *Am J Sports Med* 1977; 5:241–242.
3. Brand RL, Collins MDF. Operative management of ligamentous injuries to the ankle. *Clin Sports Med* 1982; 1(1):117–130.
4. Lauge-Hansen N. Fractures of the ankle II: combined experimental-surgical and experimental-roentgenologic investigations. *Arch Surg* 1950; 60:957–985.
5. Danis R. Les fractures malleolaires. *In* Danis R (ed). *Theorie et Pratique de l'Osteosynthese.* Paris: Mason & Cie; 1949:133.
6. Weber BG. *Die verletzungen des oberen Sprunggellenkes, Aktuelle Probleme in der Chirurgie*, 1st ed. Bern: Verlag Hans Huber; 1966.
7. Weber BG, Simpson LA. Corrective lengthening osteotomy of the fibula. *Clin Orthop* 1985; 199:61–67.
8. Muller ME, Nazarian S, Koch P. *The AO Classification of Fractures.* New York: Springer-Verlag; 1988.
9. Edeiken J, Cotler JM. Ankle trauma. *Semin Roentgenol* 1978; 13(2):145–155.
10. Yde J, Kristensen KD. Ankle fractures: supination eversion fractures, stage II. Primary and late operative and non-operative treatment. *Acta Orthop Scand* 1980; 51:695–702.
11. Canale ST, Belding RH. Osteochondral lesions of the talus. *J Bone Joint Surg* 1980; 62A:97–102.
12. Dupuytren G. Memoir sur la Fracture De L'extremite interieuve du Personé, Les Luxatrous et les Accidents qui en Vont la Suite. *Annuaire Medico-Chirurgical des Hospitaux et Hospices Civils de Paris* 1918; 1:1.
13. Pott P. *Some General Remarks on Fractures and Dislocations.* London: Hawes, Clark, Collins; 1768.
14. Maisonneuve JG. Recherches sur la fracture du perone. *Arch Gen Med* 1840; 7:165–187,433–474.
15. Rogers LF. *Radiology of Skeletal Trauma*, 2nd ed. London: Churchill Livingstone; 1992.
16. Tillaux P. *Trait de Chirurgie Clinique*, vol 2. Paris: Aselin & Houzeau; 1848.
17. Chaput V. *Les Fractures Mallolaires du Cou-de-Pied et les Accidents du Travail.* Paris: Masson & Cie; 1907.
18. Kelikian H, Kelikian AS. *Disorders of the Ankle.* Philadelphia: WB Saunders; 1985.
19. LeFort L. Note sur une variété non décrete de fracture verticale de la malléole externe par arrachement. *Bull Gen Therapy* 1886; 110:193–199.
20. Wagstaffe WW. An unusual form of fracture of the fibula. *St Thomas Hosp Rep* 1875; 6:43.
21. Henderson MS. Trimalleolar fractures of the ankle. *Surg Clin North Am* 1932; 12:867–872.
22. Cotton FJ. A new type of ankle fracture. *JAMA* 1915; 64:318–321.
23. Destot E. La troisième malléole: fracture marginale posterièure. *Lyon Chir* 1913; 9:256.
24. Lee CK, Hansen HT, Weiss AB. Supramalleolar fracture of the ankle (Malgaigne's fracture). *Am Surg* 1977; 43:589.
25. Schultz RJ. *The Language of Fractures.* Baltimore: Williams & Wilkins; 1972.
26. Destot E. *Traumatismes du Pied et Rayons X.* Paris: Masson & Cie; 1911.
27. Ovadia DN, Beals RK. Fractures of the tibial plafond. *J Bone Joint Surg* 1986; 68A:543–551.
28. Bosworth DM. Fracture-dislocation of the ankle with fixed displacement of the fibula behind the tibia. *J Bone Joint Surg* 1947; 29:130–135.
29. Olerud S. Subluxation of the ankle without fracture of the fibula. *J Bone Joint Surg* 1971; 53A:594.
30. Colville MR, Colville JM, Manoli A. Posteromedial dislocation of the ankle without fracture. *J Bone Joint Surg* 1987; 69A:706–711.
31. Harsh WN. Effects of trauma upon epiphyses. *Clin Orthop* 1957; 10:140–147.
32. MacNealy GA, Rogers LF, Hernandez R, Poznanski AK. Injuries of the distal tibial epiphysis: systematic radiographic evaluation. *AJR* 1982; 138:683–689.
33. Crenshaw AH. Injuries of the distal tibial epiphysis. *Clin Orthop* 1965; 41:98–107.
34. Goergen TG, Danzig LA, Resnick D, Owen CA. Roentgenographic evaluation of the tibiotalar joint. *J Bone Joint Surg* 1977; 59A:874–877.
35. Mandell J. Isolated fractures of the posterior tibial lip at the ankle as demonstrated by an additional projection, the "poor" lateral view. *Radiology* 1971; 101:319.
36. Kirkup JR. Ankle and tarsal joints in rheumatoid arthritis. *Scand J Rheumatol* 1974; 3:50.
37. Saunders CG, Weston WJ. Synovial mass lesions in the anteroposterior projection of the ankle joint. *J Can Assoc Radiol* 1971; 22:275–277.
38. Resnick D. Patterns of peripheral joint diseases in ankylosing spondylitis. *Radiology* 1974; 110:523–532.
39. Sholkoff SD, Glickman MG, Steinback HL. Roentgenology of Reiter's syndrome. *Radiology* 1970; 97:497–503.
40. Resnick D. Talar ridges, osteophytes, and beaks: a radiologic commentary. *Radiology* 1984; 151:329.
41. Wright V. Seronegative polyarthritis. A unified concept. *Arthritis Rheum* 1978; 21:619.
42. Clark RL, Muhletaler CA, Margulies SI. Colitic arthritis. Clinical and radiographic manifestations. *Radiology* 1971; 101:585.

TEN

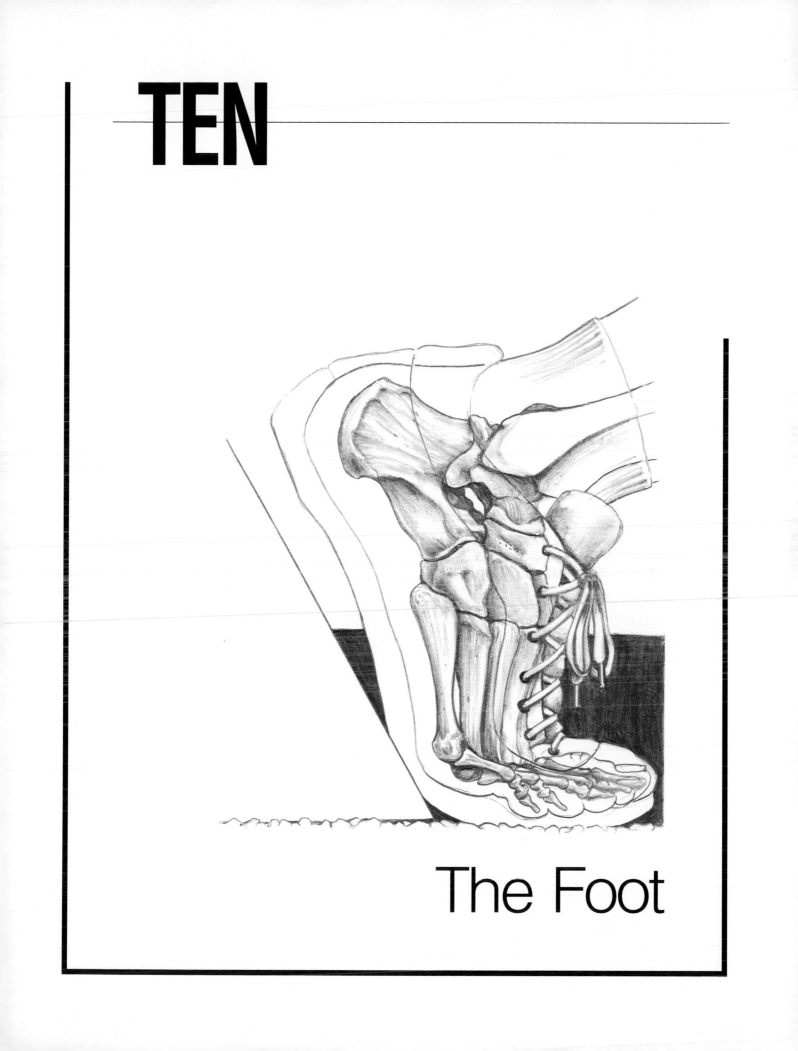

The Foot

THE FOOT: AN OVERVIEW

ROUTINE FOOT RADIOGRAPHY

Routine AP (Dorsoplantar) Foot Projection
Routine Medial (Internal) Oblique Foot Position
Routine Lateral Foot Position

SPECIALIZED FOOT RADIOGRAPHY

AP Weight-Bearing Foot Projection
Lateral (External) Oblique Foot Position
Lateral Weight-Bearing Foot Position
Tangential First MTP Joint Sesamoid Projection

SPECIALIZED TARSAL RADIOGRAPHY

Axial Dorsoplantar Calcaneus Projection
Axial Plantodorsal Calcaneus Projection
Lateral Calcaneus Position
Lateral Oblique Axial Subtalar Joint Projection
Medial Oblique Axial Subtalar Joint Projection
Medial Oblique Dorsoplantar Subtalar Joint Projection
Talar Neck Position
Tarsal Coalition Position

The Foot: An Overview

The foot is very important for normal human gait and upright stance. During the gait cycle, the foot serves as a shock absorber at heel strike, as a compliant and stable platform throughout the stance phase, and as a rigid lever to aid in toe push-off. Human ambulation is accomplished by a complex set of integrated actions. Altered function in one component may also affect the other normal components. For this reason, conditions that adversely affect the bones, articulations, or soft tissues of the foot must be accurately diagnosed and treated. Radiography has an important role in the diagnosis of many of these conditions.

All bones in the foot are subject to fracture by direct and indirect forces. In the hindfoot, both the calcaneus and talus may be fractured. The calcaneus is the most frequently fractured tarsal bone.[1, 2] In adults, 75% of such fractures are intra-articular,[3] and the fractures frequently result from landing on the feet during a fall from a height. The axial loading causes the talus to hit the calcaneus and split it. These intra-articular fractures may be evaluated with the use of special positions such as the Isherwood[4] subtalar joint positions described in this chapter. Extra-articular fractures of the calcaneus are often avulsions,[5] although the tuberosity can be fractured vertically without involving the subtalar joint. Calcaneal avulsion most commonly involves the anterior process and results from inversion–internal rotation of the foot.[6] The internal (medial) oblique foot radiograph may be useful for demonstrating this fracture. Avulsion of the posterosuperior portion of the calcaneal tuberosity is referred to as a **beak fracture** and results from avulsion by the Achilles tendon.[7] This injury is best seen on the lateral calcaneus radiograph. Avulsions may occur on the medial and lateral aspects of the plantar surface of the tuberosity. These injuries are best demonstrated on the axial projection.

The talus is the second most frequently fractured tarsal. Of tarsal fractures, osteochondral fracture of the talar dome is most common and results from an inversion or twisting injury.[8] Fracture of the talar neck, formerly called **aviator's astragalus**,[9] is second in frequency.[10] It is usually caused by hyperdorsiflexion of the foot as a result of motor vehicle accidents or significant falls.[11] A talar neck fracture can also occur with direct blows to the dorsum of the foot.[12] The talar neck position of Canale and Kelly,[13] described in this chapter, may aid in accurate diagnosis of this fracture. The head, body, and talar processes are not commonly fractured.

Injury to the midfoot is uncommon because of the high stability of this region. When such a fracture occurs, the injury often involves multiple structures. A variety of sprains, subluxations, and fracture-dislocations have been described.[14] Isolated fractures of the midfoot tarsals are uncommon; the navicular bone is most frequently involved. Of injuries to this bone, avulsion of the dorsal aspect or tuberosity is most common and may result from eversion injury.[15] Vertical or longitudinal navicular fractures are often associated with forces transmitted axially through the metatarsals. The cuboid is most frequently injured during lateral subluxation of the midtarsal joint (Chopart's joint) when the cuboid is crushed between the fourth and fifth metatarsals and the anterior calcaneus. This injury is termed a **Nutcracker fracture**.[16] Isolated cuneiform fractures are rare. They can result from direct blows but are usually associated with other injuries.

Fracture-dislocation of the tarsometatarsal joints (Lisfranc joint) is also known as the **Lisfranc fracture-dislocation**.[17] The injury may involve some or all of the joints. Displacement of the involved metatarsals may be in the same direction (medial, lateral, dorsal, plantar) or divergent (mediolateral or dorsoplantar).[18, 19] The injury typically occurs with twisting or axial loading of the plantarflexed foot.[20] The mechanism of injury is varied, ranging from floorboard impact in automobile accidents to a misstep off a curb. A Lisfranc fracture-dislocation may also result from crush injury to the foot.[21] Associated fractures are common; transverse fracture of the second metatarsal base is seen most frequently.[22] The Lisfranc joint injury may be subtle, necessitating a complete radiographic evaluation of the foot. Norfray and associates[23] reported that failure to obtain an internal oblique radiograph may lead to diagnostic error.

Fractures of the shaft and neck of the metatarsals are commonly caused by direct blows, such as a heavy object falling on the foot. Indirect twisting or shearing forces may also cause fractures. The fifth metatarsal base is frequently involved, resulting in an avulsion fracture of the tuberosity or a transverse fracture just distal to the tuberosity. This transverse fracture of the proximal fifth metatarsal is commonly referred to as **Jones' fracture**.[24] The fifth metatarsal base avulsion fractures are often caused by the same mechanism that results in ankle sprains. For this reason, the fifth metatarsal base should always be included on a lateral ankle radiograph performed to evaluate ankle inversion injuries.

Injuries to metatarsophalangeal (MTP) and interphalangeal (IP) joints are common, including sprains, subluxations, dislocations, and fracture-dislocations. An injury to the first MTP seen with increasing frequency in athletes playing on artificial turf has been termed **turf toe**.[25] The injury is usually a hyperextension sprain but may manifest as a dorsal dislocation or a fracture-dislocation.[26] Dislocation of the other MTP joints most frequently results from forces that displace the toe dorsally and laterally, such as kicking a table leg with the bare foot. Fractures or dislocations of the phalanges may result from this same mechanism. Phalangeal fracture may also occur when a heavy object falls on the toes. Radiography of the MTP joints and toes is usually limited to anteroposterior (AP) (or dorsoplantar) projection and oblique positions. A lateral position of the affected toe may be obtained with occlusal film or if the patient is able to flex the unaffected toes sufficiently to relieve superimposition.

Stress reactions or fractures occur with relative frequency in the foot. They are the result of repetitive stress, insufficient to cause an acute fracture, applied to a bone that does not have the structural strength to withstand the stress.[27] In a normal bone, this injury is referred to as a **fatigue fracture**. An **insufficiency fracture** results in the alteration of the bone's elasticity by disease. Stress reactions or fractures of the second metatarsal, third metatarsal, and calcaneus are most common and are frequently associated with marching or running.[28, 29] Stress fractures may occur in the other metatarsals, most often the first. The tarsals and sesamoids can also be involved. Radiographs are usually normal in the acute phase of stress reaction or fracture. Radioisotope bone scanning is better for early evaluation because it enables diagnosis within 2 days.[30, 31] Radiographic changes seen include trabecular condensation (common in the calcaneus), a subtle lucent line in the cortex, and slight callus formation (metatarsals).[32]

Fractures and dislocations of the foot are generally less common in children than in adults. Many of the fractures seen in adults may also be found in children. However, the distribution and frequency of injury are different. Radiographic diagnosis is more complicated because of the presence of physes and secondary ossification centers. Fractures may be incomplete or may involve the physis. Radiographic examination of the foot in children is essentially the same as in adults.

Patients with diabetes mellitus are at a greater risk for foot pathology than is the nondiabetic population. Soft tissues, bones, or joints may be involved. Stress fractures or spontaneous dislocations may result from minor traumatic episodes. A neuropathic or Charcot joint is most commonly seen in diabetic patients.[33, 34] Diabetic osteolysis may occur in the distal metatarsals and proximal phalanges.[35] A "pencil-in-cup" deformity results from pointing of the metatarsal with widening of the phalangeal base. Osteomyelitis also occurs in the diabetic foot but is more effectively diagnosed by radionuclide bone scanning because radiographic changes are late manifestations.[34] Soft-tissue pathology is frequently seen, but radiography has limited value in evaluation of the conditions.

Radiography is used to evaluate biomechanically acquired foot types and pediatric foot deformities. The AP (or dorsoplantar) and lateral foot radiographs, usually in weight-bearing, are utilized to assess the posture and interrelationships of the hindfoot, midfoot, and forefoot. The weight-bearing axial calcaneus projection of Harris and Beath[36] may be used to evaluate tarsal coalition. A lateral foot radiograph in maximal dorsiflexion can be taken to document an anterior ankle impingement of the tibia and talus.

The foot may be involved, at least to some degree, in nearly all arthritides. Routine AP, oblique, and lateral radiographs are usually sufficient to evaluate arthritis involving the joints of the foot. Rheumatoid arthritis is especially common in the forefoot, which is involved in 80%–90% of cases, and forefoot pathology is seen as the initial manifestation in 10%–20%.[37] The MTP and first IP joints are most frequently affected.[38] Radiographic manifestation in the forefoot commonly precedes that of the hand and wrist.[39] The deformities of the toes are similar to those seen in the fingers, including fibular deviation, boutonnière deformities, and swan-neck deformities. Rheumatoid arthritis in the midfoot is most common in the talocalcaneonavicular joint, especially the talonavicular joint. It also manifests in the tarsometatarsal joints and may be found in all midfoot tarsal joints.[40] Calcaneal involvement often consists of soft-tissue swelling or mass formation in the Achilles tendon area, bone erosions on the posterosuperior or posteroinferior aspects, or well-defined plantar spurs.[41]

The rheumatoid variants or seronegative spondyloarthropathies manifest in the foot. However, ankylosing spondylitis is seen much less frequently than Reiter's syndrome or psoriatic arthritis. Ankylosing spondylitis, if present, is most likely to be found in the calcaneus. Retrocalcaneal bursitis, posterior calcaneal erosions, and Achilles tendon thickening are most common.[42] The foot is involved in a high percentage of patients with Reiter's syndrome or psoriasis. The forefoot and calcaneus are most commonly affected.[43] The distal IP joints are most frequently affected in psoriatic arthritis. The joint erosions are often associated with fluffy new bone formation. The "pencil-in-cup" joint deformity is characteristic of psoriatic arthritis.[44] Calcaneal involvement of both Reiter's syndrome and psoriatic arthritis most frequently consists of erosion of the posterosuperior or posteroinferior aspects, as well as formation of an irregular plantar spur.[42]

The foot is affected in a high percentage of patients with gout. Involvement of the first MTP joint is characteristic of the disease, although any joint in the foot may be involved.[45] The foot is not frequently affected in pseudogout (crystal pyrophosphate dihydrate deposition disease [CPPD]). When present, this arthropathy most commonly affects the talonavicular and MTP joints.[46] In contrast to gout, there is absence of significant erosions in the first MTP joint.

Primary osteoarthritis may involve the foot and most commonly affects the first MTP joint. Hallux valgus or hallux rigidus may be associated with the condition. The IP joints may be affected, but the other MTP joints are seldom involved. When the TMT or intertarsal joints are affected, the changes tend to be greater medially.[47]

A great variety of other acquired conditions may affect the foot. However, for the sake of brevity, they cannot be covered in this overview.

Routine Foot Radiography

Routine AP (Dorsoplantar) Foot Projection

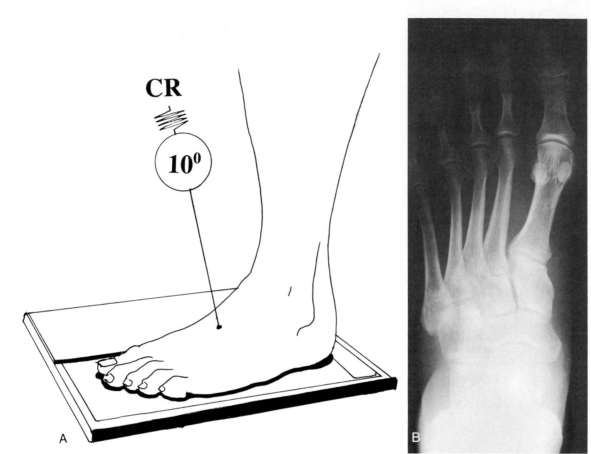

CR

10°

A

B

□ **FIGURE 10–1.**

POSITION DESCRIPTION

Part Position: The patient is supine or sitting with the knee flexed to place the plantar surface of the foot in contact with the cassette. The foot is adjusted with no medial or lateral rotation.

Central Ray: Angled 10° posteriorly (toward the heel), passing through the third metatarsal base.

Note: If only the forefoot is of interest, the central ray is directed vertically through the third metatarsal base.

IMAGE EVALUATION

An AP (dorsoplantar) projection of the foot should be demonstrated without rotation, as evidenced by equal distance between the second to fifth metatarsal shafts. The navicular, cuneiform, and cuboid bones will be visible with some superimposition. The talonavicular and calcaneocuboid joints may be visible, if exposure is sufficient.

Routine Medial (Internal) Oblique Foot Position

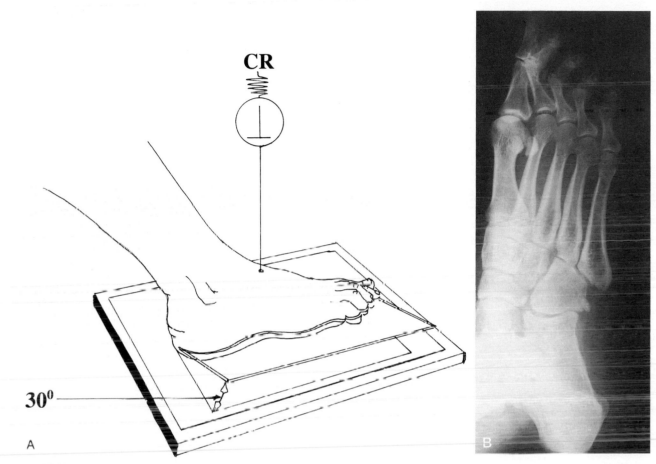

CR

30°

A

B

⊓ **FIGURE 10–2.**

POSITION DESCRIPTION

Part Position: The patient is supine or sitting with the knee flexed so that the plantar surface of the foot is in contact with the cassette. The foot is adjusted in a 30° medial (internal) oblique position.

Central Ray: Perpendicular to the cassette, passing through the third metatarsal base.

IMAGE EVALUATION

The third to fifth metatarsals should be seen without superimposition. The navicular bone, cuboid bone, third cuneiform bone, talar head, sinus tarsi, and anterior calcaneus should also be demonstrated.

Routine Lateral Foot Position

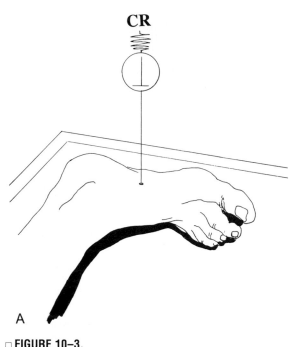

CR

A

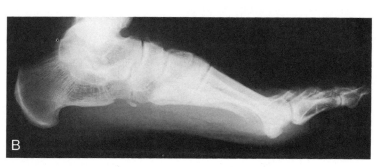

B

□ **FIGURE 10–3.**

POSITION DESCRIPTION

Part Position: The patient is recumbent on the affected side with the leg in lateral position (knee adjusted to place the transverse axis of the patella vertical). The plantar surface of the foot should be perpendicular to the plane of the cassette. The foot should be dorsiflexed, if possible.

Central Ray: Perpendicular to the cassette (vertical), entering the medial side of the foot at the level of the third metatarsal base.

IMAGE EVALUATION

The entire foot and ankle joint should be demonstrated in lateral position. The metatarsals and phalanges should be substantially superimposed. The fibula should superimpose the posterior aspect of the tibia. The sinus tarsi should be visible.

Specialized Foot Radiography

AP Weight-Bearing Foot Position

RATIONALE FOR USE

This AP foot position may be used to evaluate the *interrelationships of the tarsals and metatarsals during weight-bearing stance*. Both feet are examined.

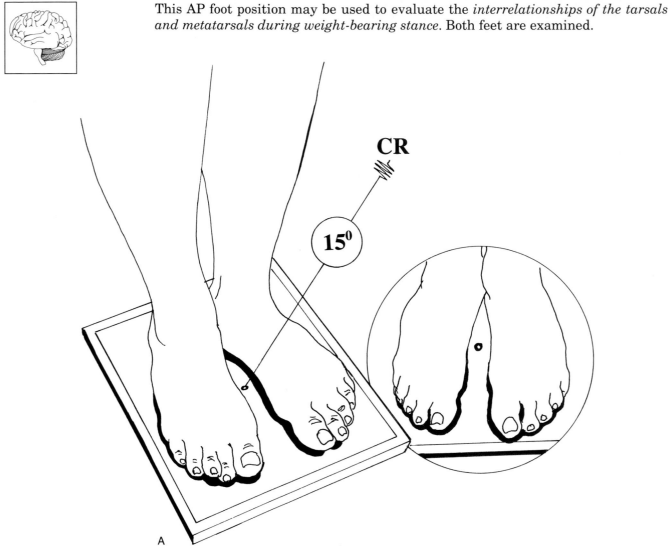

□ **FIGURE 10–4.**

POSITION DESCRIPTION

Part Position: The patient is upright, standing with both feet on a cassette. The patient's weight should be equally distributed on each foot.

Central Ray: Angled 15° posteriorly (toward the heel), passing between the feet at the level of the third metatarsal base.

AP Weight-Bearing Foot Position *(continued)*

IMAGE EVALUATION

Both feet should be demonstrated in an AP projection. The appearance of bone structures may vary, depending on abnormalities of alignment.

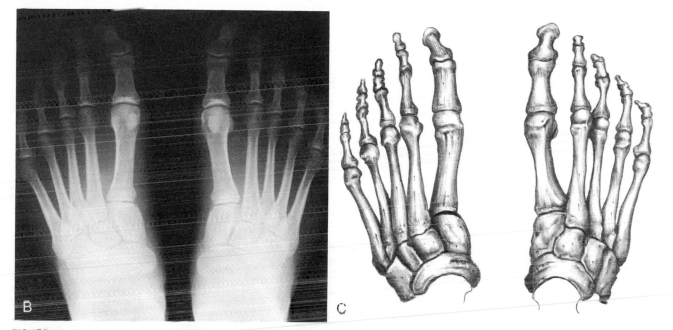

□ **FIGURE 10–4.** *(continued)*

Lateral (External) Oblique Foot Position

RATIONALE FOR USE

This external oblique position *may be used in cases in which the presence or extent of foot injury is unclear* on the routine radiographs.

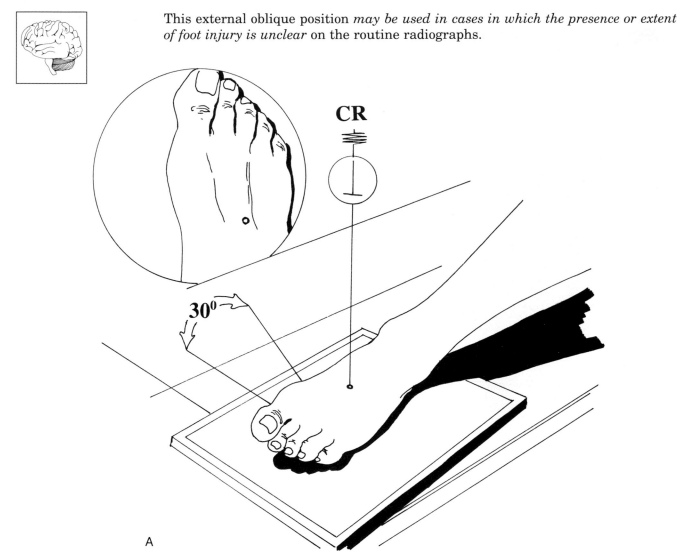

A

□ **FIGURE 10–5.**

POSITION DESCRIPTION

Part Position: The patient is supine or sitting with the knee flexed so that the plantar surface of the foot is in contact with the cassette. The foot is adjusted in a 30° lateral (external) oblique position.

Central Ray: Perpendicular to the cassette, passing through the third metatarsal base.

Lateral (External) Oblique Foot Position *(continued)*

IMAGE EVALUATION

The metatarsals should be demonstrated in an oblique position. The navicular is seen in its long axis. The first and second cuneiform bones should be demonstrated. The talar head, talonavicular joint, and calcaneocuboid joint should be visible, if the hindfoot is sufficiently exposed.

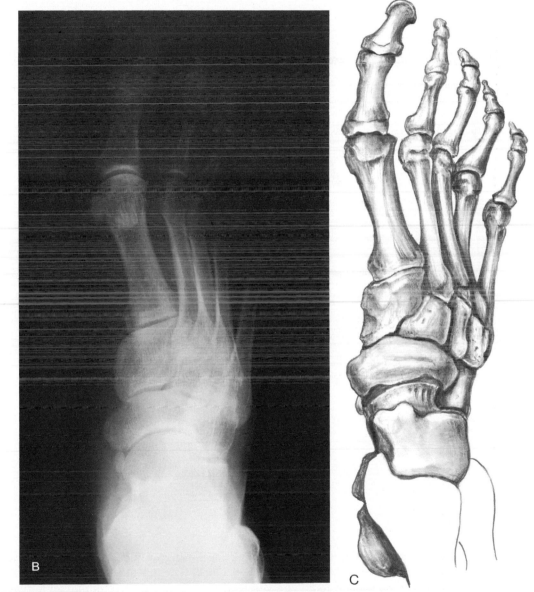

□ **FIGURE 10–5.** *(continued)*

Lateral Weight-Bearing Foot Position

RATIONALE FOR USE

This lateral foot position may be used to evaluate the *interrelationships of the tarsals and metatarsals during weight-bearing stance.* Both feet are examined.

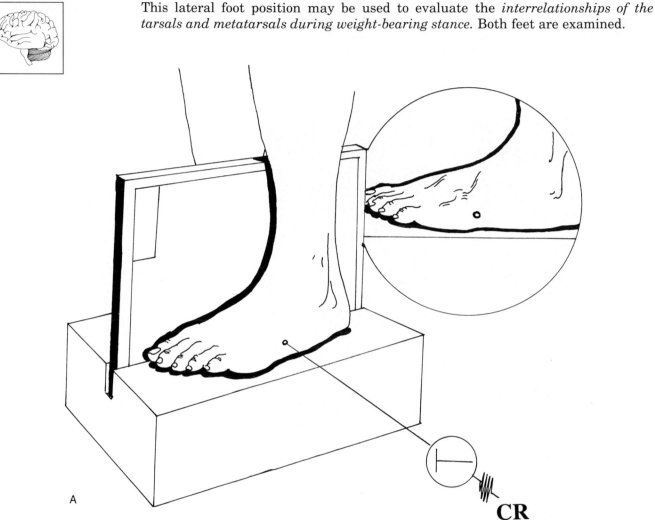

A

□ **FIGURE 10–6.**

POSITION DESCRIPTION

Part Position: The patient is upright, standing on a raised platform with a central cassette slot or with each foot on a block. The patient's weight should be equally distributed on each foot. The vertically oriented cassette is placed between the feet. The bottom of the cassette should be below the plantar surface of the foot. Both feet are exposed, either on separate cassettes or split on one cassette.

Central Ray: Perpendicular to the cassette (horizontal), entering the lateral aspect of the foot just above the fifth metatarsal base.

Lateral Weight-Bearing Foot Position *(continued)*

IMAGE EVALUATION

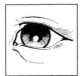

The entire foot and ankle joint should be demonstrated in lateral position. The appearance of bone structures may vary, depending on abnormalities of alignment.

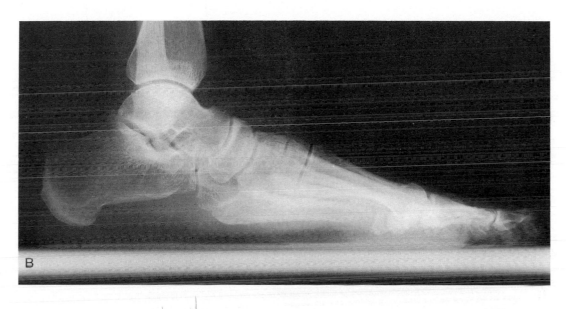

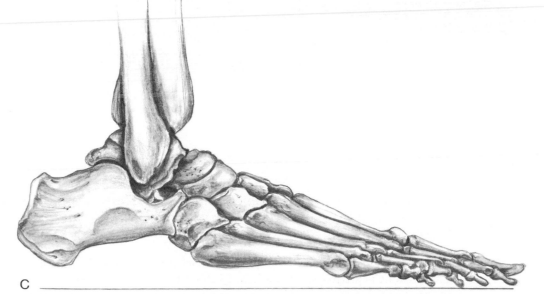

□ **FIGURE 10–6.** *(continued)*

Tangential First MTP Joint Sesamoid Projection*

RATIONALE FOR USE

This tangential projection may be used to evaluate *injury to the sesamoids of the first metatarsophalangeal (MTP) joint.*

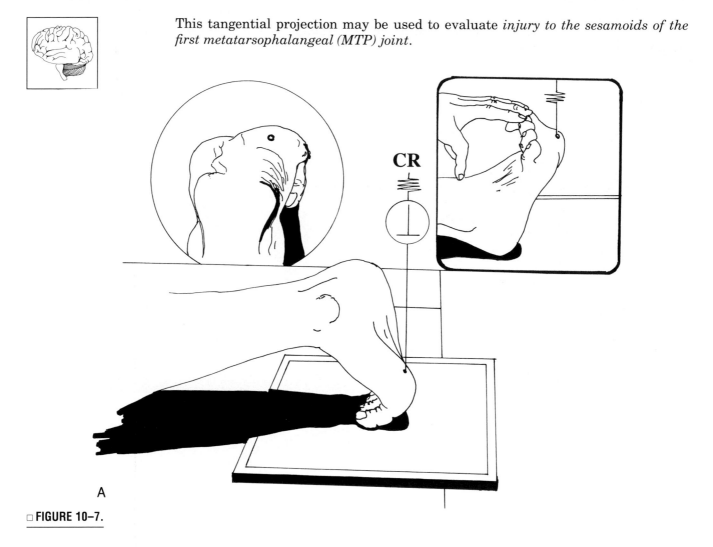

A

□ **FIGURE 10–7.**

POSITION DESCRIPTION

Part Position: The patient is prone with the dorsiflexed toes of the affected foot resting on a cassette. The degree of dorsiflexion of the great toe is adjusted to place the plantar surface of the first MTP joint perpendicular to the cassette.

Note: Holly† described a reverse of this position that may be easier for the patient: The patient is sitting with the heel of the affected foot resting on the cassette, and the toes are dorsiflexed by placing a strap around the toes and adjusting the degree of foot flexion so that the plantar surface of the first MTP joint is perpendicular to the cassette.

Central Ray: Perpendicular to the cassette (vertical), passing through the plantar surface of the first MTP joint.

Tangential First MTP Joint Sesamoid Projection* *(continued)*

IMAGE EVALUATION

The sesamoids of the first MTP joint should be projected free of bone superimposition.

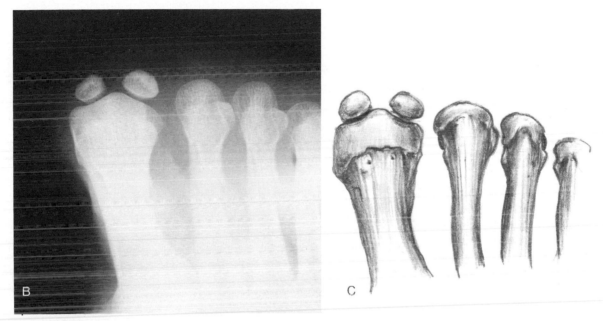

□ **FIGURE 10–7.** *(continued)*

---

*Lewis RW. Non-routine views in roentgen examination of the extremities. *Surg Gynecol Obstet* 1938; 69:38–45.
†Holly EW. Radiography of the tarsal sesamoid bones. *Med Radiog Photog* 1955; 31:73.

Specialized Tarsal Radiography

Axial Dorsoplantar Calcaneus Projection

RATIONALE FOR USE

This projection may be used to obtain an *axial projection of the entire calcaneus and talocalcaneal joint.* The dorsoplantar projection results in less distortion than the plantodorsal projection, but is not appropriate for patients with severe trauma, who should not be moved from the supine position.

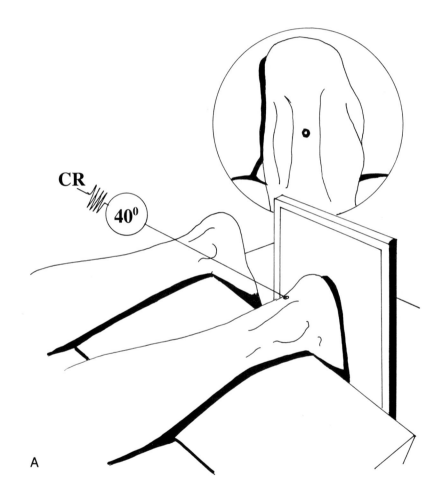

A

□ **FIGURE 10–8.**

POSITION DESCRIPTION

Part Position: The patient is prone with the affected ankle elevated so that the long axis of the foot is oriented vertically and the toes just contact the table top. The vertically oriented cassette is placed in contact with the plantar surface of the affected foot.

Central Ray: Angled 40° caudad, oriented with the long axis of the foot and entering the Achilles tendon 2 inches proximal to the plantar surface of the heel.

Axial Dorsoplantar Calcaneus Projection *(continued)*

IMAGE EVALUATION

An axial projection of the entire calcaneus and the talocalcaneal joint should be demonstrated. When the talocalcaneal joint is well demonstrated, the posterior portion of the calcaneus is often overexposed. A second exposure may be required to demonstrate both areas.

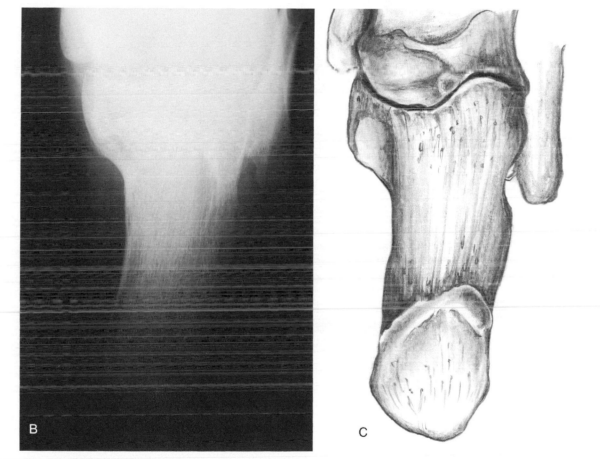

□ **FIGURE 10–8.** *(continued)*

Axial Plantodorsal Calcaneus Projection

RATIONALE FOR USE

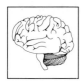

This projection may be used to obtain an *axial projection of the entire calcaneus and talocalcaneal joint.* The plantodorsal projection is commonly used in cases of severe trauma when the patient should not be moved from the supine position.

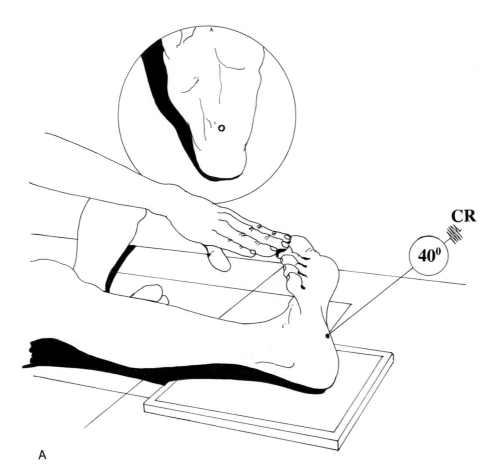

CR

40°

A

□ **FIGURE 10–9.**

POSITION DESCRIPTION

Part Position: The patient is supine with the leg extended and the long axis of the foot oriented vertically (toes pointing straight up). The cassette is placed under the foot and ankle. The foot is dorsiflexed to place the plantar surface perpendicular to the cassette.

Note: If sufficient dorsiflexion is not possible, the leg can be elevated to adjust the plantar surface perpendicular to the cassette.

Central Ray: Angled 40° cephalad, oriented with the long axis of the foot and entering the plantar surface of the foot 3 inches anterior to the posterior surface of the heel.

Axial Plantodorsal Calcaneus Projection *(continued)*

IMAGE EVALUATION

An axial projection of the entire calcaneus and the talocalcaneal joint should be demonstrated. When the talocalcaneal joint is demonstrated, the posterior portion of the calcaneus is often overexposed. A second exposure may be required to demonstrate both areas.

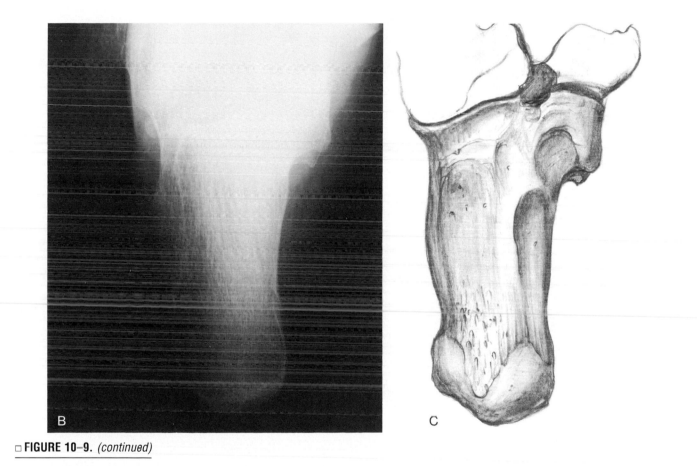

□ **FIGURE 10–9.** *(continued)*

Lateral Calcaneus Position

RATIONALE FOR USE

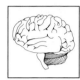

This position may be used to demonstrate the *calcaneus and its articulations in a lateral position.*

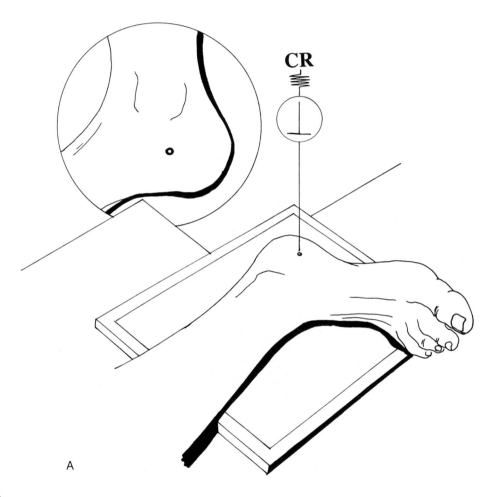

A

□ **FIGURE 10–10.**

POSITION DESCRIPTION

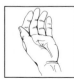

Part Position: The patient is recumbent on the affected side with the leg in a lateral position (knee adjusted to place the transverse axis of the patella vertical). The plantar surface of the foot should be perpendicular to the plane of the cassette. The foot should be dorsiflexed, if possible.

Central Ray: Perpendicular to the cassette, entering at the midcalcaneus.

Lateral Calcaneus Position *(continued)*

IMAGE EVALUATION

The calcaneus and its articulations with the talus, navicular, and cuboid bones should be demonstrated in lateral position. The sinus tarsi should be seen between the posterior and middle talocalcaneal joints. The tibiotalar joint should also be included on the radiograph.

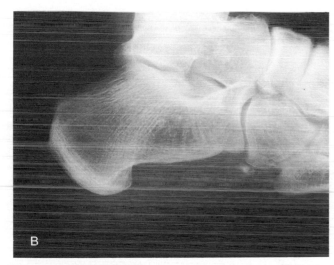

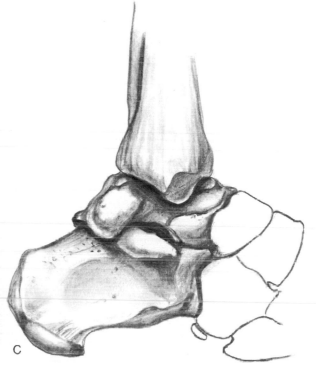

□ **FIGURE 10–10.** *(continued)*

Lateral Oblique Axial Subtalar Joint Projection*

RATIONALE FOR USE

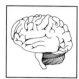

This projection may be used to demonstrate the *posterior subtalar joint* for evaluation of joint surface involvement in fractures of the calcaneus or talus. Also, bone fusion (bridge or coalition) between the talus, calcaneus, or navicular may be demonstrated.

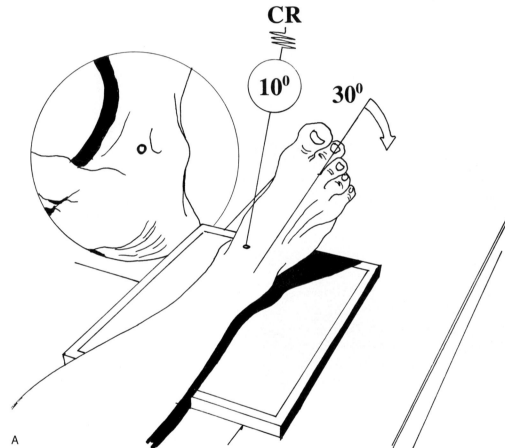

□ **FIGURE 10–11.**

POSITION DESCRIPTION

Part Position: The patient is supine with the leg extended and rotated outward so that the ankle is in a 30° external oblique position. The foot should be dorsiflexed and everted, if possible.

Central Ray: Angled 10° cephalad, oriented with the long axis of the tibia and entering the ankle 1 inch distal to the medial malleolus.

Lateral Oblique Axial Subtalar Joint Projection* *(continued)*

IMAGE EVALUATION

The posterior subtalar joint should be well demonstrated. The middle and anterior subtalar joints will be obscured by superimposition of the inferior aspect of the talar neck and head.

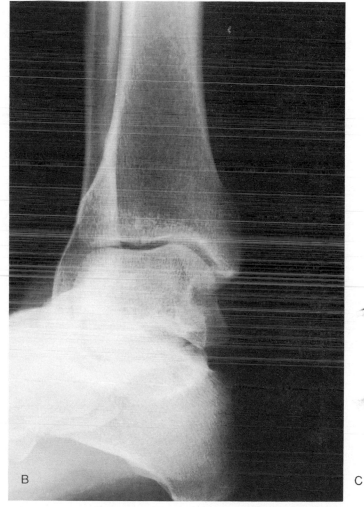

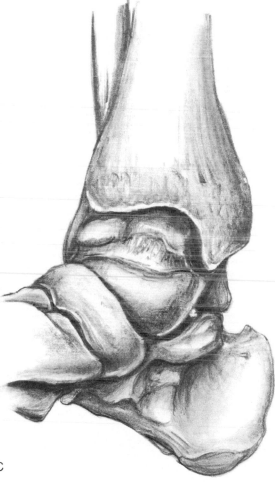

B   C

□ **FIGURE 10–11.** *(continued)*

*Isherwood I. A radiological approach to the subtalar joint. *J Bone Joint Surg* 1961; 43B(3):566–574.

Medial Oblique Axial Subtalar Joint Projection*

RATIONALE FOR USE

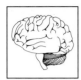

This projection may be used to demonstrate the *middle and posterior subtalar joints* for evaluation of joint surface involvement in fractures of the calcaneus or talus. Also, fusion (bridge or coalition) between the talus, calcaneus, or navicular bones may be demonstrated.

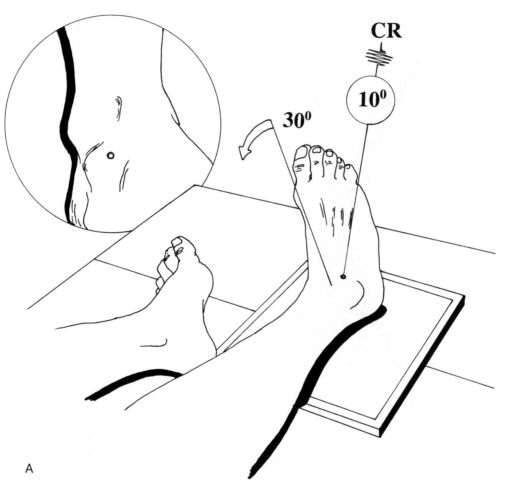

A

□ **FIGURE 10–12.**

POSITION DESCRIPTION

Part Position: The patient is supine with the leg extended and rotated inward so that the ankle is in a 30° internal (medial) oblique position. The foot should be dorsiflexed and inverted, if possible.

Central Ray: Angled 10° cephalad, oriented with the long axis of the tibia and entering the ankle at a point 1 inch distal and 1 inch anterior to the lateral malleolus.

Medial Oblique Axial Subtalar Joint Projection* *(continued)*

IMAGE EVALUATION

The sinus tarsi should be open with the middle subtalar joint seen anterior to it and the posterior subtalar joint seen posterior to it.

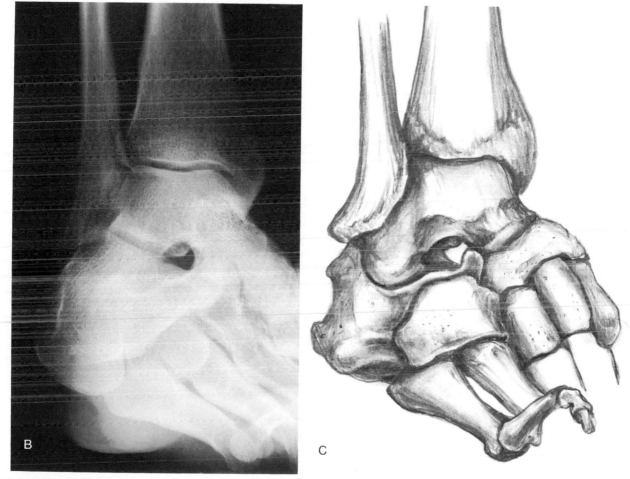

□ **FIGURE 10–12.** *(continued)*

---

*Isherwood I. A radiological approach to the subtalar joint. *J Bone Joint Surg* 1961; 43B(3):566–574.

Medial Oblique Dorsoplantar Subtalar Joint Projection*

RATIONALE FOR USE

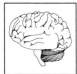

This projection may be used to demonstrate the *anterior subtalar joint* for evaluation of joint surface involvement in fractures of the calcaneus or talus. Also, fusion (bridge or coalition) between the talus, calcaneus, or navicular bones may be demonstrated.

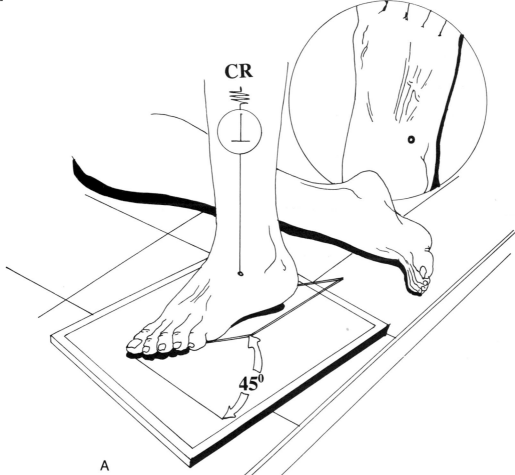

□ **FIGURE 10–13.**

POSITION DESCRIPTION

Part Position: The patient is supine or sitting with the knee flexed so that the plantar surface of the foot is in contact with the cassette. The foot is adjusted in a 45° medial (internal) oblique position.

Central Ray: Perpendicular to the cassette, entering at a point 1 inch distal and 1 inch anterior to the lateral malleolus.

Medial Oblique Dorsoplantar Subtalar Joint Projection* *(continued)*

IMAGE EVALUATION

The anterior subtalar joint should be well demonstrated. The talonavicular and calcaneocuboid joints are also demonstrated. The posterior subtalar joint is seen through the superimposed shadow of the distal fibula.

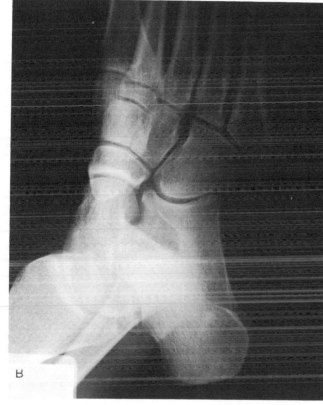

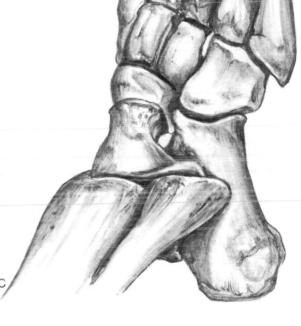

□ **FIGURE 10–13.** *(continued)*

---

*Isherwood I. A radiological approach to the subtalar joint. *J Bone Joint Surg* 1961; 43B(3):566–574.

Talar Neck Position*

RATIONALE FOR USE

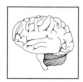

This position may be used to demonstrate the *entire talar neck* for evaluation of fractures or to assess anatomical reduction after fracture treatment.

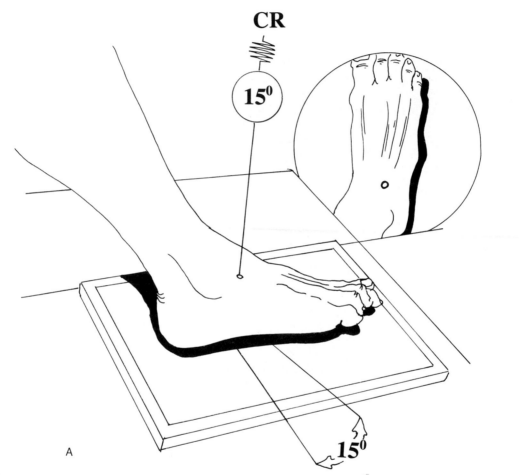

□ **FIGURE 10–14.**

POSITION DESCRIPTION

Part Position: The patient is seated on the table with the knee flexed so that the plantar surface of the foot is in contact with the cassette. The foot is adjusted in a 15° medial (internal) oblique position.

Central Ray: Angled 15° posteriorly (toward the heel), oriented with the long axis of the foot and entering the dorsum of the foot at the level of the talar neck.

Talar Neck Position* *(continued)*

IMAGE EVALUATION

The entire neck of the talus should be demonstrated. The posterior portion of the talar neck will be superimposed over the calcaneus. The talonavicular and calcaneocuboid joints are also demonstrated.

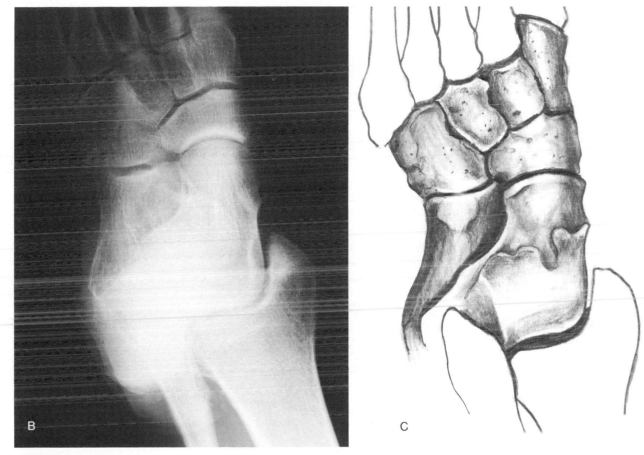

□ **FIGURE 10–14.** *(continued)*

---

*Canale ST, Kelly FB. Fractures of the talar neck: long-term evaluation of seventy-one cases. *J Bone Joint Surg* 1978; 60A(2):143–156.

Tarsal Coalition Position*

RATIONALE FOR USE

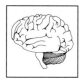

This position may be used to obtain an *axial projection of the talocalcaneal articulations* to assess the presence of *talocalcaneal coalition.*

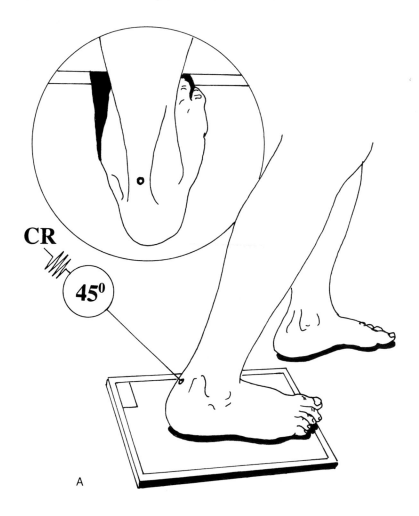

□ **FIGURE 10–15.**

POSITION DESCRIPTION

Part Position: The patient stands with the plantar surface of the affected foot on the cassette and the other foot one step forward. The heel of the affected foot should be in contact with the cassette.

Central Ray: Directed toward the posterior surface of the ankle at an angle of 45°, entering the Achilles tendon approximately 3 inches proximal to the plantar surface of the heel.

Tarsal Coalition Position* *(continued)*

IMAGE EVALUATION

An axial projection of the calcaneus and the talocalcaneal articulations should be demonstrated. When the talocalcaneal region is well demonstrated, the posterior portion of the calcaneus is often overexposed.

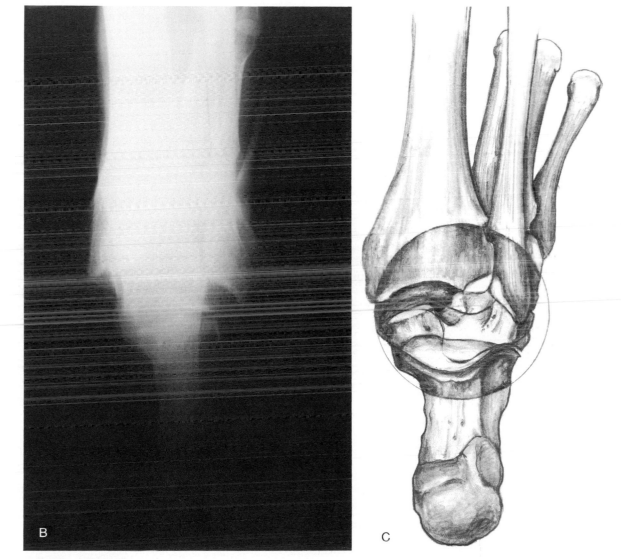

□ **FIGURE 10–15.** *(continued)*

---

*Harris RI, Beath T. Etiology of peroneal spastic flat foot. *J Bone Joint Surg* 1948; 30B:624–634.

References

1. Cave EF. Fracture of the os calsis—the problem in general. *Clin Orthop* 1963; 30:64–66.
2. Essex-Loprestie P. The mechanism, reduction technique, and results in fractures of the os calcis. *Br J Surg* 1952; 39:395–419.
3. Aaron DAR, Howat TW. Intra-articular fractures of the calcaneum. *Injury* 1976; 7:205.
4. Isherwood I. A radiologic approach to the subtalar joint. *J Bone Joint Surg* 1961; 43B:566–574.
5. Rowe CR, Sakellarides HT, Freeman PA, Sorbie C. Fractures of the os calcis. A long-term follow-up study of 146 patients. *JAMA* 1963; 184:920–923.
6. Renfrew DL, El-Khoury GY. Anterior process fractures of the calcaneus. *Skeletal Radiol* 1985; 14:121–125.
7. Lowy M. Avulsion fractures of the calcaneus. *J Bone Joint Surg* 1969; 51B:494–497.
8. Anderson IF, Crichton KJ, Grattan-Smith T, et al. Osteochondral fractures of the talar dome. *J Bone Joint Surg* 1989; 71A:1143–1152.
9. Coltart WD. Aviator's astragalus. *J Bone Joint Surg* 1952; 34B:545–566.
10. Adelaar RS. The treatment of complex fractures of the talus. *Orthop Clin North Am* 1989; 20:691–707.
11. Penny JN, Davis LA. Fractures and fracture-dislocations of the neck of the talus. *J Trauma* 1980; 20:1029–1037.
12. Lorentzen JE, Christensen SB, Krogsoe O, Sneppen O. Fractures of the neck of the talus. *Acta Orthop Scand* 1977; 48:115–120.
13. Canale ST, Kelly FB. Fractures of the talar neck: long-term evaluation of seventy-one cases. *J Bone Joint Surg* 1978; 60A(2):143–156.
14. Main BJ, Jowett RL. Injuries of the mid-tarsal joint. *J Bone Joint Surg* 1975; 57B:89–97.
15. Eichenholtz SN, Levene DB. Fracture of the tarsal navicular bone. *Clin Orthop* 1964; 34:142–157.
16. Hermel MB, Gershon-Cohen J. The Nutcracker fracture of the cuboid by indirect violence. *Radiology* 1953; 60:850–854.
17. Foster SC, Foster RR. Lisfranc's tarsometatarsal fracture-dislocation. *Radiology* 1976; 120:79–83.
18. Hardcastle PH, Reschauer R, Kutscha-Lissberg E, Schoffmann W. Injuries to the tarsometatarsal joint. *J Bone Joint Surg* 1982; 64B:349–356.
19. Myerson MS, Fisher RT, Burgess AR, Kenzora JE. Fracture-dislocations of the tarsometatarsal joints: end result correlated with pathology and treatment. *Foot Ankle* 1986; 6(5):225–242.
20. Wiley JJ. The mechanism of tarsometatarsal joint injuries. *J Bone Joint Surg* 1971; 53B:474–482.
21. Myerson MS. The diagnosis and treatment of injuries to the Lisfranc joint complex. *Orthop Clin North Am* 1989; 20(4):655–664.
22. Wilson DW. Injuries of the tarsometatarsal joints: etiology, classification, and results of treatment. *J Bone Joint Surg* 1972; 54B:677–686.
23. Norfray JF, Geline RA, Steinberg RI, et al. Subtleties of Lisfranc fracture-dislocations. *AJR* 1981; 137:1151–1156.
24. Jones R. Fracture of the base of the fifth metatarsal bone by indirect violence. *Am J Surg* 1902; 35:697–700.
25. Rodeo SA, O'Brien S, Warren RF, et al. Turf toe: an analysis of metatarsophalangeal joint sprains in professional football players. *Am J Sports Med* 1990; 18:280.
26. Clanton TO, Butler JE, Eggert A. Injuries to the metatarsophalangeal joints in athletes. *Foot Ankle* 1986; 7(3):162–176.
27. Santi M, Sartoris DJ, Resnick D. Diagnostic imaging of tarsal and metatarsal stress fractures (Part 1). *Orthop Rev* 1989; 18(2):178–185.
28. Daffner RH. Stress fractures. *Skeletal Radiol* 1987; 2:221–229.
29. Greaney RB, Gerber FH, Laughlin RL. Distribution and natural history of stress fractures in U.S. marine recruits. *Radiology* 1983; 146:339–346.
30. Geslian GE, Thrall JH, Espinosa JL, Older RA. Early detection of stress fractures using ^{99m}Tc-polyphosphate. *Radiology* 1976; 121:683–687.
31. Wilcox JR, Moniot AL, Green JP. Bone scanning in the evaluation of exercise-related stress injuries. *Radiology* 1977; 123:699–703.
32. Wilson ES, Katz FN. Stress fractures. An analysis of 250 consecutive cases. *Radiology* 1969; 92:481–486.
33. Beidleman B, Duncan GG. Charcot joints and infectious-vascular lesions of bone in diabetes mellitus. *Am J Med* 1952; 12:43–52.
34. Jacobs AM. Radiographic evaluation of the diabetic foot. *In* Weissman SD (ed). *Radiology of the Foot,* 2nd ed. Baltimore: Williams & Wilkins; 1989:262–288.
35. Schwarts GS, Berenyl MR, Siegel MW. Atrophic arthropathy and diabetic neuritis. *Am J Roentgenol* 1969; 106:523.
36. Harris RI, Beath T. Etiology of peroneal spastic flat foot. *J Bone Joint Surg* 1948; 30B:624–634.
37. Calabro JJ. A critical evaluation of the diagnostic features of the feet in rheumatoid arthritis. *Arthritis Rheum* 1962; 5:19.
38. Resnick D. The interphalangeal joint of the great toe in rheumatoid arthritis. *J Can Assoc Radiol* 1975; 26:255.
39. Martel W. Acute and chronic arthritis of the foot. *Semin Roentgenol* 1970; 5:391.
40. Resnick D. Roentgen features of the rheumatoid mid and hindfoot. *J Can Assoc Radiol* 1976; 27:99.
41. Gerster JC, Vischer TL, Bennani A, Fallet GH. The painful heel. Comparative study in rheumatoid arthritis, ankylosing spondylitis, Reiter's syndrome, and generalized osteoarthrosis. *Ann Rheum Dis* 1977; 36:343.
42. Resnick D, Feingold ML, Card J, et al. Calcaneal abnormalities in articular disorders. rheumatoid arthritis, ankylosing spondylitis, psoriatic arthritis, and Reiter's syndrome. *Radiology* 1977; 125:355.
43. Schumacher TM, Genant HK, Kellet MJ, et al. HLA-B27 associated arthropathies. *Radiology* 1978; 126:289–297.
44. Bartolomei FJ. Pedal radiographic manifestations of the seronegative spondyloarthritides. Part II. Psoriatic arthritis. *JAPA* 1986; 76:266–274.
45. Barthelemy CR, Nakayama DA, Carrerra GF, et al. Gouty arthritis: a prospective radiographic evaluation of sixty patients. *Skeletal Radiol* 1984; 11:1–8.
46. Resnick D. Niwayama G, Goergen TG, et al. Clinical, radiographic, and pathologic abnormalities in calcium pyrophosphate dihydrate deposition disease (CPPD): pseudogout. *Radiology* 1977; 122:1–15.
47. McLeod RA. Arthritis. *In* Berquist TH (ed). *Radiology of the Foot and Ankle.* New York: Raven Press; 1989:213–246.

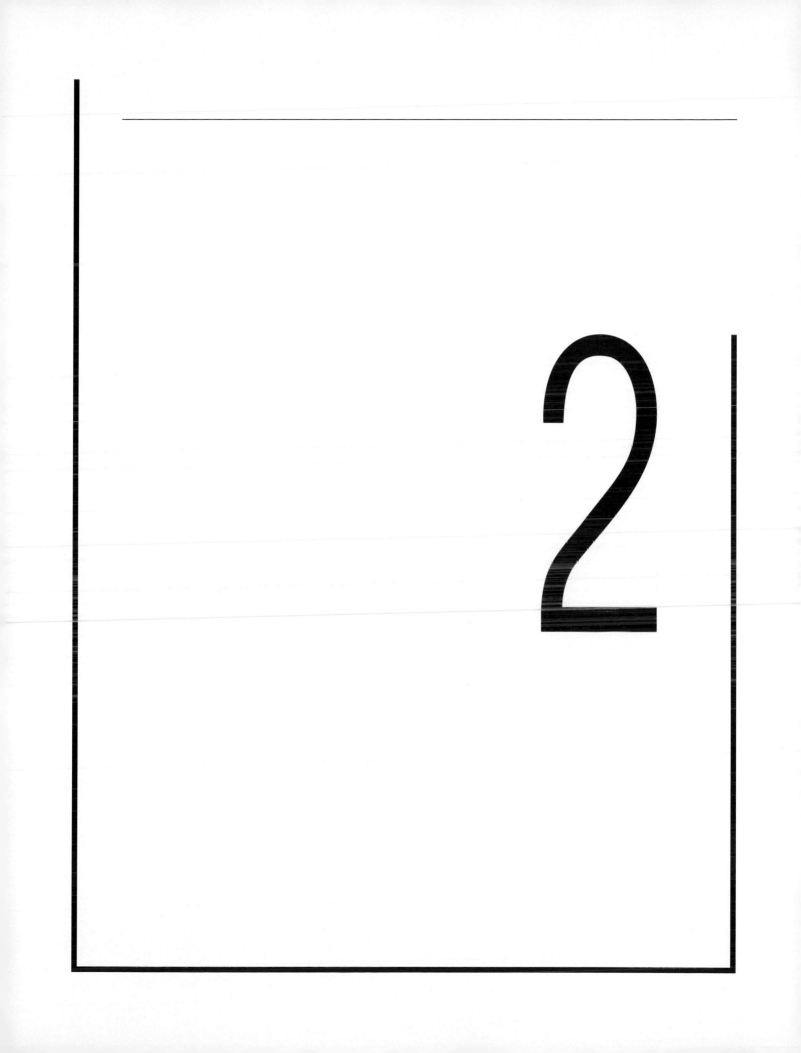

2

ELEVEN

Fractures

CLASSIFICATION OF FRACTURES

DESCRIPTION OF FRACTURES

Location
Direction of Fracture Lines
Alignment of Fracture Fragments
Other Special Features

FRACTURES IN CHILDREN

RADIOGRAPHIC EVALUATION OF FRACTURES

FRACTURE HEALING

RADIOGRAPHIC EVALUATION OF FRACTURE HEALING

EPONYMIC (NAMED) FRACTURES

FRACTURES WITH DESCRIPTIVE NAMES

Proper imaging of fractures requires more than knowledge of radiographic positioning for the injured part. The radiographic examination must be performed in a manner that will yield maximal information regarding the injury. To accomplish this consistently requires a more complete understanding of fractures. This chapter discusses classification and descriptions of fractures, fractures in children, radiographic evaluation of new and healing fractures, and stages of fracture healing.

Classification of Fractures

Skeletal fractures are classified as either closed or open and as either incomplete or complete. They are also classified by mode of injury, including traumatic, stress, and pathological fractures.

With the *closed* fracture, previously termed *simple*, there is no associated skin wound. The fracture is therefore not subject to bacterial contamination by external exposure. In the *open* fracture, sometimes termed *compound*, there is an associated wound to overlying skin and soft tissue that allows exposure to bacteria from the external environment (Fig. 11–1). Radiographically, air is often seen in the soft tissues immediately adjacent to the fracture.

The *incomplete* fracture, found predominantly in the more elastic bones of children, is the result of a partial disruption of bony trabeculae. These bony injuries are classified as follows:

Greenstick: fracture of one cortex (Fig. 11–2)
Torus: buckling of one cortex (Fig. 11–3)
Bowing (acute plastic): bending without cortical disruption

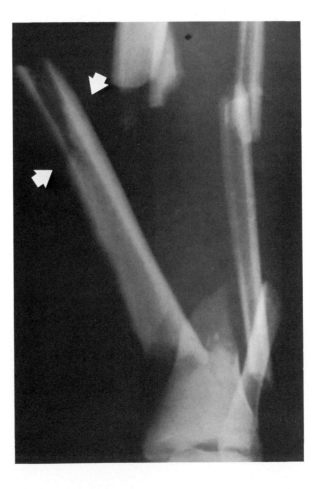

□ **FIGURE 11–1.**

Open fracture of the tibia. Segmented fractures of the tibia and fibula are demonstrated, with the proximal end of the tibial segment protruding through the skin of the leg (arrows).

Classification of Fractures *(continued)*

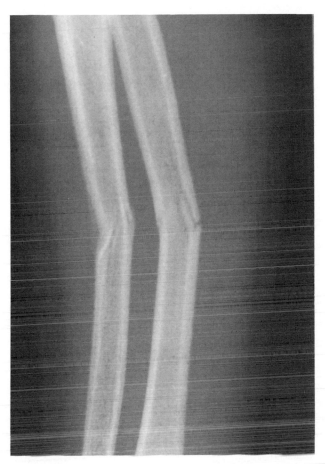

□ **FIGURE 11–2.**

Greenstick fracture of the radius and ulna of a child. The mid-shafts of the radius and ulna are incompletely fractured; only one cortical line in each bone is completely disrupted.

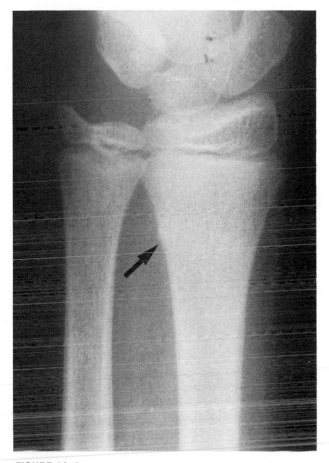

□ **FIGURE 11–3.**

Torus fracture of the distal radius in a child. There is a slight outward buckling of the cortex of the distal radius (arrow).

Classification of Fractures *(continued)*

The *complete* fracture is the result of full trabecular disruption with creation of at least two bone fragments. This category is further divided in relation to number of fragments present. One fracture line with two fragments is termed a *simple* fracture (Fig. 11–4). A fracture with more than two fragments is called *comminuted* (Fig. 11–5). The degree of comminution is described in a range from slight (few fragments) to severe (many fragments).

Traumatic fractures are caused by a single specific causative injury. The fracture may be caused by direct or indirect forces. Direct forces include low-impact strike with a hard object (tapping), crushing, and penetration. Most fractures are caused by forces indirectly affecting the site of injury. These forces include tension (pulling), angulation (bending), compression, and rotation. They often occur in combination. The appearance of the fracture is a result of the amount and types of force that acted on the bone.

Stress fractures are usually caused by repeated minor injury with no single specific causative injury. They are most prevalent in the metatarsals (walking/marching) and tibia-fibula (running/dancing). Strenuous, frequently repeated activities are a common cause of these fractures. Less frequently, a stress fracture results from a single extreme muscular contraction such as throwing a ball.

Pathological fractures occur in a bone already weakened by disease. The most common cause is a metastatic tumor. Other causes include benign bone tumors or cysts, congenital disease such as osteogenesis imperfecta, and bone-wasting disorders. Pathological fractures occur most often in the spine, humerus, femur, and tibia.

Classification of Fractures *(continued)*

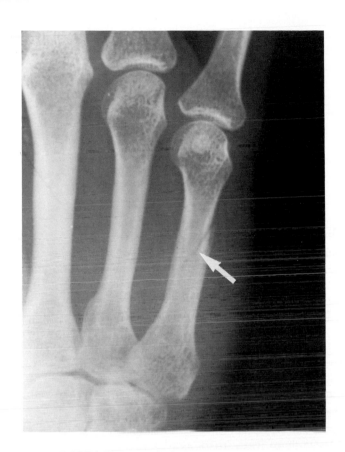

□ FIGURE 11–4.

Simple oblique fracture of the fifth metacarpal (arrow) divides the bone into two fragments.

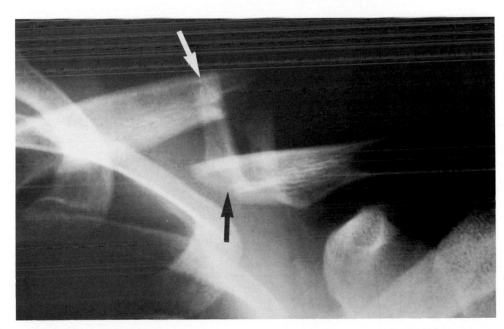

□ FIGURE 11–5.

Comminuted fracture of the clavicle (arrows) divides the bone into more than two fragments.

Description of Fractures

Fractures are described by location, direction of the fracture line or lines, alignment of fragments, and other special features. These descriptions are important to the orthopaedic surgeon when method of treatment is considered. The radiographer needs to be familiar with the terminology to facilitate communication with the surgeon or radiologist. The fracture description may also provide valuable information for guiding the radiographic procedure, especially during follow-up examination after treatment has been completed.

Location

Location of the fracture indicates the portion of bone involved. The description may include the general portion of the bone, indicate association with a particular bony structure, or refer to anatomical orientation. This information is particularly useful when the radiographer decides what portion of a long bone to include on follow-up films.

Location of fractures in short and long bones is usually described in relation to a general portion of bone. For descriptive purposes, these bones are divided in half or into thirds. The commonly used terms are *midshaft* and *proximal, middle,* or *distal third.*

Fracture location may be associated with specific anatomical structures. *Malleolar* (Fig. 11–6), *condylar, trochanteric* (Fig. 11–7), *articular* (Fig. 11–8), and *physeal* (Fig. 11–9) are examples.

Location of fractures may also be described by anatomical orientation. Examples of this include *volar surface* and *medial border.*

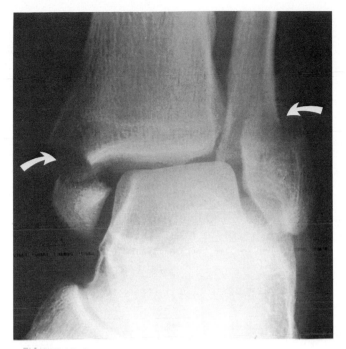

□ FIGURE 11–6.

Tri-malleolar fractures of the tibial and fibular malleoli (arrows). Note the talotibial subluxation associated with this group of fractures.

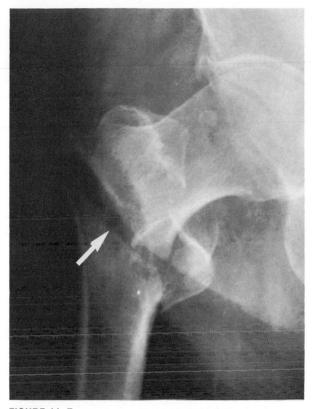

□ FIGURE 11–7.

Intertrochanteric fracture of the femur (arrow). The fracture line runs between the greater and lesser trochanters.

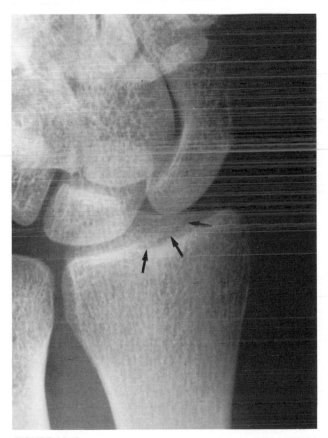

□ FIGURE 11–8.

A subtle fracture through the articular surface of the distal radius is demonstrated (arrows). The fracture is nondisplaced and was originally seen in only one projection from the multiple-angle scaphoid series.

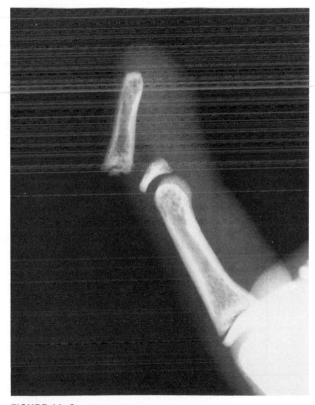

□ FIGURE 11–9.

Physeal fracture. There is a fracture-dislocation through the physis of the distal phalanx.

421

Description of Fractures *(continued)*

Direction of Fracture Lines

Direction of fracture lines is important to the surgeon for assessing the relative stability of a fracture. Some fractures are stable after reduction; others require internal fixation to maintain stability until healing is complete. Orientation of the fracture line is usually described in relation to the long axis of long/short bones, longest axis of irregular bones, or the long axis of the body. The descriptors include the following:

Transverse fractures are perpendicular to the long axis (Fig. 11–10). They are commonly caused indirectly by tension or angulation forces and directly by a blow from a hard object (tapping fracture).

Longitudinal fractures are parallel to the long axis (Fig. 11–11). They are not commonly seen alone, usually occurring in a complex fracture.

Oblique fractures are oriented approximately 45° to the long axis (see Fig. 11–4). They commonly result from compressive forces directed along the long axis of long and short bones.

Spiral fractures are obliquely oriented, but the fracture lines are longer and more parallel to the long axis than are those of the oblique fracture (Fig. 11–12). The spiral fracture results from the addition of twisting or torsion forces during injury.

Fractures may also be described as *horizontal* (see Fig. 11–10) or *vertical* (see Fig. 11–11) in relation to the long axis of the body.

Alignment of Fracture Fragments

Alignment of fracture fragments is described in relation to orientation of one fragment to the other or orientation to the long axis of the body. Common descriptors include the following:

Displacement: A fragment may be described as medially or laterally displaced.

Angulation: This term may describe the direction of both fragments (i.e., medial angulation of midshaft humeral fracture) or only one fragment (i.e., lateral angulation of distal humeral fragment).

Rotation: A fragment may be described as being rotated internally or externally from its normal position.

Overriding: Overlapping of fracture fragments results in foreshortening.

Distraction: This term means separation or loss of contact between fragments.

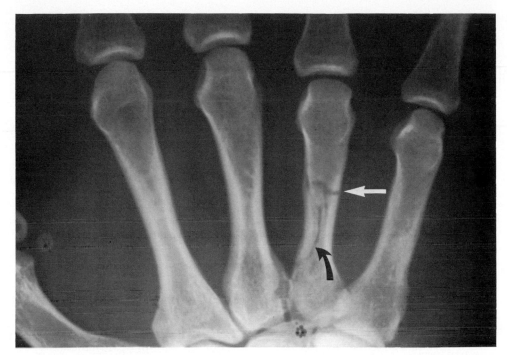

□ FIGURE 11-10.

Transverse fracture through the midshaft of the fourth metacarpal (white arrow). There is also a longitudinal fracture component directed proximally along the axis of the metacarpal (black arrow).

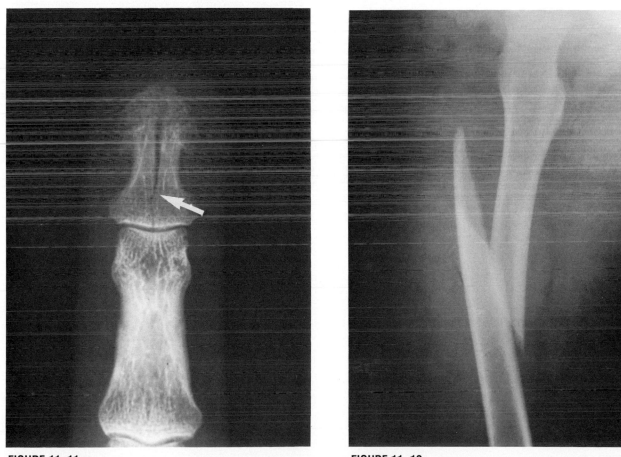

□ FIGURE 11-11.

Longitudinal fracture of the distal phalanx (arrow) resulted from a crush injury (finger trapped in a garage door).

□ FIGURE 11-12.

Spiral fracture of the midshaft of the femur in a child as a result of torsional force.

Description of Fractures *(continued)*

Other Special Features

Bone shape and certain modes of injury result in characteristic fractures:

Impacted fractures occur when one fragment is driven into another: for example, when the femoral neck is driven into the femoral head (Fig. 11–13).

Depressed fractures are caused by compression forces and result in a step-off or depression at the bone surface. These are often described in the skull and tibial plateau (Fig. 11–14).

Compression fractures are caused by compression forces and result in wedging (as in a vertebral body) (Fig. 11–15) or a troughlike depression (as in the humeral or femoral head).

Avulsion fractures are small fragments pulled from bony prominences as a result of excessive tension in the attached ligaments or tendons (Fig. 11–16). Also, this term may be applied to small fragments (chips) caused by a direct blow from a hard object.

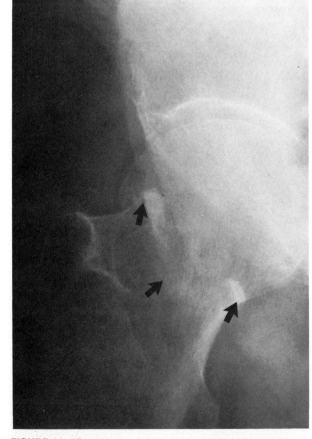

□ **FIGURE 11–13.**

Impacted fracture. A subcapital femoral fracture demonstrates the femoral neck driven into the femoral head (arrows).

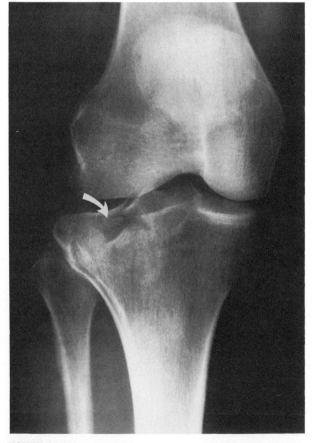

□ **FIGURE 11–14.**

Depressed fracture of the tibial plateau is seen on the lateral aspect of the tibia (arrow). This fracture was caused by the impact of the lateral femoral condyle on the tibial plateau.

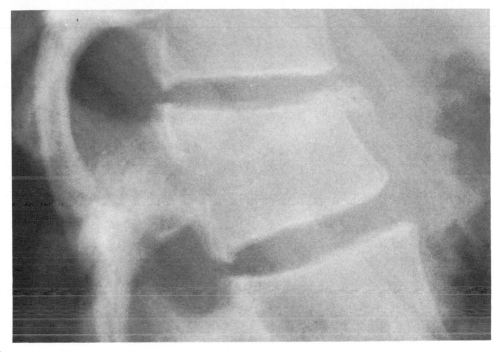

□ FIGURE 11–15.

Compression fracture of a thoracic vertebra is seen. The fracture displays the classic wedge shape.

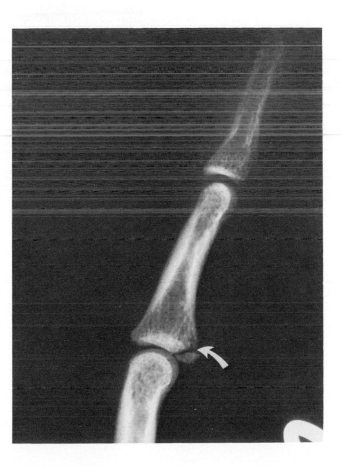

□ FIGURE 11–16.

Avulsion fracture of the middle phalanx. This type of fracture is commonly called a volar plate fracture and is the result of hyperextension of the finger.

Fractures in Children

The manifestations and consequences of fractures in children are different from those of fractures in adults. These fractures vary from those in adults in prevalence of type and location. The presence of active growth centers (epiphyses and apophyses) adds an additional consideration for the evaluation of the pediatric injury.

The skeleton of a child is more elastic than that of an adult. According to Rogers,[1] this is because of greater porosity and water content, as well as a slightly lower mineral content. Events that cause complete fractures in adults often cause incomplete fractures in children. For example, the cortex bends or buckles but does not fully fracture. These injuries are often radiographically subtle and challenge both the radiographer and the radiologist or orthopaedist. However, the diagnostic picture is not as bleak as it may appear. In spite of this greater elasticity, complete fractures involving the shaft of the long and short bones are the most common fractures in children[2] and are readily apparent on radiographs.

In addition to the tendency for incomplete fracture in juvenile bone, the presence of epiphyseal growth plates further complicates the radiographic evaluation. The epiphyseal plate (physis) is cartilaginous and thus radiolucent. Injury to this structure may not be visible on the radiograph, as in the case of a Salter-Harris type I epiphyseal separation.[3] The growth centers of bony processes (apophyses), such as the medial epicondyle of the distal humerus, may also be separated without radiographic evidence. However, a piece of the metaphysis usually accompanies the epiphysis as it separates[4] (Salter-Harris type II) and thus provides radiographic evidence of the injury. Trueta and Amato[5] demonstrated that an epiphyseal plate injury may have serious consequences if the vascular supply to the cartilage has been disrupted. Growth of the affected bone may be altered or disrupted entirely. It is extremely important that this type of injury be recognized and treated.

Radiographic Evaluation of Fractures

It is not enough to merely image a fracture. Each radiographic examination should include information on fracture classification, fragment alignment or displacement, how long the fracture has been present, and evidence of adjacent or associated injury. All these factors affect the course of treatment.

A complete examination requires imaging the entire affected bone, if possible. Radiographers satisfy this requirement by including both joints on long and short bones. The affected part should also be images in two 90° planes, if possible. Satisfying these two requirements allows effective evaluation of apposition, angulation, displacement, and rotation of fracture fragments.

In addition, exposure factors should be appropriate for evaluation of associated soft-tissue injury and evidence of fracture healing. The selected kilovoltage should be sufficient to penetrate the bone and visualize the fracture line but not overpenetrate the adjacent soft tissues. The number of milliampere-seconds should not lead to overexposure of the soft tissues. A properly exposed image allows evaluation of overlying skin integrity and displacement of fat pads or fascial planes. If a lipohemarthrosis (fat-blood level in joint) is suspected, a horizontal beam radiograph is required.

The radiographer should be cognizant of possible growth plate trauma when a child's injury involves the end of a long bone. The physeal cartilage is weaker than the associated bone, muscle, and fibrous joint structures. According to Salter and Harris[3], injuries that would cause a dislocation or ligament tear in adults may result in epiphyseal separation or apophyseal avulsion in children. Great care should be taken to obtain optimal images of both bone and soft tissues. The first clue to a subtle fracture may be the associated soft-tissue swelling. Rockwood and associates[6] stated that when an epiphyseal plate injury is suspected after the routine films are viewed, additional images may be taken with the central ray placed to pass through and parallel to the plate. This minimizes parallax distortion and optimizes image evaluation of subtle injury. Just as in the adult, two projections at 90° are usually necessary to fully evaluate the injury. In addition, images of the opposite side may be needed for comparison. It is important that these images duplicate the positions of the original examination, if they are to be of value.

Postreduction or post-treatment radiographs must provide slightly different information. The images should demonstrate changes in apposition or angulation of the fracture fragments. The position or condition of fixation devices must be evaluated by comparison with the previous images. This requires viewing the previous projections to ensure the positioning has been duplicated in the current examination. The images should also document the stage of fracture healing, such as callus formation or obliteration of the fracture line or lines.

Fracture Healing

The extent of fracture healing is primarily a clinical determination. The fracture is considered to be united when it is stable, when there is no pain at the site, and when use of the affected part is restored. The fracture healing process is approaching the intermediate stage before it is seen radiographically. However, an understanding of the complete process enhances the radiographer's evaluation of the radiographic examination and ensures that complete information has been obtained.

The process of fracture healing is an incompletely understood phenomenon. Discussion of the process is often divided into three overlapping stages: inflammatory, reparative, and remodeling. According to Hulth,[7] the inflammatory stage is relatively brief, whereas the majority of the fracture healing process is encompassed by the reparative and remodeling stages. The process may also be described through a chronology of significant events. Either manner of discussion is correct, because they describe the same progression of events. The following is a description of the healing events common to closed treatment (cast, brace, and so forth) of long bone diaphysis fractures.

The early (inflammatory) stage of fracture healing begins with formation of a hematoma at the fracture site. Inflammatory cells migrate to the site, and a fracture exudate forms. The fragment ends begin to necrose, as osteocytes die from loss of blood supply.[8]

In the reparative phase of fracture healing, granulation tissue forms. Vasodilation occurs, increasing blood flow to the area. New blood vessels proliferate from within the bone and from the overlying periosteum. A fracture callus is formed, as the granulation tissue matures. This immature callus is present both within the bone (endosteal) and on the surface of the bone (periosteal). It is composed primarily of fibrous tissue, cartilage, and woven bone.

Remodeling is the most lengthy phase of fracture healing. The endosteal and periosteal callus continues to mature. Excess repair tissue and remaining dead bone are reabsorbed. The woven bone is replaced by laminar (mature) bone, and the bony matrix is reorganized along lines of stress. The bone is concurrently revascularized as the blood vessel proliferation started in the reparative stage is organized.

This description of the fracture healing process is a generalization and does not accurately chronicle the events that take place in all types of bone. Small irregular bones, such as the scaphoid, and bony prominences, such as a malleolus, develop very few external (periosteal) calluses. They heal primarily by endosteal callus formation. It is more difficult to radiographically document intermediate stages of fracture healing in these bones.

Radiographic Evaluation of Fracture Healing

As previously mentioned, fracture healing is primarily a clinical determination. However, radiographic evaluation is useful for visually documenting the stage of healing. Radiography is especially important in cases in which delay or failure of the healing process is suspected.

The earliest radiographic evidence of fracture healing is widening of the fracture line with loss of definition at the fracture ends. This is caused by absorption of necrotic bone at the fragment ends, which occurs late in the initial (inflammatory) stage of healing. This radiographic appearance is usually seen between 1 and 2 weeks after the fracture incident.

The second radiographic sign of fracture healing is appearance of an external callus (Figs. 11–17A, 11–17B). This callus is rather translucent, because it contains immature woven bone. Initially, the callus does not appear to contact the fracture site. As it matures, the callus appears to proceed toward the fracture margins. With continued maturation, the woven bone is replaced by lamellar bone, and the callus exhibits the radiographic appearance of mature bone.

The endosteal callus is difficult to visualize radiographically. However, the completion of this aspect of the healing process is evidenced by disappearance of the fracture line. This finding signals completion of bony bridging between the fracture fragments.

Rigid internal fixation alters fracture healing and therefore the radiographic appearance of healing. There is usually no appreciable widening of the fracture line in the early stage of healing. The only evidence seen radiographically may be gradual disappearance of the fracture line. Perren and associates[9] warned that radiographic examinations of internally fixed fractures displaying formation of a significant external callus or widening of the fracture line may indicate an abnormality in the healing process, such as excessive fracture movement or infection.

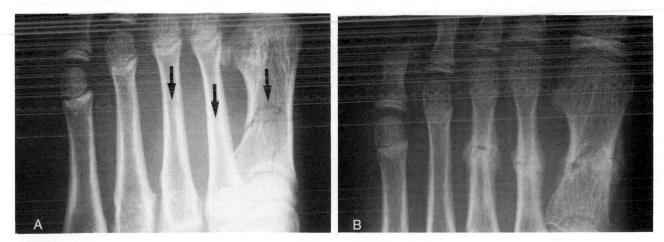

□ **FIGURE 11–17.**

A, Multiple metatarsal fractures (arrows) are seen in a patient who dropped a heavy object on the foot. Note the faint nondisplaced fracture lines seen in the second and third metatarsals. B, Follow-up radiograph of case seen in part A, taken 1 month after the injury, shows well-defined callus formations at the fracture sites. Note the widening of the fracture lines.

Eponymic (Named) Fractures

Barton's fracture: fracture of the distal end of the radius into the wrist joint; unstable oblique intra-articular fracture of the dorsal or ventral surface of the distal radius.

Bennett's fracture: fracture of the base of the first metacarpal bone, running into the carpometacarpal joint and complicated by subluxation.

Bosworth's fracture: spiral fracture of the distal fibula with posterior dislocation and entrapment of the proximal fragment posterior to the tibia.

Colles' fracture: hyperextension fracture of the distal radius in which the distal fragment is displaced or angulated posteriorly and the radioulnar joint is disrupted. The ulnar styloid may also be fractured by avulsion forces.

Cotton's fracture: also called a tri-malleolar fracture. Refers to a combination of fractures involving the medial malleolus, the lateral malleolus, and the posterior lip of the tibia (posterior malleolus).

Dupuytren's fracture: fracture of the distal fibula with rupture of the deltoid ligament, lateral subluxation of the talus, and disruption of the distal tibiofibular syndesmosis.

Duverney's fracture: fracture of the ilium just below the anterior superior iliac spine.

Essex-Lopresti fracture: comminuted, impacted fracture of the radial head and neck with associated distal radioulnar joint dislocation.

Galeazzi's fracture: fracture of the radius above the wrist (junction of middle and distal thirds) with distal radioulnar joint subluxation or dislocation.

Gosselin's fracture: a V-shaped fracture of the distal tibia that extends into the joint.

Hutchinson's fracture: also called the chauffeur's fracture. A sagittally oriented, intra-articular fracture of the radial styloid. Historically associated with sudden unwinding of the engine crank in early automobiles.

Jefferson's fracture: a burst (compression) fracture involving both anterior and posterior arches of the atlas.

Jones' fracture: proximal diaphyseal fracture of the fifth metatarsal.

LeFort's fracture I: transverse fracture at the base of the maxillary antra, resulting in separation of the alveolar process. Also called Guerin's fracture.

LeFort's fracture II: pyramidal fracture of the central portion of the face.

LeFort's fracture III: extensive transverse fracture resulting in complete craniofacial separation.

Lisfranc's fracture-dislocation: fracture-dislocation of the tarsometatarsal joints (Lisfranc joint).

Maisonneuve's fracture: fracture of the proximal fibula with rupture of the deltoid ligament, lateral subluxation of the talus, and disruption of the distal tibiofibular syndesmosis.

Malgaigne's fracture: a supramalleolar transverse, oblique, or comminuted fracture of the distal tibia. Also refers to fracture of the anterior and posterior pelvic arches on the same side.

Monteggia's fracture: a fracture involving the proximal half of the shaft of the ulna and associated dislocation of the radiohumeroulnar joint (often the head of the radius). Sometimes called a parry fracture because it may be caused by attempts to fend off blows with the forearm.

Moore's fracture: fracture of distal radius with ulnar head dislocation and entrapment of the ulnar styloid beneath the annular ligaments.

Pott's fracture: Dupuytren's fracture with intact tibiofibular syndesmosis.

Eponymic (Named) Fractures *(continued)*

Quervain's fracture: fracture of the scaphoid with volar dislocation of the lunate.

Rolando's fracture: comminuted Bennett's fracture.

Segond's fracture: avulsion fracture on the margin of the lateral tibial condyle at the attachment of the lateral capsular ligament.

Skillern's fracture: complete fracture of distal radius with incomplete (greenstick) fracture of distal ulna.

Smith's fracture: reverse Colles' fracture; hyperflexion fracture of the distal radius with anterior displacement and anterior angulation of the distal fragment.

Steide's fracture: fracture of the medial femoral condyle.

Tillaux fracture: avulsion fracture of either the anterior or posterior tubercle of the lateral tibial articular surface, associated with disruption of the distal tibiofibular syndesmosis.

Wagstaffe-LeForte fracture: avulsion of the anterior fibular tubercle by the anterior tibiofibular ligament.

Fractures with Descriptive Names

Beak fracture: avulsion of the posterosuperior portion of the calcaneal tuberosity by the Achilles tendon.

Blow-out fracture: orbital floor caused by a sudden increase in intraorbital pressure resulting from traumatic force.

Boxer's fracture: a transverse fracture through the metacarpal neck, resulting in volar angulation of the head. The fracture name is derived from the common mechanism of injury; punching a solid object with a bare fist.

Bucket-handle fracture: fracture of the anterior and posterior pelvic arches on the opposite sides.

Bumper fracture: fracture of one or both legs caused by impact of an automobile bumper. Often occurs just below the knees and involves the tibial plateau.

Butterfly fracture: comminuted fracture with a main fragment shaped in such a way that the fragments on either side resemble the wings of a butterfly.

Buttonhole fracture: perforation of the bone by a missile (bullet or other small, rapidly moving object).

Chance fracture: thoracolumbar distraction injury involving transverse fracture through the posterior elements, which may extend into the posterosuperior or posteroinferior portion of the vertebral body.

Clay-shoveler's fracture: avulsion fracture of a spinous process, most often of the seventh cervical vertebra.

Fulcrum fracture: thoracolumbar distraction injury involving transverse fracture through the posterior elements and transverse fracture of the vertebral body.

Hangman's fracture: bilateral avulsion fractures through the pedicles of the axis (C2) with or without subluxation of the second cervical vertebra on the third.

Insufficiency fracture: results in bone with altered elasticity resulting from disease.

March fracture: also called a fatigue fracture; fracture of a bone in the lower extremity, developing after repeated stresses, as seen in soldiers.

Nutcracker fracture: crushing of the cuboid between the fourth or fifth metatarsal and the anterior calcaneus during lateral subluxation of the midtarsal joint (Chopart's joint).

Paratrooper fracture: fracture of the posterior articular margin of the tibia and/or of the internal or external malleolus.

Pilon fracture: a comminuted fracture of the tibial plafond involving the medial malleolus, lateral malleolus, anterior tibial lip, and the distal tibia proximal to the articular surface. It results from impact of the talus against the plafond. A hallmark of the pilon fracture is an anteriorly displaced fracture of the anterior tibial lip, often maintained in association with the talus.

Ping-pong fracture: depressed skull fracture resembling the indentation made by pressing a finger into a ping-pong ball.

Sprinter's fracture: avulsion fracture of the anterosuperior or anteroinferior iliac spine, caused by violent muscular action.

Straddle fracture: bilateral fracture of both pubic rami.

Teardrop fracture: hyperflexion fracture-dislocation in the cervical spine with a characteristic "teardrop" fragment of the anteroinferior vertebral body.

Tripod fracture: trimalar fracture involving fracture of the three processes of the zygoma: zygomatic arch, orbital process, and maxillary process.

References

1. Rogers LF. *Radiology of Skeletal Trauma.* London: Churchill Livingstone; 1982:67–87.
2. Silverman FN. Problems in pediatric fractures. *Semin Roentgenol* 1978; 13:167.
3. Salter RB, Harris WR. Injuries involving the epiphyseal plate. *J Bone Joint Surg Am* 1963; 45A(3):587–622.
4. Rogers LF. The radiography of epiphyseal injuries. *Radiology* 1970; 96:289–299.
5. Trueta J, Amato VP. The vascular contribution to osteogenesis III. Changes in the growth cartilage caused by experimentally induced ischemia. *J Bone Joint Surg* 1960; 42B:571–587.
6. Rockwood CA, Wilkins KE, King RE. *Fractures in Children,* vol 3. Philadelphia: JB Lippincott; 1984:125–127.
7. Hulth A. Current concepts of fracture healing. *Clin Orthop* 1989; 249:265–284.
8. Cruess RL, Dumont J. Fracture healing. *Can J Surg* 1975; 18:403–410.
9. Perren SM, Matter P, Ruedi R, et al. Biomechanics of fracture healing after internal fixation. *Surg Annu* 1975; 7:361–390.

Bibliography

Adams JC. *Outline of Fractures,* 8th ed. London: Churchill Livingstone; 1983.

Berquist TH. *Imaging of Orthopedic Trauma,* 2nd ed. New York: Raven Press; 1992.

Greenspan A. *Orthopedic Radiology: A Practical Approach.* Philadelphia: JB Lippincott; 1988.

Rockwood CA, Green DP, Buckholz RW. *Rockwood and Green's Fractures in Adults,* vols 1 and 2. Philadelphia: JB Lippincott; 1991.

Rogers LF. *Radiology of Skeletal Trauma.* London: Churchill Livingstone; 1982.

Weissman BNW, Sledge CB. *Orthopedic Radiology.* Philadelphia: WB Saunders; 1986.

TWELVE

Orthopaedic Hardware

TYPES OF FIXATION HARDWARE

Wires
Pins
Screws
Plates
Nails
Arthroplastic Components
External Fixation
Spinal Instrumentation

RADIOGRAPHY OF FIXATION HARDWARE

Numerous items of orthopaedic hardware may be seen on radiographs. They are used to fix fractures, provide stability, replace joints, and correct malalignment, deformity, or limb length discrepancies. Radiography of anatomy that includes orthopaedic hardware requires attention to the integrity of both the bone and the hardware. Proper imaging necessitates at least a cursory understanding of the form and function of these hardware components.

Types of Fixation Hardware

Wires

Wires have several uses for fracture fixation. They may be used as pins, for application of skeletal traction in children, to wrap around the shaft of a long bone, or to tie selected fracture fragments together.

Kirschner wires (K-wires) are thin wire pins used to fix fractures in short bones (such as in the hands or feet) and near joints where the load on the fractures is expected to be light (Figs. 12–1A, 12–1B). K-wires are also used for provisional approximation of complex fractures before definitive fixation with other devices such as screws and plates. They may be used with a traction bow to apply skeletal traction, especially in children.

Cerclage wiring is a technique in which wire is wrapped around a bone for temporary approximation to aid definitive fixation or for definitive fixation in combination with other hardware such as plates or rods. Cerclage wiring may also be applied to provide fracture protection when prosthetic joints are placed in osteopenic bone (Fig. 12–2).

Tension band wiring may be used in selected locations to provide definitive fixation of fractures by "tying" the fractured ends of the bone together. The wire is passed in and out of the cortex of each fragment and then twisted together. Addition of two parallel K-wires is often necessary to provide rotational stability. Transverse patellar or olecranon fractures are most frequently treated in this manner (Fig. 12–3). Fractures of the greater trochanter and distal clavicle may also be treated with tension band wiring.

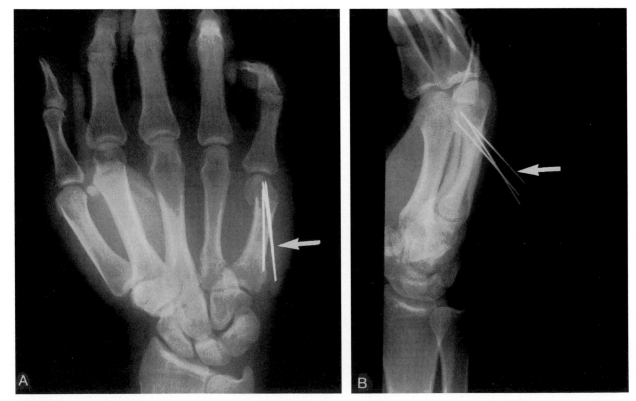

□ **FIGURE 12–1.**

A, Multiple Kirschner wire (arrow) fixation of a distal fifth metacarpal fracture. *B,* The volar angulation of the distal fragment is demonstrated on the lateral radiograph. The anteroposterior orientation of the Kirschner wires is also evident (arrow).

Types of Fixation Hardware *(continued)*

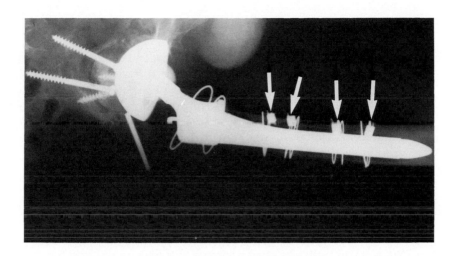

□ **FIGURE 12–2.**

Cerclage wiring (arrows) as an adjunct to total hip arthroplasty. The wires provide additional support to prevent fracture of bone adjacent to the prosthesis stem.

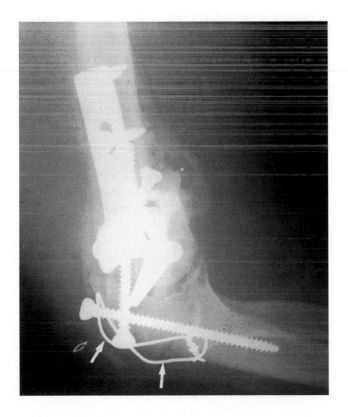

□ **FIGURE 12–3.**

Tension band wiring (arrows) of an olecranon fracture. In addition, cancellous screws and a compression plate were used to repair this extensively fractured elbow.

Types of Fixation Hardware *(continued)*

Pins

Pins are metallic cylinders that are larger in diameter than wires but smaller than nails. The Steinmann pin is used for transfixion to achieve skeletal traction and may be used with external fixators. The Knowles pin is a special screw used to treat nondisplaced or impacted subcapital fractures of the femoral head (Fig. 12–4). Full or half pins with a screw component have been developed for use with external fixation systems (Fig. 12–5).

Screws

Screws are used to fix bone to bone, to attach plates and implants to bone, and to attach soft tissues (ligaments. tendons) to bone. Screws are usually either cortical or cancellous to match the type of bone structure in which they will reside. Cortical screws have fine threads the full length of the shaft. These are the screws commonly used to attach plates to bone (see Fig. 12–4). Cortical screws may also be used to fix bone to bone, as in interfragmentary compression, but a gliding hole must be drilled adjacent to the screw head to produce the compressing (lag screw) effect.

Cancellous screws have larger threads with more surface area to improve purchase in the softer cancellous bone (Fig. 12–6). The shaft is usually smooth adjacent to the screw head to allow interfragmentary compression (pulling together the fragments) without the need to drill a gliding hole. Washers or plates may be needed to prevent the screw head from burying into the thin cortex over the cancellous bone.

A great number of screws are designed for use in special situations. Cannulated screws are hollow to allow passage over a fluoroscopically placed guide wire for percutaneous fixation (Fig. 12–7). These screws are frequently used to treat nondisplaced or impacted femoral neck fractures. Herbert screws are threaded differently at each end and have no screw head, and so they can be inserted through articular surfaces without protruding. Large screws with a smooth central shaft and threads at both ends are used to "lock" intramedullary nails. Dynamic or sliding hip screws with side plates are used to treat intertrochanteric and some subtrochanteric fractures in elderly patients (see Fig. 12–4). The dynamic condylar screw with side plate is used to fix supracondylar and intercondylar fractures of the distal femur.

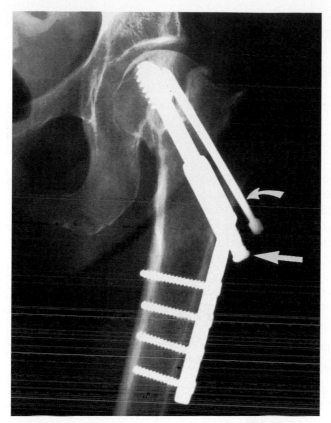

□ FIGURE 12–4.

A Knowles pin (curved arrow) and a sliding hip screw with side plate (straight arrow) were used to repair this subcapital femoral fracture. Cortical screws were used to attach the side plate to the femoral shaft.

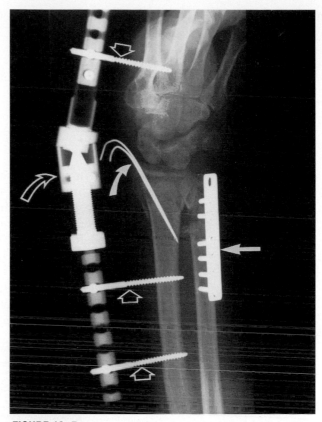

□ FIGURE 12–5.

An external fixation device (open curved arrow) with threaded half pins (open straight arrows) used in conjunction with Kirschner wires (curved solid arrow) and a dynamic compression plate (straight solid arrow) for the repair of a distal radius and ulnar fracture.

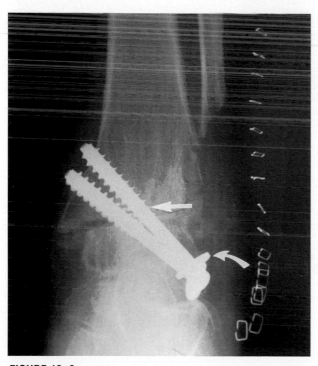

□ FIGURE 12–6.

Two large cancellous screws were used to secure this tibiotalar arthrodesis (straight arrow). Washers (curved arrow) were added to the screws to prevent the screw heads from breaking through the talar cortex.

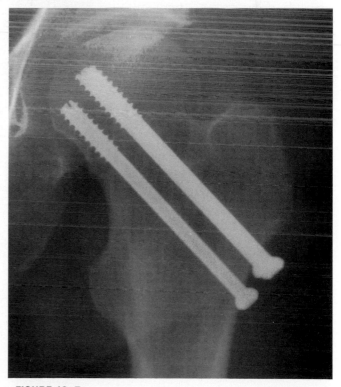

□ FIGURE 12–7.

Two cannulated screws were used to fix this femoral neck fracture.

Types of Fixation Hardware *(continued)*

Plates

Plates come in a variety of shapes and sizes for use in very diverse situations. Dynamic compression plates are commonly used to provide interfragmentary compression or to protect an interfragmentary lag screw fixation (see Fig. 12–5). Buttress plates are used to fix large articular fragments to the shaft and to support, or buttress, the metaphyseal portion during healing. Reconstruction plates are specially constructed to allow bending or molding to the contour of a bony surface. The angled blade plate is used to treat subcondylar fractures of the proximal femur and supracondylar or intercondylar fractures of the distal femur. T-, U-, or L- shaped plates are used in a variety of special situations and locations (Fig. 12–8).

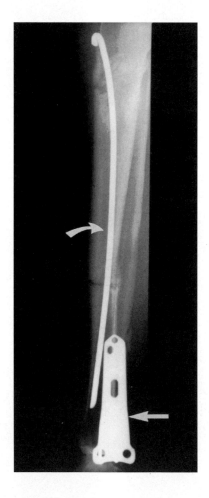

□ **FIGURE 12–8.**

A specially shaped compression plate (straight arrow) used to fix a distal tibial fracture. A Rush rod (curved arrow) was used to stabilize the midshaft fracture of the tibia.

Types of Fixation Hardware *(continued)*

Nails

Nails are primarily used for intramedullary fixation of diaphyseal fractures in long bones. The most common indication for use is in closed fractures in which early mobility is desired (Fig. 12–9A, 12–9B). Some nails require enlarging the medullary canal by reaming to improve the nail contact with the bone. Intramedullary nails may be "locked" with cross screws to increase rotational stability (Fig. 12–10). Smaller diameter nails such as Hackethal nails, Rush rods, and Ender pins may be used in groups. A great variety of nails are designed for treatment of specific fractures.

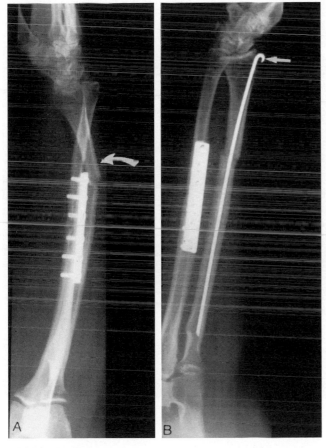

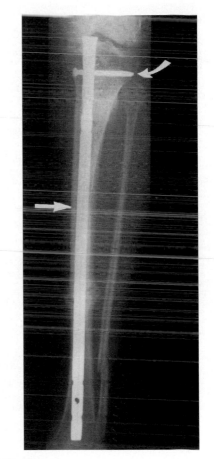

□ **FIGURE 12–9.**

□ **FIGURE 12–10.**

A, A dynamic compression plate was used for the initial repair of a forearm injury. However, a postoperative lateral radiograph demonstrated significant anterior angulation of the distal radial fragment (arrow). *B,* The alignment of the radius was corrected during a second surgical procedure with the addition of a Rush rod (straight arrow).

An intramedullary nail (straight arrow) with a proximal locking screw (curved arrow) was used to stabilize this midshaft fracture of the tibia.

Types of Fixation Hardware *(continued)*

Arthroplastic Components

Components for joint arthroplasty have been developed for most joints. They are commonly used in the hip and knee (Figs. 12–11A, 12–11B; also see Fig. 12–2). In addition, they may be used to reconstruct the joints of the shoulder, elbow, wrist, ankle, and phalanges (Figs. 12–12, 12–13). All or part of the joint components may be replaced. The components may be fixed to bone with cement or form fitted (noncemented) (Fig. 12–14). Some components are nonmetallic (plastic, ceramic) and may be radiolucent.

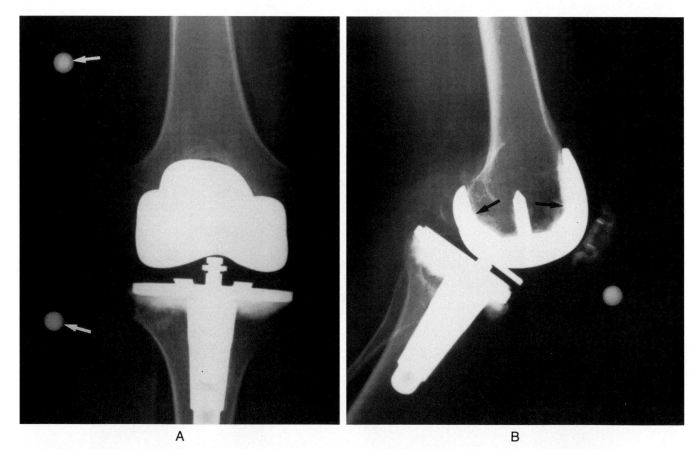

A   B

□ **FIGURE 12–11.**

Total knee arthroplasty. Both femoral and tibial components are well demonstrated. *A*, 100-mm magnification marker balls (arrows) are demonstrated. These markers are used to determine the percentage of magnification of each radiograph. *B*, A perfect lateral radiograph is needed for accurately assessing the integrity of the bone/component interface (arrows).

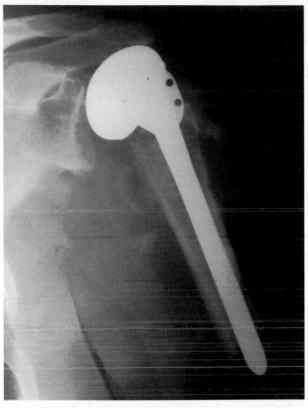

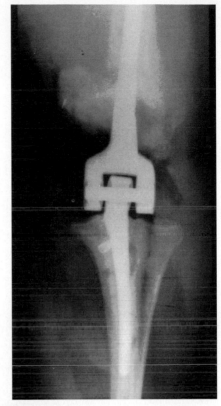

□ **FIGURE 12–12.**

A total shoulder arthroplasty demonstrating cephalad migration.

□ **FIGURE 12–13.**

Intraoperative radiograph of a total elbow arthroplasty.

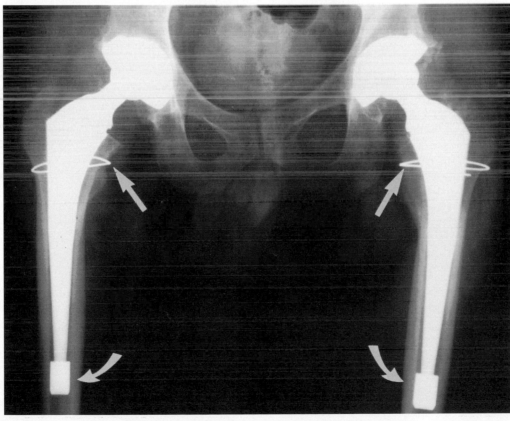

□ **FIGURE 12–14.**

Bilateral total hip arthroplasty. These are cementless femoral components, as indicated by the shape of their distal tips (curved arrows). Cerclage wiring (straight arrows) is also demonstrated.

Types of Fixation Hardware *(continued)*

External Fixation

External fixation devices are commonly used to stabilize fractures in situations in which internal fixation is contraindicated or must be delayed. They are also used for limb lengthening or for correcting malalignment. The frame may consist of longitudinal members, rings, or arcs. The bone may be held by half pins, full transfixion pins, or transfixion wires (Figs. 12–15*A*, 12–15*B*). The Hoffmann frame is the most common pin and frame (longitudinal) device and is used for fracture stabilization. The Ilizarov device is the most common ring fixator and is used primarily for limb lengthening; it may also be used for fracture treatment. The Ace-Fischer frame is a hybrid device in which arcs or half rings are used as frame components.

Types of Fixation Hardware *(continued)*

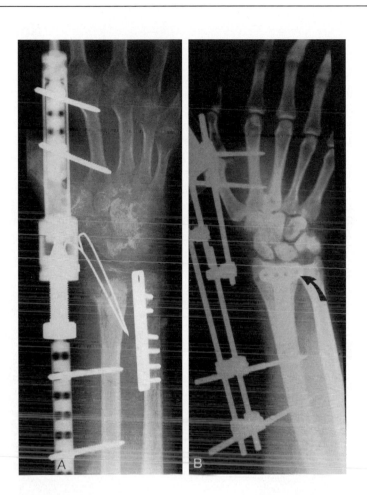

□ **FIGURE 12–15.**

Two types of external fixation devices. *A,* This centrally articulated, tubular fixator with threaded half pins was used in conjunction with a dynamic compression plate and two Kirschner wires to fix the distal radius and ulna fractures. *B,* This Hoffmann frame fixator was used with a T-shaped compression plate (arrow) to stabilize the distal radius fracture.

Types of Fixation Hardware *(continued)*

Spinal Instrumentation

Spinal fractures may be fixed with a variety of plates, screws, and wiring techniques. In addition, a number of instrumentation systems have been developed to provide spinal stabilization, as well as correction of deformities such as scoliosis. The posterior distraction systems (e.g., Harrington, Jacobs) consist of distraction rods with laminar and transverse process hooks (Fig. 12–16). The posterior transverse loading systems (e.g., Luque, Galveston technique, unit rod) include smooth rods and sublaminar wiring (Fig. 12–17). The posterior de-rotation systems (e.g., Cotrel-Dubousset, Isola, TSRH) consist of malleable rods, lamina and pedicle hooks, sacral or pedicle screws and connecting cross-members (Figs. 12–18*A*, 12–18*B*, 12–19*A*, 12–19*B*). Ventral de-rotation systems (e.g., Zielke) include vertebral body screws and flexible threaded rods (Fig. 12–20). Other spinal instrumentation systems that do not fit these categories have been developed (Fig. 12–21*A*, 12–21*B*).

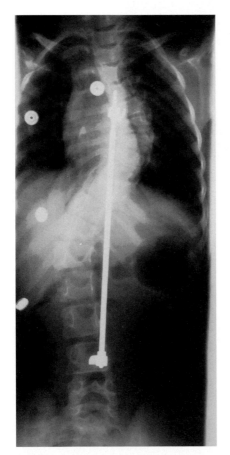

□ **FIGURE 12–16.**

Single Harrington rod used to treat this thoracolumbar scoliosis.

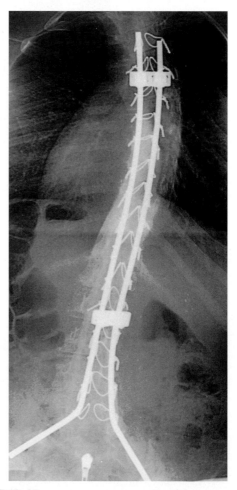

□ **FIGURE 12–17.**

Luque instrumentation with sublaminar wiring and Galveston pelvic fixation technique were used to treat this thoracolumbar scoliosis.

Types of Fixation Hardware *(continued)*

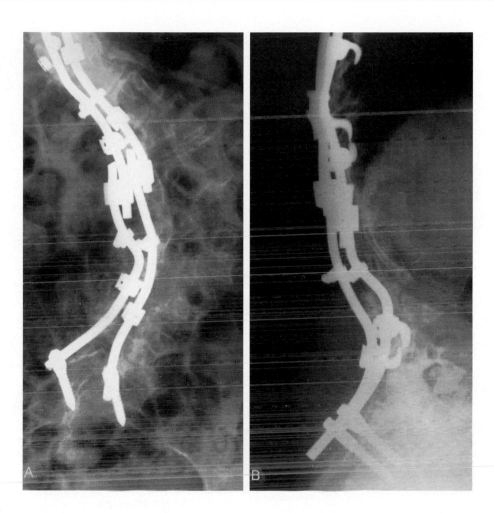

□ **FIGURE 12-18.**

Anteroposterior (A) and lateral (B) radiographs of Cotrel-Dubousset spinal instrumentation for treatment of severe scoliosis.

Types of Fixation Hardware *(continued)*

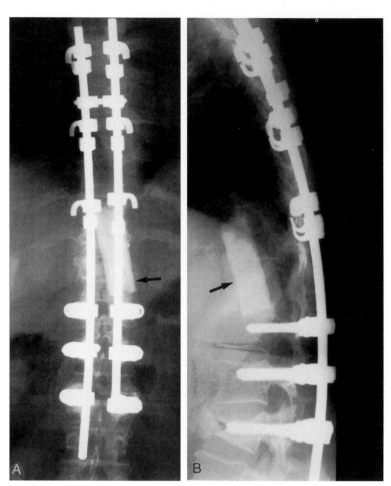

□ **FIGURE 12–19.**

Anteroposterior (*A*) and lateral (*B*) radiographs of Isola spinal instrumentation for stabilization of a lower thoracic osteoporotic burst fracture. A bone graft (arrows) is also demonstrated in each.

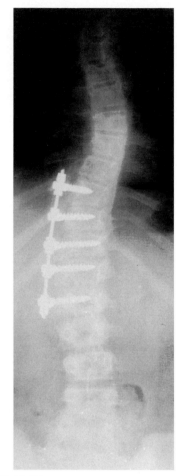

□ **FIGURE 12–20.**

Zielke instrumentation used to ventrally de-rotate this thoracolumbar scoliosis.

Types of Fixation Hardware *(continued)*

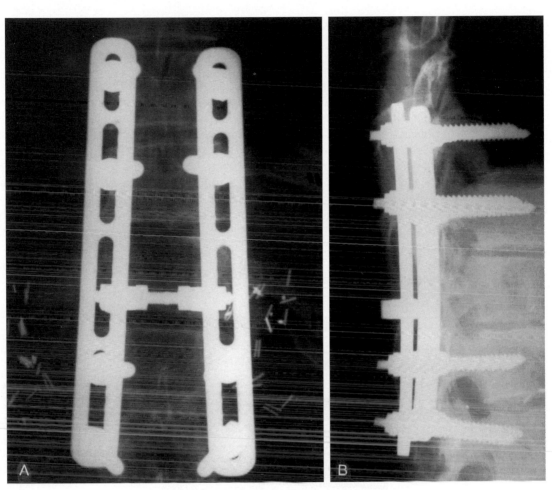

□ **FIGURE 12–21.**

Anteroposterior (*A*) and lateral (*B*) radiographs of a Steffee plate with transpedicular screw fixation for spinal stabilization after resection of a tumor.

Radiography of Fixation Hardware

Radiography of a body part treated by application of orthopaedic hardware requires attention to both the anatomical components and the hardware. Positioning and exposure factors that allow evaluation of bone, soft tissues, and fixation components must be chosen.

Fracture fragments must be assessed for both anatomical alignment and approximation. Standard positions or projections for the particular anatomical region are often sufficient. However, when special positions are necessary, they should be used for both the initial assessment and postreduction, if possible. As treatment progresses, radiographic evidence of fracture healing should be demonstrated. The presence and extent of fracture callus may be affected by numerous factors such as time lapsed since injury, rigidity of fixation, and degree of adjacent soft-tissue trauma.

The hardware components themselves are often subject to stresses during the healing process, and as a result, they may fail. The components can break, loosen, or fail to maintain proper fixation or alignment. Assessment of hardware integrity is an important part of radiography for evaluation of fractures treated by hardware placement (Figs. 12–22, 12–23, 12–24).

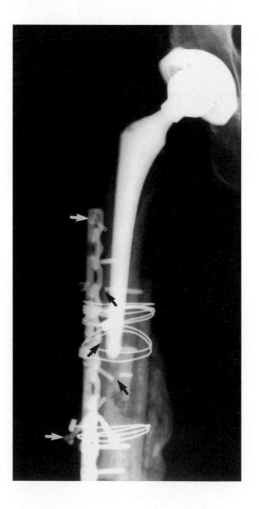

□ **FIGURE 12–22.**

Multiple broken (black arrows) and loosened (white arrows) compression plate screws in a total hip arthroplasty. Cerclage wiring was added to augment the plate fixation.

Radiography of Fixation Hardware *(continued)*

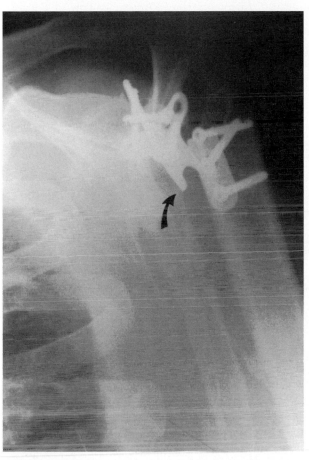

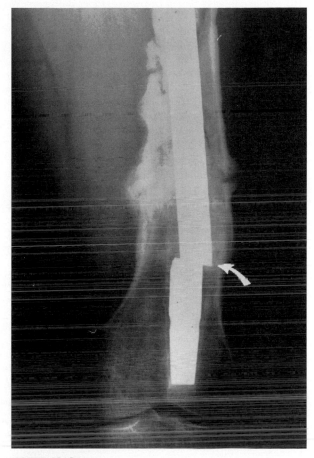

□ **FIGURE 12–23.**

Failure of a compression plate used for treatment of a humeral neck fracture. The plate has broken across one of the screw holes (arrow).

□ **FIGURE 12–24.**

Failure of an intramedullary rod (arrow) at the distal end of the femur.

Bibliography

An HS, Cotler JM (eds). *Spinal Instrumentation.* Baltimore: Williams & Wilkins; 1992.

Browner BD, Edwards CC. *The Science & Practice of Intramedullary Nailing.* Philadelphia: Lea & Febiger; 1987.

Chapman MW, Madison M (eds). *Operative Orthopaedics,* 2nd ed, vol 1. Philadelphia: JB Lippincott; 1993.

Hansen ST, Swiontkowski MF (eds). *Orthopaedic Trauma Protocols.* New York: Raven Press; 1993.

Mears DC. *External Skeletal Fixation.* Baltimore: Williams & Wilkins; 1983.

Muller ME, Allgower M, Schneider R, Willenegger H. *Manual of Internal Fixation,* 3rd ed. New York: Springer-Verlag; 1991.

Petty W. *Total Joint Replacement.* Philadelphia: WB Saunders; 1991.

Seligson D (ed). *Concepts in Intramedullary Nailing.* Orlando, FL: Grune & Stratton; 1985.

THIRTEEN

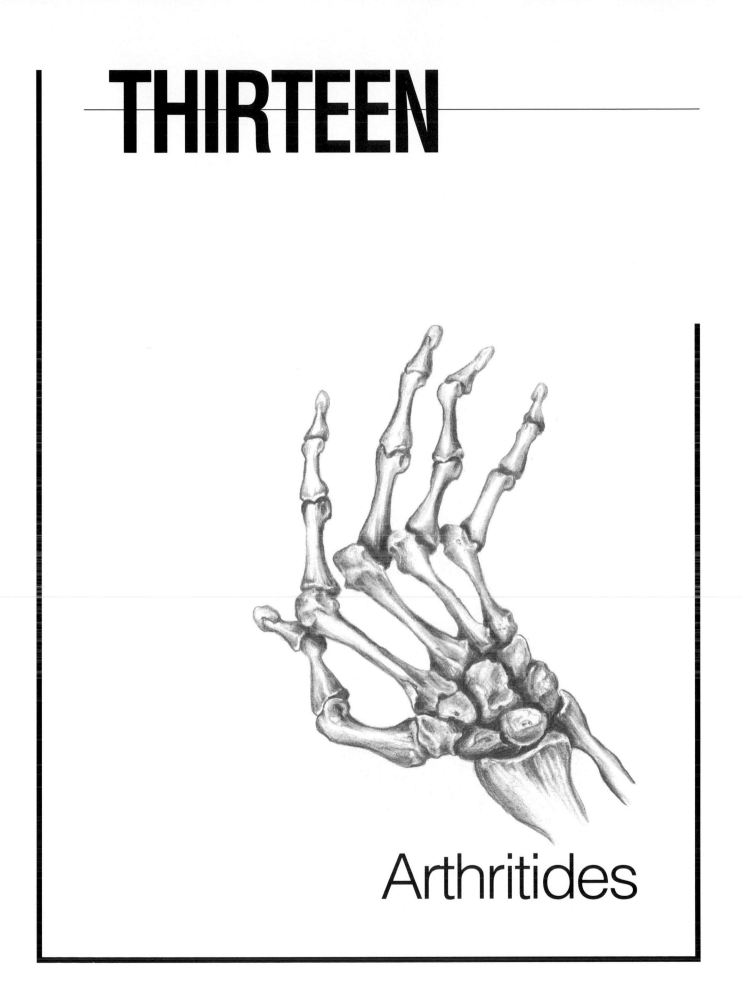

Arthritides

OSTEOARTHRITIS

RHEUMATOID ARTHRITIS

SERONEGATIVE SPONDYLOARTHROPATHIES

Ankylosing Spondylitis
Reiter's Syndrome/Reactive Arthritis
Psoriatic Arthritis
Enteropathic Arthritis

CRYSTAL DEPOSITION ARTHRITIDES

Gout
Calcium Pyrophosphate Dihydrate Deposition Disease
(Pseudogout)

CONNECTIVE TISSUE ARTHRITIDES

ARTHRITIS IN CHILDREN

OTHER ARTHRITIDES

Arthritis is an abnormality of the joints that is often, but not exclusively, inflammatory in nature. It may result from degenerative, inflammatory, or metabolic processes. Joint involvement may be one of many manifestations of a rheumatic disease. Radiography has a varied role in the diagnosis and treatment of arthritides. Initial images may be used both to narrow the number of differential diagnoses and to stage the degree of joint and soft-tissue involvement. During the course of treatment, radiography may be used to evaluate progression or regression of the disease. However, clinical manifestations and radiographic findings are not always correlated. In addition, some rheumatic diseases are accompanied by no radiographic findings. Because the focus of this book is orthopaedic radiography, discussion in this chapter has been limited to rheumatic conditions with radiographic manifestations.

Osteoarthritis

Osteoarthritis (OA), also called degenerative joint disease or osteoarthrosis, is a common noninflammatory disorder of movable joints. OA is not a single disease but is instead a heterogeneous group of conditions characterized by articular cartilage deterioration and by new bone formation at the articular margin and in the subchondral region. When a causative factor cannot be identified, the condition is classified as *primary or idiopathic* OA. If a direct cause (i.e., trauma) for the degenerative articular changes can be identified, it is classified as *secondary* OA. The condition usually progresses slowly over a period of years. More rapid progression of OA in the hands and wrists is frequently associated with inflammatory episodes and is termed *erosive* OA (Fig. 13–1).

Primary OA commonly affects specific sites in the hands, wrists, feet, and spine, as well as the knees, hips, acromioclavicular joints, and temporomandibular joints.

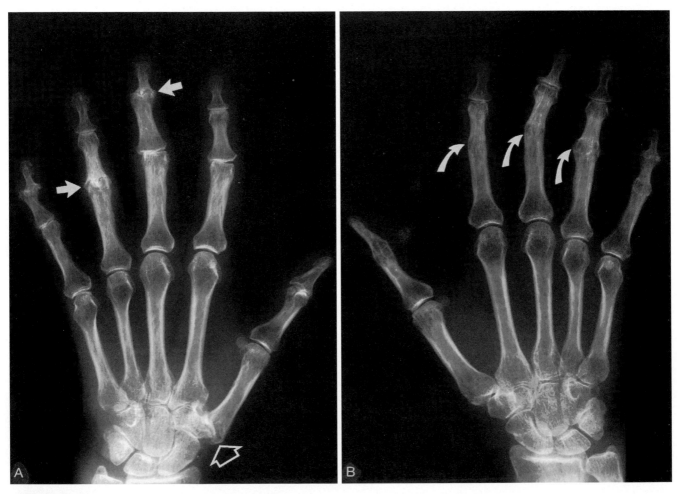

□ **FIGURE 13–1.**

Erosive osteoarthritis. *A,* Gullwing deformities are evident in the left third distal interphalangeal joint and the fourth proximal interphalangeal joint (solid arrows). There is left trapeziometacarpal joint destruction and subluxation (open arrow). *B,* Bony ankylosis is present in the right second, third, and fourth proximal interphalangeal joints (curved arrows).

Osteoarthritis *(continued)*

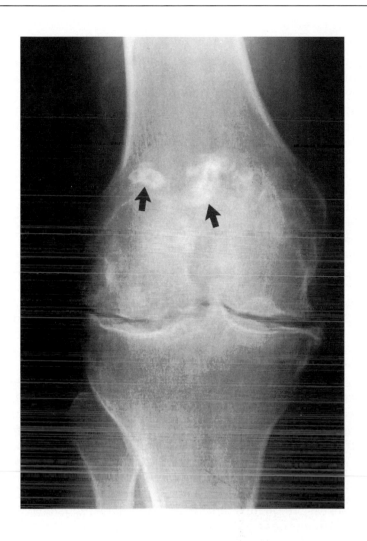

□ **FIGURE 13–2.**

Osteoarthritis of the knee with joint space narrowing, marginal osteophytes, and loose bodies (arrows).

The distal interphalangeal (DIP) joint is the common site of finger involvement and is manifested as *Heberden's nodes*, which are osseous and cartilaginous enlargements on the dorsomedial and dorsolateral aspects. The carpometacarpal (CMC) joint is the most frequently involved thumb joint. In the wrist, OA most commonly affects the scaphotrapezoid joint. OA involving the foot is commonly seen in the first metatarsophalangeal (MTP) joint. The weight-bearing portions of the hip (superior) and knee (medial femorotibial compartment) usually demonstrate the initial and greatest degenerative changes. Both the apophyseal and intervertebral joints of the spine may be affected. Degenerative changes in the spine may occur at any level but are more frequently seen at the sites of greatest spinal motion.[1]

The radiographic appearance of OA consists of non-uniform joint-space narrowing, subchondral sclerosis (osteocondensation), subchondral cysts, pseudocysts or "geodes," and osteophytes at the articular margins (Fig. 13–2). Bone loss, remodeling, and joint incongruity may be seen. There are some differences in radiographic appearance, depending on the specific joint involved. The radiographic features of OA specific to each joint are discussed in the overviews of Chapters 1 to 10.

Rheumatoid Arthritis

Rheumatoid arthritis (RA) is a chronic, inflammatory disease. It is a systemic illness including articular manifestations, involvement of various organs, and constitutional features such as fatigue, weight loss, anemia, anorexia, and low-grade fever. The cause of RA is unknown but has been and continues to be extensively investigated. The identification of multiple causal factors has given rise to current theory that the disease may have no single cause but instead results from a complex sequence of biochemical and cellular events related to the patient's genetic makeup, environment, or hormonal status.[2, 3]

The articular manifestation consists of a symmetrical polyarthritis; the small joints of the hands and feet are involved early in the course of the disease. Specifically, the metacarpophalangeal (MCP) and proximal interphalangeal (PIP) joints of the hands and feet are commonly affected. In addition, there is a predilection for RA to affect the intercarpal joints, the radiocarpal joint, and the distal radioulnar joint. RA also affects large joints such as the hip, knee, elbow, and shoulder. The ankle, calcaneus, temporomandibular joint, acromioclavicular joint, and sternoclavicular joint can be involved. In the spine, RA is usually limited to the cervical region but occasionally affects the dorsolumbar spine and sacroiliac joints.

A number of organs may be involved in RA, including the skin (in which the manifestation is ulceration), muscles (wasting), eyes (scleritis, keratoconjunctivitis), lungs (fibrosis, nodules, pleural effusion), heart (pericarditis, myocarditis, nodules, valvulitis, vasculitis), spleen (enlargement), kidneys (amyloidosis), gastrointestinal tract (amyloidosis), bone marrow (anemia, thrombocytosis), blood vessels (vasculitis), lymph nodes (enlargement), exocrine glands (Sjögren's syndrome), and nerves (peripheral neuropathy, myelopathy). This extra-articular involvement of organs occurs in a significant number of RA patients, and it appears to be associated with more severe rheumatoid disease.[4]

The diagnosis of RA is sometimes difficult in the early stage because the patient may have constitutional symptoms but no joint involvement. The onset of articular manifestations in this early stage commonly consists of a slowly progressing tenosynovitis, frequently accompanied by joint effusions. Patient complaints include pain, tenderness, swelling, and morning stiffness in the involved joints, commonly in the MCP and PIP joints of the hands and the analogous joints in the feet. Radiographic findings in the early stage rheumatoid joint are limited to soft-tissue swelling and periarticular osteoporosis (Fig. 13–3).

As RA progresses, cartilage and bone destruction begins. The cartilage destruction is seen on radiographs as a symmetrical narrowing of the joint space. Bone destruction often begins on the "bare" intra-articular cortical surface at the junction of the articular cartilage and the inflamed synovium, resulting in breaks in the cortical line ("dot-dash" appearance). Over time, the cortical destruction extends into the underlying trabecular bone and may result in significant bone erosions (Fig. 13–4). The characteristic hand deformities begin to occur, including ulnar deviation of the phalanges at the MCP joints and the boutonnière and swan-neck deformities of the interphalangeal joints. Foot deformities follow a pattern similar to those of the hand and commonly include hallux valgus deformity of the great toe, fibular deviation of the second to fourth toes, a "cocked-up" flexion deformity of the toes, and collapse of the transverse (metatarsal) arch. Involvement of joints other than the hands, wrists, and feet may begin to occur, if it has not already.

Rheumatoid Arthritis *(continued)*

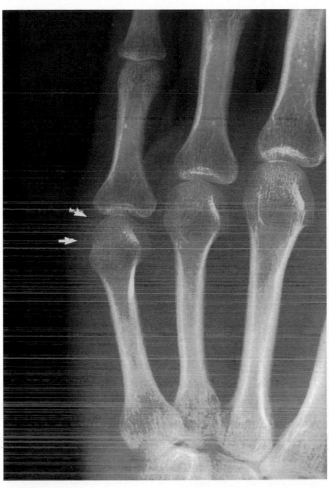

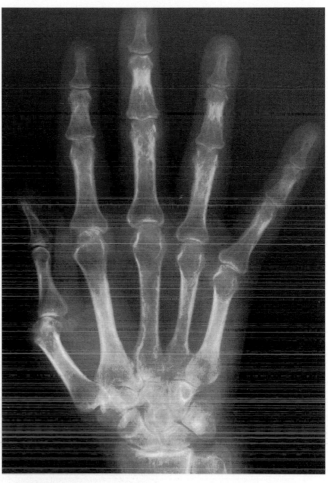

□ **FIGURE 13–3.**

Early rheumatoid arthritis. Capsular distension of the fifth metacarpophalangeal joint (arrows).

□ **FIGURE 13–4.**

Rheumatoid arthritis of the hand and wrist demonstrating diffuse osteoporosis, joint space narrowing, and marginal erosions.

Rheumatoid Arthritis *(continued)*

RA features in these other joints are discussed in the chapter overviews specific to each joint. Extra-articular and constitutional manifestations also worsen. Rheumatoid nodules may appear or increase, and muscle atrophy becomes marked. The patient may exhibit increased weight loss and fatigue. Joint stiffness may no longer be limited to morning. In some patients, the disease continues to progress to the point of severe deformity and loss of function in the involved joints (Fig. 13–5).

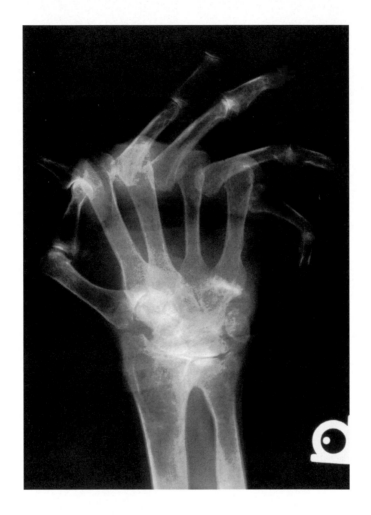

□ **FIGURE 13–5.**

Severe rheumatoid arthritis with extensive deformities, including subluxation and ulnar deviation of the second to fifth digits, boutonnière deformities of the thumb and fifth finger, ankylosis of the carpus, and destruction of the radiocarpal joint with ulnar translation of the carpus.

Seronegative Spondyloarthropathies

The seronegative spondyloarthropathies, or rheumatoid variants, are a group of inflammatory joint diseases that include ankylosing spondylitis, Reiter's syndrome/reactive arthritis, psoriatic arthritis, and enteropathic arthritis. These conditions are termed *seronegative* because in affected patients, results of tests for rheumatoid factor are negative. There is an association between the seronegative spondyloarthropathies and the presence of the histocompatibility antigen HLA-B27: more than 95% of patients with ankylosing spondylitis and approximately 50%–75% in patients with the other conditions.[5] Patients with this group of arthritides often display common features, including ocular involvement, spondylitis, and sacroiliitis.

Seronegative Spondyloarthropathies *(continued)*

Ankylosing Spondylitis

Ankylosing spondylitis (AS) is the most prevalent of the seronegative spondyloar-thropathies. AS is a chronic inflammatory arthritide affecting primarily the sacro-iliac joints and the spine. In addition, peripheral joints such as the shoulders, hips, knees, ankles, costovertebral joints, costotransverse joints, manubriosternal joints, and symphysis pubis may be involved. Less frequently, AS affects the hands, wrists, and feet. Enthesitis (inflamed tendon or ligament insertion) may occur at the ischial tuberosities, iliac crests, greater trochanters, and heels. Extra-articular organs involved include the eyes (uveitis, iridocyclitis), heart (conduction defects), aorta (incompetence), lungs (fibrosis), and kidneys (immunoglobulin A [IgA] nephropathy, amyloidosis).

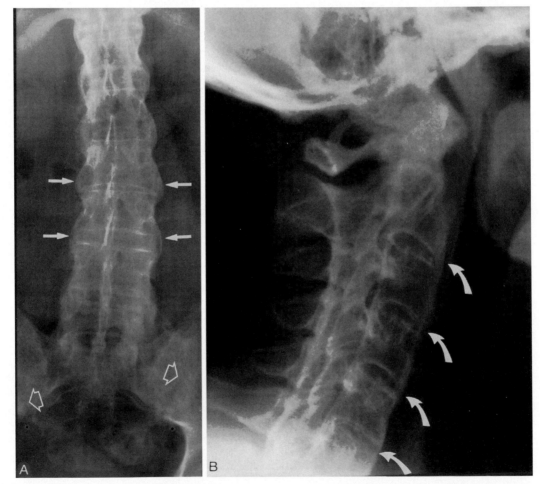

□ **FIGURE 13–6.**

Ankylosing spondylitis. *A,* Anteroposterior radiograph of the lumbar spine, demonstrating bilateral syndesmophytes (solid arrows) and bilateral sacroiliitis (open arrows). *B,* Lateral radiograph of the cervical spine, demonstrating anterior syndesmophytes (curved arrows) and apophyseal joint ankylosis. This appearance is referred to as a "bamboo spine."

Seronegative Spondyloarthropathies *(continued)*

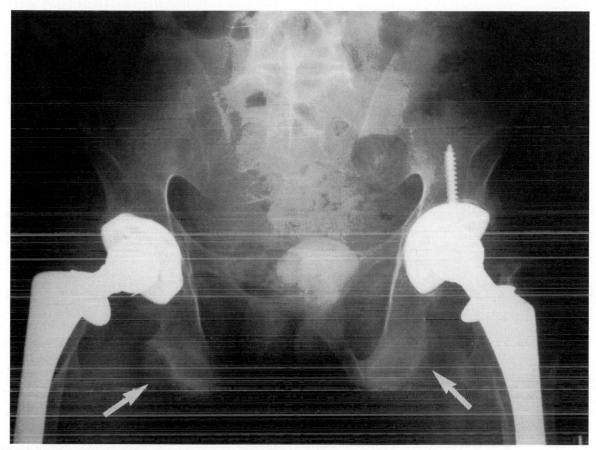

□ **FIGURE 13–7.**

Ankylosing spondylitis. Anteroposterior pelvis radiograph demonstrating bilateral sacroiliac ankylosis and ischial enthesopathy at the adductor origins (arrows). Bilateral total hip prostheses are evident.

Radiographic features of AS are demonstrated in the spine, the sacroiliac joints, and the peripheral joints. Osteitis of the lower thoracic and lumbar vertebra is an early manifestation and results in the characteristic squaring of the vertebral bodies. Spine involvement also results in osseous bridging of adjacent vertebral bodies by vertically oriented syndesmophytes. Inflammatory synovitis affects the apophyseal joints and may proceed to bony ankylosis. The classic "bamboo spine" is the result of ankylosis of the intervertebral and apophyseal joints of an entire spinal segment (Fig. 13–6A). The cervical spine is involved later in the course of the disease (see Fig. 13–6B). The sacroiliitis is usually bilateral and symmetrical. The radiographic appearance is of a widened joint space and periarticular sclerosis. The sacroiliitis may progress to ankylosis of the sacroiliac joints (Fig. 13–7). The inflammatory process seen in the peripheral joints is similar to that of rheumatoid arthritis but with less osteoporosis and more reactive sclerosis. The enthesitis at tendon or ligament attachments on the ischial tuberosities, iliac crests, and heels may result in irregular new bone formation at the cortical margin termed *whiskering* (see Fig. 13–7).

Seronegative Spondyloarthropathies *(continued)*

Reiter's Syndrome/Reactive Arthritis

Reiter's syndrome and the other forms of reactive arthritis manifest as sterile inflammatory arthropathies occurring after an infection but at a site remote from the initial infection. Both enteric infections (*Shigella, Salmonella, Yersinia, Campylobacter*) and sexually acquired infections (*Chlamydia, Ureaplasma,* human immunodeficiency virus [HIV]) have been established as predisposing factors.[6, 7, 8] Reiter's syndrome is most commonly found in young men. It is characterized by the classic triad of urethritis, conjunctivitis, and arthritis. However, many patients do not manifest all three features.[9] Other mucocutaneous features include gastroenteritis, penile ulcerations or plaques (balanitis circinata), oral ulcerations, and a characteristic dermatitis (keratoderma blennorrhagicum). In addition, an enthesitis commonly involves the calcaneus at the insertions of the Achilles tendon and plantar fascia. Other sites of enthesis inflammation include the digits (toes and fingers), ischial tuberosities, iliac crests, symphysis pubis, and anterolateral chest wall (insertions of serratus anterior muscles).

The extra-articular manifestations usually occur first, and the arthritis that follows characteristically involves the lower extremities. Typically, the articular component of Reiter's syndrome manifests as an acute, asymmetrical, inflammatory oligoarthritis (involving few joints). There is a predilection for involvement of the foot, particularly the MTP and interphalangeal (IP) joints of the great toe (Fig. 13–8A) and of the calcaneus. In addition, the other joints of the forefoot, the ankle, and the knee are sites of frequent involvement. The arthritis may ascend to involve the hips, sacroiliac joints, dorsolumbar spine, and upper extremities (usually hands and wrists). The inflammatory process may affect entire digits (dactylitis) of the foot or hand, resulting in a "sausage digit."

The radiographic features of Reiter's syndrome arthritis include soft-tissue swelling, joint-space narrowing, marginal or central erosions of the articular surface, erosions of involved entheses, and reactive new bone formation. The reactive bony proliferation may occur as linear or "fluffy" ossification in the periosteum of involved bones and as a sclerotic or irregular appearance at the sites of articular or enthesis erosions (see Fig. 13–8B). The bony proliferation may progress to ankylosis in the sacroiliac joints. In the dorsolumbar spine, the reactive ossification is manifested by formation of asymmetrical, nonmarginal syndesmophytes and perivertebral ossification.

Seronegative Spondyloarthropathies *(continued)*

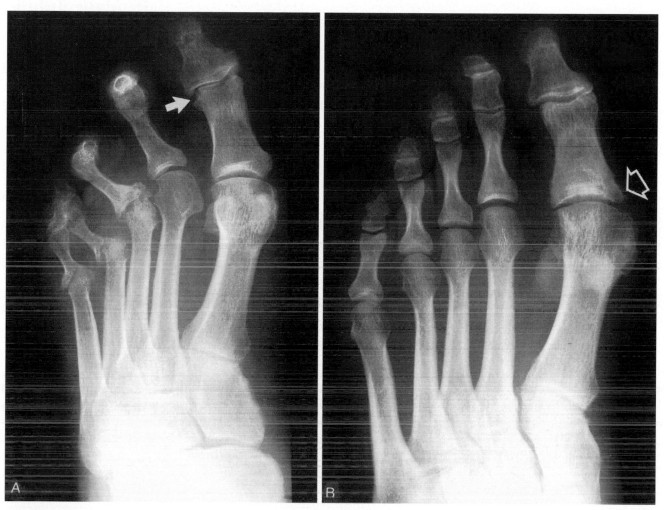

☐ **FIGURE 13–8.**

Reiter's syndrome arthritis. *A,* Erosion of the interphalangeal joint of the great toe (arrow) is present. Joint destruction and deformities involve the metatarsophalangeal joints of the third to fifth toes. Fluffy new bone formation is evident. *B,* Early involvement of the metatarsophalangeal joint of the first toe with marginal erosions and fluffy new bone formation (arrow).

Seronegative Spondyloarthropathies *(continued)*

Psoriatic Arthritis

Psoriatic arthritis (PSA) is an inflammatory joint disease associated with the skin condition psoriasis. The percentage of patients with psoriasis and an associated arthritis is low, but a strong correlation between PSA and psoriatic finger or toe nail dystrophy has been established.[10, 11] In the majority of patients, PSA has been found to be delayed for approximately two decades after onset of psoriasis.[12] Multiple patterns of joint involvement have been identified, resulting in formulation of five clinical subgroups of PSA.[13] Group 1 is characterized by predominant involvement of the hand DIP joints. Group 2 is characterized by arthritis mutilans caused by destruction of the phalanges and metacarpal joints, usually in the hands. Group 3 is characterized by a symmetrical polyarthritis very similar to RA. Group 4, which affects the largest number of patients, is characterized by an asymmetrical oligoarticular arthritis of the DIP, PIP, MCP, and MTP joints. Group 5 is characterized by spondylitis and sacroiliitis.

The radiographic appearance of joint involvement in PSA is similar to that of RA. However, several characteristics aid in differentiation, including an asymmetrical, oligoarticular distribution of the lesions and the involvement of the DIP joints and the sacroiliac joints. Other characteristics in peripheral joints include a predilection for the DIP and PIP joints, osteolysis, "pencil-in-cup" deformity of joints, and bony ankylosis (Fig. 13–9). On occasion, large peripheral joints may be involved. PSA involvement in the dorsolumbar spine may include asymmetrical nonmarginal syndesmophytes, perivertebral ossification, and ankylosis. Unlike Reiter's syndrome arthritis, PSA may involve the cervical spine, and patients may exhibit syndesmophyte formation, disc-space narrowing, apophyseal joint sclerosis, ankylosis, and atlanto-axial subluxation. One or both sacroiliac joints can be affected and may exhibit marginal erosions, joint-space narrowing, reactive sclerosis, and ankylosis.

Enteropathic Arthritis

There is a well-established association between inflammatory bowel conditions and the seronegative spondyloarthropathies.[14] The manifestation and distribution of joint involvement vary with the causative condition. Crohn's disease and ulcerative colitis are associated with a spondyloarthropathy very similar to uncomplicated AS. When the bowel inflammation is caused by a bowel infection, the joint involvement manifests as a reactive arthritis. Whipple's disease, a rare systemic syndrome, has both an inflammatory bowel component and a polyarticular arthritic component.

Seronegative Spondyloarthropathies *(continued)*

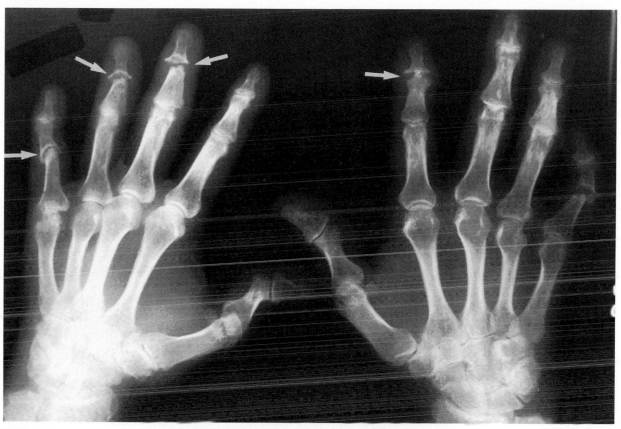

□ **FIGURE 13–9.**

Psoriatic arthritis. Pencil-in-cup deformities are present in the left third and fourth distal interphalangeal joints, the left fifth proximal interphalangeal joint, and the right second distal interphalangeal joint (arrows). Fuzzy indistinct erosions are present in numerous other joints in both hands and in the left wrist.

Crystal Deposition Arthritides

The crystal deposition arthritides are a group of inflammatory joint diseases resulting from a periarticular and intra-articular accumulation of monosodium urate monohydrate crystals (gout), calcium pyrophosphate dihydrate (CPPD) crystals (pseudogout), or numerous other crystals.

Gout

Gout is characterized by acute and extremely painful attacks of oligoarticular inflammation caused by deposition of monosodium urate monohydrate crystals in and around the involved joints. The MTP joint of the great toe is the most common site of involvement (Fig. 13–10).[15] Other commonly affected joints include the calcanei, ankles, knees, elbows, wrists, and fingers (Figs. 13–11A, 13–11B). The crystal deposition results from hyperuricemia, which may have numerous causes, including drug therapies (i.e., diuretics, cyclosporine), alcoholism, lead poisoning, hypertension, renal insufficiency, heredity, and obesity.[16] Gout occurs predominantly in males over 40 years of age.[17] The early stage of gout consists of acute attacks of oligoarticular arthritis without joint destruction. As the disease pro-

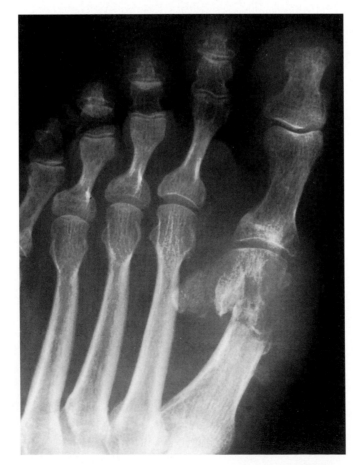

☐ **FIGURE 13–10.**

Gout. Significant soft-tissue swelling and bone destruction at the distal end of the first metatarsal are evident. The first metatarsophalangeal joint space is essentially normal.

Crystal Deposition Arthritides *(continued)*

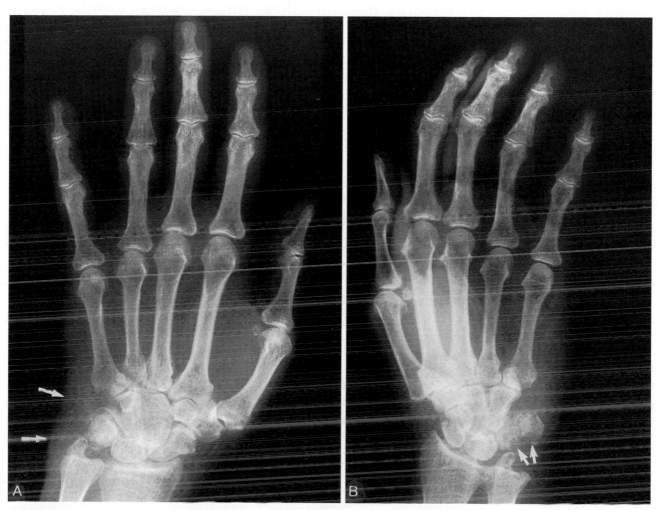

□ **FIGURE 13–11.**

Gout. *A,* This posteroanterior hand radiograph is unremarkable except for soft-tissue swelling on the ulnar side of the wrist (arrows). *B,* The Nørgaard position radiograph demonstrates erosion of the pisiform and triquetrum (arrows). This case demonstrates the value of the Nørgaard, or "ballcatcher," position when imaging the hand for arthritis.

gresses, the arthritis becomes erosive, and nodules of urate crystals (tophi) form around the joint, subcutaneously and within bone. Chronic tophaceous gout may result in joint destruction and bony lysis in association with the presence of the tophi. The arthritis tends to be polyarticular at this later stage. However, it can be differentiated from the polyarthritis of RA because the erosions are asymmetrical and exhibit overhanging margins.[18] These manifestations of long-standing gout are less frequently seen in compliant patients in whom the disease was correctly diagnosed and effectively treated.

The radiographic features of gout differ with the duration of the disease. Early findings are soft-tissue swelling and joint effusions, often limited to one (MTP) or a few joints. As the disease progresses, marginal erosions with sclerotic and overhanging borders are seen. However, the joint space is often normal even when extensive erosions are present. Tophi are seen as soft-tissue masses, most frequently in the feet, ankles, knees, elbows, and hands. Bone erosions remote from the joint are associated with tophi in these locations (see Fig. 13–10).

Crystal Deposition Arthritides *(continued)*

Calcium Pyrophosphate Dihydrate Deposition Disease (Pseudogout)

CPPD disease is a condition resulting from the presence of calcium pyrophosphate dihydrate crystals in articular cartilage, fibrocartilage, ligaments, tendons, bursae, and joint capsules. The severity and pattern of joint involvement is quite variable, ranging from acute attacks in isolated joints to chronic degenerative or inflammatory manifestations in multiple joints.[19] An acute episode restricted to one or a few peripheral joints is termed *pseudogout* because it mimics a gouty arthritic attack. CPPD disease may manifest as a progressive degeneration of multiple joints that is similar to osteoarthritis. It is differentiated from primary osteoarthritis, not only by the presence of CPPD crystals in the synovial fluid of the involved joints, but also by the involvement of joints not characteristically affected by osteoarthritis, such as the MCP joints, wrists, elbows, and shoulders. The condition may occasionally mimic the inflammatory polyarthritis of RA.

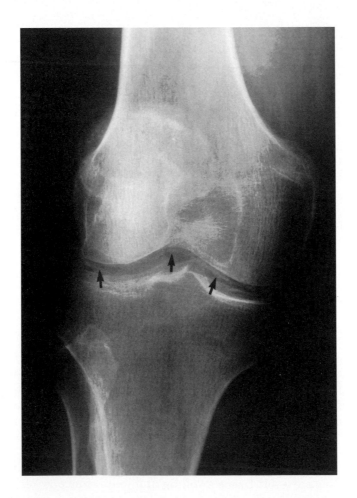

□ **FIGURE 13–12.**

Calcium pyrophosphate dihydrate (CPPD) crystal arthropathy. Anteroposterior knee radiograph demonstrating chondrocalcinosis as punctate calcification of the menisci. This is seen as a line of calcification within and parallel to the joint space (arrows).

Crystal Deposition Arthritides *(continued)*

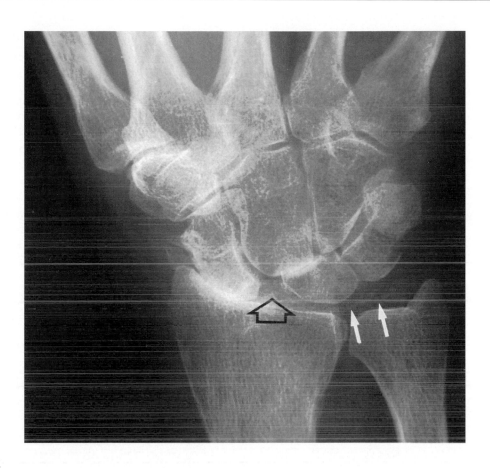

□ **FIGURE 13-13.**

Calcium pyrophosphate dihydrate (CPPD) crystal arthropathy. The posteroanterior wrist radiograph demonstrates loss of the radiocarpal joint space and calcification of the triangular fibrocartilage (solid white arrows). Scapholunate accelerated collapse (SLAC wrist) is also evident, with significant widening of the scapholunate joint (open black arrow).

Radiographic findings differ with the manifestation of the disease. Characteristic calcifications may be seen in hyaline (articular) cartilage, fibrocartilage, ligaments, tendons, bursae, and joint capsules. The calcification of articular cartilage appears as a thin radiopaque line parallel to the subchondral bone. Fibrocartilaginous structures, such as the menisci of the knee, exhibit a punctate (dotted) pattern of calcification (Fig. 13–12). Joint-space narrowing, subchondral sclerosis, subchondral cysts and marginal osteophytes may be seen (Fig. 13–13). Specific degenerative findings, such as large subchondral cysts[20] and patellofemoral joint-space narrowing,[21] have been reported as suggestive for CPPD arthropathy. Articulations commonly affected by CPPD disease include the knees (most common), wrists, elbows, shoulders, hips, symphysis pubis, sacroiliac joints, and intervertebral joints. Intra-articular CPPD deposition may represent a common final pathway of a series of metabolic disorders, including hemochromatosis and ochronosis.

Many other crystals may be deposited in and around the joints. These include basic calcium phosphate (BCP: hydroxyapatite, octocalcium phosphate, tricalcium phosphate), calcium oxalate, and numerous other less frequently occurring crystals. Radiographs may demonstrate calcifications periarticularly and sometimes intra-articularly. The arthritis associated with BCP or calcium oxalate deposition may mimic gout or pseudogout if an acute episode occurs. The chronic form may result in joint destruction.

Connective Tissue Arthritides

A number of connective tissue disorders produce joint manifestations. Among these disorders are systemic lupus erythematosus (SLE), scleroderma, and polymyositis/dermatomyositis.

SLE is a chronic, inflammatory connective tissue disorder that affects many organ systems. The disease is characterized by the presence of autoantibodies that are involved in tissue damage. The disease is often associated with the characteristic butterfly rash on the face. Joint involvement is common in SLE and includes joint effusions, juxta-articular osteoporosis, joint subluxations, hand deformities, osteonecrosis, and soft-tissue wasting.[22] Joint erosions occur infrequently (Fig. 13–14).

Scleroderma is a connective tissue disorder characterized by skin thickening and fibrosis. In addition to musculoskeletal involvement, other organs may be affected, including the gastrointestinal tract, lungs, heart, peripheral vascular system, and kidneys. Radiographic findings include resorption of the distal phalangeal tufts; erosions of the DIP, PIP, and CMC joints; and periarticular (Fig. 13–15) and intra-articular calcifications.[23]

Polymyositis and dermatomyositis are chronic inflammatory disorders of striated muscle that result in muscle weakness. Dermatomyositis is differentiated from polymyositis by the presence of a characteristic rash. Radiographic findings are usually limited to soft-tissue calcifications.

Connective Tissue Arthritides *(continued)*

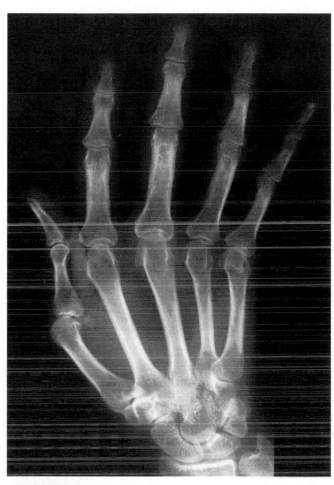

□ **FIGURE 13–14.**

Systemic lupus erythematosus (SLE). Posteroanterior hand radiograph demonstrating ulnar deviation of the second to fifth digits without evidence of joint erosions.

⊓ **FIGURE 13–15.**

Scleroderma. Periarticular calcifications are evident on this posteroanterior hand radiograph.

Arthritis in Children

Many types of arthritis may be seen in children. An arthritis is generally considered to be of juvenile onset if it occurs on or before the 16th birthday. Juvenile rheumatoid arthritis (JRA), or juvenile chronic arthritis, is the most common rheumatic disease affecting children. Three forms of the disease have been identified: pauciarticular, polyarticular, and systemic. Patients with JRA exhibit a range of features, including systemic manifestations and involvement of a varied number of joints. Joint involvement is usually symmetrical and commonly affects the knees, ankles, and wrists.[24] In addition, the elbows, hands, feet, hips, shoulders, and cervical spine are often involved.[25] The sacroiliac joints, sternoclavicular joints, and temporomandibular joints have also been found to be affected.[25, 26] Abnormalities of growth and development are frequently seen in children with JRA. Retardation of linear growth (stature) may result,[27] and localized growth disturbances, such as mandibular hypoplasia,[28] leg length discrepancies,[29] and brachydactyly (a shortened digit), may occur. Another characteristic localized growth disturbance is broadening (overgrowth) of bone ends, especially the distal end of the proximal phalanx in the hand.[30]

Early radiographic changes in all forms of JRA include periarticular soft-tissue swelling and osteoporosis. Periosteal new bone formation adjacent to the joint is another early manifestation, but it is limited to the polyarticular and systemic forms.[31] Late radiographic changes include joint-space narrowing, bone erosions at joint margins, subluxation of large joints (especially the hip and atlanto-axial joints), and compression fractures of vertebral bodies and epiphyses.[25] Bony ankylosis may occur, especially in the carpus[32] and in the apophyseal joints of the cervical spine (Figs. 13–16, 13–17).[33]

The pauciarticular form of JRA involves four or fewer joints, usually of the lower extremities.[34] The knee is most frequently affected, especially in a monarticular manifestation.[35] Systemic features are rare, with the exception of eye disease (anterior uveitis).[36]

Polyarticular-onset JRA is characterized by arthritis in five or more joints, and in affected patients, test results for the rheumatoid factor are most commonly negative. The rheumatoid factor–positive polyarticular form of JRA tends to have a late onset and a clinical pattern very similar to that of adult RA.[37] Systemic manifestations may be present in patients with polyarticular JRA but are mild in comparison to those of systemic-onset JRA.

Children with systemic-onset JRA, also called Still's disease, present with a high spiking fever and a characteristic rash. Hepatosplenomegaly, lymphadenopathy, and cardiopulmonary complications are also common.[38] Joint involvement may follow either a pauciarticular course (most common) or a polyarticular course, and joint manifestations mirror those forms.[34]

In addition to JRA, a significant number of other arthritides and conditions with arthritic components affect the pediatric population. Among these conditions are connective tissue diseases (SLE, scleroderma, dermatomyositis, vasculitis), the seronegative spondyloarthropathies (AS, psoriatic arthritis, Reiter's syndrome, enteropathic arthritis), septic arthritis, and numerous metabolic, endocrine, and neuropathic disorders. Many of these diseases are similar to those found in adults. It is not yet understood whether the differences between the adult and pediatric forms of these equivalent rheumatic diseases are related to the rapid growth and development of the involved tissues or related to distinct disease states.

Arthritis in Children *(continued)*

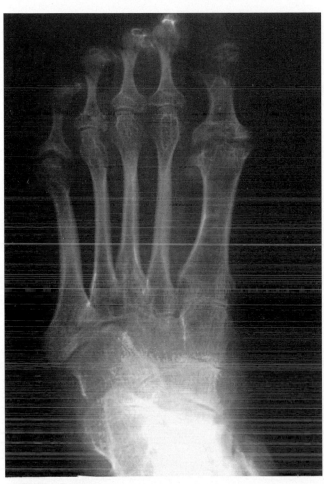

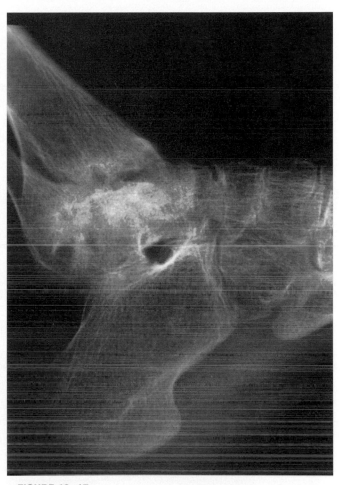

□ **FIGURE 13–16.**

Juvenile rheumatoid (or juvenile chronic) arthritis. Thinning of the metatarsal shafts, ankylosis of the tarsus, and erosions of the first metatarsophalangeal joint are seen on this anteroposterior foot radiograph.

□ **FIGURE 13–17.**

Juvenile rheumatoid (or juvenile chronic) arthritis. This lateral ankle radiograph demonstrates tibiotalar erosions.

Other Arthritides

In addition to those causes of arthritis previously discussed, a significant number of conditions and causative agents may result in an arthritis. The most prevalent of these are infections (bacterial, viral, fungal, parasitic) that may result in joint effusion, osteoporosis, and rapid joint-space loss and may progress to ankylosis (Fig. 13–18). Other conditions and causes of an arthritis include trauma, neuropathy, hematologic disorders, vasculitis, rheumatic fever, endocrine disorders, and genetic disorders. The radiographic appearances of these arthritides are variable, but careful attention to imaging principles enables demonstration of pathological changes in the involved structures.

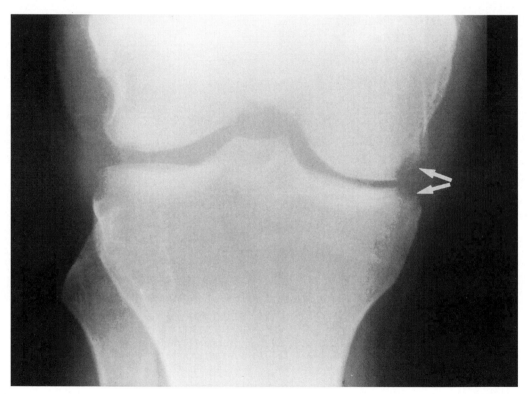

□ **FIGURE 13–18.**

Septic arthritis. Evidence of joint effusion and erosions on both surfaces of the medial joint margins (arrows) are seen in this anteroposterior knee radiograph.

References

1. Moskowitz RW. Clinical and laboratory findings in osteoarthritis. *In* McCarty DJ, Koopman WJ (eds). *Arthritis and Allied Conditions: A Textbook of Rheumatology*. Philadelphia: Lea & Febiger, 1993:1746.
2. Harris ED. Excitement in synovium: the rapid evolution of understanding of rheumatoid arthritis and expectations for therapy. *J Rheumatol* 1992; 19(Suppl 32):3–5.
3. Zvaifler N. New perspectives on the pathogenesis of rheumatoid arthritis. *Am J Med* 1988; 85(Suppl 4A):12.
4. Bhardwaj N, Paget SA. Rheumatoid arthritis. *In* Paget SA, Fields TR (eds). *Rheumatic Disorders*. Boston: Andover, 1992:19–58.
5. Khan MA, van der Linden SM. Ankylosing spondylitis and other spondyloarthropathies. *Rheum Dis Clin North Am* 1990; 16(3):551–579.
6. Amor B. Suspected infectious agent and host environment interactions in spondyloarthropathies. *Clin Exp Rheumatol* 1987; 5(Suppl 1):19–24.
7. Inman RD. Reiter's syndrome and reactive arthritis. *In* Khan MA (ed). *Ankylosing Spondylitis & Related Spondyloarthropathies*. Philadelphia: Hanley & Belfus, 1990.
8. Winchester R, Bernstein DH, Fischer HD, et al. The co-occurence of Reiter's syndrome and acquired immunodeficiency. *Ann Intern Med* 1987; 106:19–26.
9. Arnett FC. Seronegative spondyloarthropathies. *Bull Rheum Dis* 1987; 37:1–12.
10. Moll JM, Wright V. Psoriatic arthritis. *Semin Arthritis Rheum* 1973; 3:55–78.
11. Scarpa R, Oriente P, Pucino A, et al. Psoriatic arthritis in psoriatic patients. *Br J Rheumatol* 1984; 23:240–250.
12. Biondi Oriente C, Scarpa R, Pucino A, Oriente P. Psoriasis and psoriatic arthritis. Dermatological and rheumatological co-operative clinical report. *Acta Derm Venereol Suppl (Stockh)* 1989; 146:69–71.
13. Gerber LH, Espinosa LR (eds). *Psoriatic Arthritis*. Orlando, FL: Grune & Stratton, 1985.
14. Mielants H, Veys EM. The gut in the spondyloarthropathies [editorial]. *J Rheumatol* 1990; 17:7–10.
15. Grahame R, Scott JT. Clinical survey of 354 patients with gout. *Ann Rheum Dis* 1970; 29:461–468.
16. Roubenoff R. Gout and hyperuricemia. *Rheum Dis North Am* 1990; 16(3):539–549.
17. Lawrence RC, Hochberg MC, Kelsey JL, et al. Estimates of the prevalence of selected arthritis and musculoskeletal diseases in the United States. *J Rheumatol* 1989; 16:427–441.
18. Martel W. The overhanging margin of bone: a roentgenologic manifestation of gout. *Radiology* 1968; 91:755–756.
19. McCarty DJ. Diagnostic mimicry in arthritis: patterns of joint involvement associated with calcium pyrophosphate dihydrate crystal deposits. *Bull Rheum Dis* 1975; 25:804–809.
20. Resnick D, Niwayama G, Goergen TG, et al. Clinical, radiographic, and pathologic abnormalities in calcium pyrophosphate dihydrate deposition disease (CPPD): pseudogout. *Radiology* 1977; 122:1–15.
21. Dieppe PA, Alexander GJ, Jones HE, at al. Pyrophosphate arthropathy: a clinical and radiographic study of 105 cases. *Ann Rheum Dis* 1982; 41:371–376.
22. Noonan CD, Odone DT, Engelman EP, et al. Roentgen manifestations of joint disease in systemic lupus erythematosis. *Radiology* 1963; 80:837–843.
23. Bassett LW, Blocka KLN, Clements PJ, et al. Skeletal findings in progressive systemic sclerosis (scleroderma). *AJR* 1981; 136:1121–1126.
24. Ansell BM. Joint manifestations in children with juvenile chronic polyarthritis. *Arthritis Rheum* 1977; 20:204.
25. Martel W, Holt JF, Cassidy JT. Roentenologic manifestations of juvenile rheumatoid arthritis. *AJR* 1962; 88:400–423.
26. Stabrun AE, Larheim TA, Hyeraal HM. Temporomandibular joint involvement in juvenile rheumatoid arthritis. *Scand J Rheumatol* 1989; 18.197–204.
27. Bernstein BH, Stobie D, Singsen BH, et al. Growth retardation in juvenile rheumatoid arthritis (JRA). *Arthritis Rheum* 1977; 20:212.
28. Ganik R, Williams FA. Diagnosis and management of juvenile rheumatoid arthritis with TMJ involvement. *Cranio* 1986; 4:254.
29. Simon S, Whiffen J, Shapiro F. Leg-length discrepancies in monoarticular and pauciarticular juvenile rheumatoid arthritis. *J Bone Joint Surg* 1981; 63A:209.
30. Poznanski AK. *The Hand in Radiologic Diagnosis: with Gamuts and Pattern Profiles*, 2nd ed. Philadelphia: WB Saunders, 1984:823–838.
31. Cassidy JT, Martel W. Juvenile rheumatoid arthritis: clinicoradiologic correlations. *Arthritis Rheum* 1977; 20:207.
32. Maldonada-Cocco JA, Garcia-Morteo O, Spindler AJ, et al. Carpal ankylosis in juvenile rheumatoid arthritis. *Arthritis Rheum* 1980; 23(11):1251–1255.
33. Hensinger RN, DeVito PD, Ragsdale CG. Changes in the cervical spine in juvenile rheumatoid arthritis. *J Bone Joint Surg* 1986; 68A:189.
34. Cassidy JT, Levinson JE, Bass JC, et al. A study of classification criticria for a diagnosis of juvenile rheumatoid arthritis. *Arthritis Rheum* 1986; 29(2):274–281.
35. Cassidy JT, Brody GL, Martel W. Monoarticular JRA. *J Pediatr* 1967; 70:867.
36. Chylack LT. The ocular manifestations of juvenile rheumatoid arthritis. *Arthritis Rheum* 1977; 20:217–230.
37. Cassidy JT, Valkenburg HA. A five year prospective study of rheumatoid factor tests in juvenile rheumatoid arthritis. *Arthritis Rheum* 1967; 10:83.
38. Calabro JJ. Other extraarticular manifestations of juvenile rheumatoid arthritis. *Arthritis Rheum* 1977; 20:237–240.

Index